"Medic"

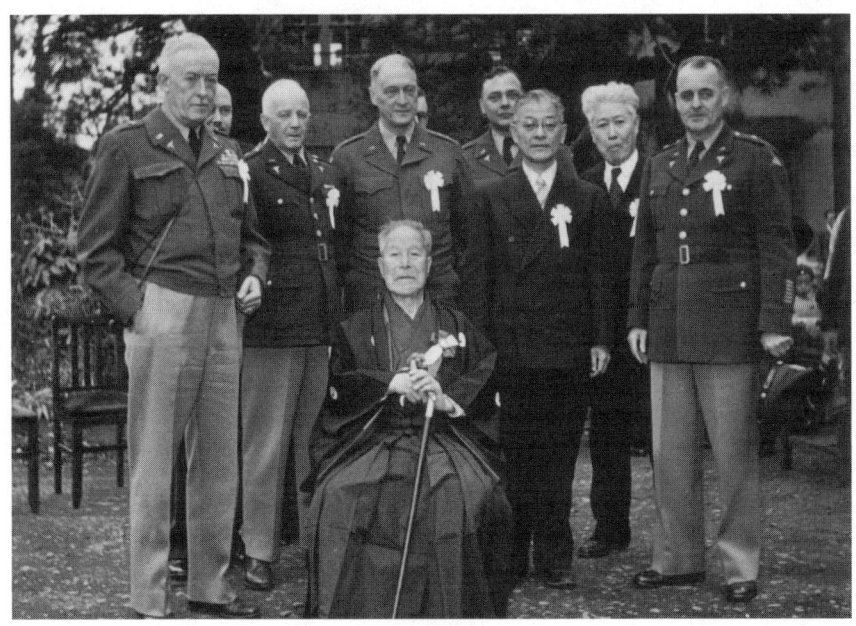

Crawford F. Sams with distinguished physicians of the Institute of Infectious Diseases and the U.S. Army shortly before he left Japan in 1951. Tokyo, 6 April 1951. Seated: Dr. Shiga Kiyoshi (Vice President, Institute). Standing, left to right: Gen. James S. Simmons, obstructed, Gen. Raymond Bliss (Surgeon General of the U.S. Army), Gen. Edgar Erskine Hume (Theater Surgeon, Far East Command), obstructed, obstructed, Dr. Kitasato, unidentified, Brig. Gen. C.F. Sams. (Courtesy of the Hoover Institution Archives, Stanford University.)

"*Medic*"

The Mission of an American
Military Doctor in Occupied
Japan and Wartorn Korea

Crawford F. Sams

Edited, with an
Introduction and Notes, by
Zabelle Zakarian

An East Gate Book

M.E. Sharpe
Armonk, New York
London, England

An East Gate Book

Copyright © 1998 by M. E. Sharpe, Inc.

All rights reserved. No part of this book may be reproduced in any form without written permission from the publisher, M. E. Sharpe, Inc., 80 Business Park Drive, Armonk, New York 10504.

This book is based on the manuscript, "Medic," by Crawford F. Sams, from the Crawford F. Sams Collection, Hoover Institution Archives, Stanford University. All portions of the manuscript included in this book are published with permission of Stanford University. All of the photographs in this book are from the Crawford F. Sams Collection, Hoover Institution Archives, Stanford University. They are published with permission of Stanford University. Figure 19 is also published with permission of the Radiation Effects Research Foundation, Hiroshima, Japan.

Library of Congress Cataloging-in-Publication Data

Sams, Crawford F.
Medic : the mission of an American military doctor in occupied Japan and wartorn Korea / Crawford F. Sams : edited by Zabelle Zakarian.
p. cm.
"An East gate book."
Includes bibliographical references (p.   ) and index.
ISBN 0-7656-0030-7 (hardcover : alk. paper)
1. Sams, Crawford F. 2. United States. Army—Officers—Biography. 3. United States. Army—Medical personnel—Biography. 4. Japan—History—Allied occupation, 1945–1952. 5. Korea—History—Allied occupation, 1945–1948. I. Zakarian, Zabelle, 1950-   . II. Title.
UH347.S36A3   1998
355'0092—dc21
[B]
97-35989
CIP

Printed in the United States of America

The paper used in this publication meets the minimum requirements of American National Standard for Information Sciences— Permanence of Paper for Printed Library Materials, ANSI Z 39.48-1984.

MV (c)   10   9   8   7   6   5   4   3   2   1

Contents

List of Illustrations	vii
Introduction	ix
Chronology of Sams's Life and Work	xvii
Dedication	1
Epigram	2
Preface	3
The Move	5

Japan

1. The Perimeter	9
2. Tokyo	25
3. The Decision: SCAP	32
4. First Reconnaissance of Japan	44
5. Food Relief and Nutrition	54
6. The Reorganization of Health and Welfare	68
7. Statistics: A Health and Welfare Tool	77
8. The Preventive Medicine Program, Part I: Controlling Wildfire Diseases	81
9. The Preventive Medicine Program, Part II: Environmental Sanitation and Viral Diseases	92
10. The Preventive Medicine Program, Part III: Treatment and Prevention	102
11. The Veterinarians	114
12. Medicine and Dentistry	120
13. Pharmacy and the Pharmaceutical Industry	132
14. Nursing	140
15. Hospitals	144
16. The Atomic Bomb Casualty Commission	150

17. Narcotics Control	153
18. Welfare	157
19. Social Security	167
20. The Communist Activities	174
21. The Big Question	183
22. Summation of the Occupation	188
23. Life in Japan	189

Korea

24. 1945–1948	203
25. 1950–1951	209
26. The Breakout	223
27. North Korea	231
28. The New War	236
29. A Complication	243
30. A Korean Episode	246
31. The Relief of General MacArthur	255
32. The Twenty-second of April Offensive	258

Coming Home

Return to the United States	261
Notes	265
Appendix I: Editorial Decisions	295
Appendix II: Photographs	299
Index	301
About the Editor	313

List of Illustrations

1. Burned-out Streetcar. Occupation of Japan, circa September 1945.   13
2. Remains of the Yamato Department Store. Occupation of Japan, circa September 1945.   13
3. Col. C.F. Sams at General Headquarters, SCAP. Tokyo, circa October 1945.   26
4. Col. C.F. Sams at General Headquarters, SCAP. Tokyo, circa October 1945.   26
5. Col. C.F. Sams at General Headquarters, SCAP. Tokyo, circa October 1945.   26
6. Temporary Shelters Built Along the Roadbeds of Railroads. Occupation of Japan, circa September 1945.   31
7. Brig. Gen. C.F. Sams Reviews an Organizational Chart of the Public Health and Welfare Section of SCAP. Tokyo, 11 January 1949.   40
8. Brig. Gen. C.F. Sams Visits with Japanese Children. Occupation of Japan, circa 1951.   46
9. Japanese Children Crowd Around Brig. Gen. C.F. Sams. Occupation of Japan, circa 1951.   47
10. Members of the United States Food Mission on a Visit to Japan. Tokyo, 6 February 1947.   61
11. The Promulgation of the Japanese Constitution at the House of Peers. Tokyo, 3 May 1947.   69
12. The Emperor and Empress of Japan at the Mass Celebration of the Promulgation of the Constitution. Tokyo, May 1947.   70

13. Staff of the Toyonaka Model Health Center with Gen. James S. Simmons and Brig. Gen. C.F. Sams. Toyonaka, Japan, 1951. 74

14. A Demonstration of the Cox Method of Producing Typhus Vaccine at the Institute of Infectious Diseases. Tokyo, 16 April 1947. 86

15. Two Women Receive Typhus Vaccinations at Yurakucho Station. Japan, circa May 1947. 87

16. Brig. Gen. C.F. Sams Reviews the Japanese B Encephalitis Research Project at Komagome Hospital. Tokyo, 31 August 1948. 99

17. A Social Worker at the Suginami Model Health Center Interviews a Woman with Tuberculosis. Tokyo, 4 October 1948. 112

18. Brig. Gen. C.F. Sams Presents the Legion of Merit Medal to Grace E. Alt. Tokyo, 21 August 1947. 142

19. Officers of SCAP and the Atomic Bomb Casualty Commission on a Visit to the ABCC's Facilities. Hiroshima, 14 July 1949. 151

20. SCAP's Social Work Consultants Confer with Leaders of Japan's Social Work and Welfare Organizations. Tokyo, 7 October 1948. 162

21. Members of Japan's Imperial Family Attend the First Postwar Meeting of the International Red Cross of Japan Following its Reorganization. Tokyo, 10 December 1948. 198

Introduction

When the atomic bombs were dropped on Hiroshima and Nagasaki on the sixth and ninth of August 1945, Crawford Sams was on his way to the Philippines. Having served as chief of the Planning Branch of the War Department in Washington, D.C., Sams was eager to get back into "the fray." It had been two years since he had served in combat operations as theater surgeon in the Middle East. When the war in Europe had finally ended in May 1945, he not only had expected to be deployed to the Pacific theater for the conclusion of that phase of the war but also had been offered two assignments on General MacArthur's staff: one as a staff officer; another as a medical officer. After rounds of consultations and given the requisite concurrences, he felt he could be of "greater service to the Army and the Medical Department" as the chief medical officer of the military government section of the Far East Command; thus, with utmost courtesy, he had respectfully requested reassignment from Gen. Russell Maxwell's staff to the Pacific theater in July 1945.[1]

Despite the rumors of surrender that followed the bombings, fighting continued in the Philippines, and Sams did not believe Japan's surrender was imminent. Since May 1945, the U.S. Army had assumed Japan would not surrender without a large-scale ground invasion. Such an invasion was planned for November 1945 and March 1946, which would allow time to prepare for the occupation. But the quirks of military history soon changed these assumptions.

Following Japan's surrender on the second of September 1945, occupation forces encountered tragedy—not triumph. During the war, the Japanese people had endured a heavy burden of disease. The toll of tuberculosis on civilian populations had been harsh, and owing to damaged sewage systems and interrupted vaccination programs, dysentery, typhoid, typhus, smallpox, and parasitic infections were raging. To safeguard the security and health of occupation forces in Japan, Sams, as head of the Public Health and Welfare Section of the military government, would have to control "wildfire" epidemics among the Japanese people as well as administer food and relief to millions of homeless evacuees and destitute repatriates.

Rapid progress in controlling communicable diseases occurred during the occupation of Japan, from September 1945 to April 1952. Drawing upon recent advances in public health research and his formative experiences with disease control and prevention in Panama and the Middle East, Sams directed the Public Health and Welfare (PHW) Section of the Supreme Commander for the Allied Powers (SCAP) to mobilize public health and welfare services from a wartime standstill to a nationwide system. To treat and prevent the major causes of death and disease, the PHW Section set up nationwide programs for immunization, sanitation, and disease surveillance. It also administered food and relief supplies and reformed the pre-existing local health centers into a network of health and welfare information and services. These programs were gradually integrated with reforms in medical care and professional training, welfare and social insurance programs, and the disease and vital statistic-reporting system; the rehabilitation of the medical supply industry; and the resumption of public health training. The scope of these reforms included raising the standards of knowledge and practice for doctors, nurses, pharmacists, dentists, veterinarians, laboratory scientists, dieticians, and social workers. By establishing standards for professional training, and by drafting the legal authority to justify and sustain these programs in Article 25 of the Constitution, Sams also secured a new framework for public health and welfare administration and practice in Japan.

Gen. James S. Simmons (1890–1954), who served as Dean of the Harvard School of Public Health from 1946 to 1954, and whom Sams considered his mentor in the field of preventive medicine, described these achievements in Japan during the occupation as unprecedented and unsurpassed in public health and military medical history.[2] Dr. Hashimoto Michio, who, as a young physician, witnessed these reforms and who later became an official of Japan's Ministry of Health and Welfare and Environment Agency, characterized the institutional memory of Sams's contribution as a turning point in the development of modern public health administration in Japan: "In the history of public health in Japan, the achievement and contribution of Dr. Sams is the great contribution to modern public health administration backed by [the] nationwide system of health center[s] during the chaotic postwar days."[3] Despite their perspectives from within the field of public health, little has been written outside of Japan about public health and welfare reforms during the occupation; or about their implications for social, economic, and political change in postwar Japan; or even about the person who led them.[4] Nor have we begun to assess the record that Sams himself has left.

The Manuscript and the Book

This book is based on the manuscript, "Medic," by Crawford F. Sams (1902–1994). Dr. Sams wrote "Medic" between 1955 and 1958, after he retired from military service. He wrote the manuscript with a general reader in mind and later included it in his collection of papers and photographs that he granted to the Hoover Institution Archives in 1979. The manuscript consists of over 734 typewritten pages. No drafts are known to exist.

"Medic" bridges autobiography and history in a narrative that embodies the archetypal notion of an odyssey or quest that culminates in service to society. By its method and tone, "Medic" resembles what James Atlas calls "an act of remembrance."[5] Sams uses this device to signify the results of a career that combined an interest in medicine with military service—one which began with World War I and culminated in the cold war—and to confirm and justify his convictions regarding public health and democracy. He also memorializes friendships between fellow officers and physicians not simply as a matter of military protocol or professional etiquette, but to preserve a meaning of friendship between officers and among nations that had been forged during the rigors of training and in the uncertainties of world war. Above all, his claim to the title "Medic" reflects a sense of irony and nostalgia.

"Medic" has five parts. Part I spans the period from 1910 to 1941, and includes Sams's recollections of his youth; his medical training; his training as an army officer; his first tour of duty outside the forty-eight states, in Panama, where he first had responsibility for public health activities; and his experience as an instructor at the Infantry School in the period leading up to World War II. In part II, Sams recalls his then classified mission in North Africa to set up U.S. military headquarters prior to the declaration of war by the United States. He also surveys the medical problems he encountered in the Middle East theater from 1941 to 1943. In part III, he describes his tasks at the Medical Field Service School and in the War Department in Washington, D.C., from 1943 to 1945. He also recounts his tour of the European theater in the winter of 1944–45. These three parts describe Sams's apprenticeship for what he referred to as "the 'big job' later on."[6]

In part IV, Sams discusses what he considered to be his greatest challenge: the reforms in public health and welfare that he led in Japan from 1945 to 1951. His account of the occupation describes the programs and activities of the PHW Section of SCAP. It contains information that closely adheres to unclassified official reports of the PHW Section of SCAP. In length, part IV constitutes over forty percent of the manuscript and is at least twice as long as each of the other parts.

Part V covers Sams's missions in Korea from 1945 to 1951, where he served as a health and welfare advisor to the U.S. Army forces that occupied Korea south of the thirty-eighth parallel between 1945 and 1948, and as chief of health and welfare of the United Nations Command during the Korean War from June 1950 to June 1951. He describes how, as a "medic" during the Korean War, he not only studied the evacuation of wounded soldiers and the operations of the MASH units (the Mobile Army Surgical Hospitals) in the combat zones to determine why the rates of missing-, wounded-, or killed-in-action were so high, but also braved a military intelligence mission to confirm reports of "plague" among North Koreans, in order to protect United Nations troops. He also describes his concluding assignments in the United States between 1951 and 1955. Part V covers most of the same period as part IV but is only one-third as long.

This book reproduces parts IV and V, which cover the last ten years of Sams's military service and which conclude with his return to his own country, his family, and civilian life. In length, they represent over half of "Medic." They are preceded by Sams's Dedication and Preface and are reproduced with minor revisions, which are discussed in appendix I. Occasional quotations from the earlier parts appear in this Introduction and in the notes. This book also includes a chronology of Sams's life and work, which is based in part on the manuscript, as well as a number of photographs from the occupation of Japan, the selection of which is discussed in appendix II.

The publication of Sams's account of his missions in Japan and Korea is intended to serve three broad aims. First, Sams's recollections of the occupation of Japan not only add to the dearth of publications available in western languages on public health and welfare reforms in Japan during the occupation but also enlarge our perspective of continuity and change in debates over the organization of medical care, the financing of health insurance, and the design of social insurance and welfare policies in industrial democracies. Second, in addressing the unanticipated role of public health reforms in the decision to resume industrialization in Japan, Sams presents a point of reference for comparative perspectives of the role of public health in patterns of economic development. He also invites us to consider whether the integrated methods used in the health and welfare field in Japan—the "multi-angle approach"—should be applied elsewhere in foreign aid programs.

Third, in contrast to Sams's peacetime work in Japan, his account of the strenuous efforts to control disease among civilians, refugees, and troops in Korea offers a "medic's" view of the cold war. Sams's depiction of this turning point in international relations can not only broaden our understanding of the unresolved conflict between Koreans but also challenge us to examine our policies concerning the conduct of subsequent and perhaps future occupations, if not wars; for in recounting the military, humanitarian, and ideological reasons to control diseases during the occupation of Korea and the Korean War, he also reveals the convictions and ideals that guided his generation of U.S. military leaders.

Sams's Apprenticeship and Transformation

Two decisions set the course of Sams's odyssey: his decision to combine a career in medicine with military service; and his decision to set aside a longstanding interest in neurosurgery and neurosciences in favor of preventive medicine. Sams, like his father, pursued a dual career. (His father, who died when Sams was fifteen years old, was a lawyer who preferred the more humble profession of teaching and public school administration.) Upon completing high school in East Saint Louis, Illinois, in 1918, Sams enlisted in the army at the age of sixteen and served for fourteen months during World War I. He later found mentors in Col.

Marshall Randol and David Prescott Barrows, the President of the University of California, who was also a commanding general of the California National Guard in which Sams served while he was an undergraduate student in psychology at the Berkeley campus in the early 1920s. Colonel Randol had dual status in the U.S. Army and the National Guard and had selected Sams for training as an army line officer. Between 1925 and 1929, Sams interrupted his military service to attend medical school at Washington University in Saint Louis. Later, however, he noted that his transition as an officer of the army medical corps was not difficult because he had had training as an army officer and had learned to fit into a military organization before studying medicine.

From about 1904 to 1930, medical education and the practice of medicine in the United States had been undergoing major reforms. Although medical specialties as we know them today did not formally exist, Sams worked on the cutting edge of new developments in the fields of neurosurgery and neurosciences. In medical school, he worked closely with Dr. Ernest Sachs, an eminent neurosurgeon. He published three scientific papers by the time he had completed medical school and introduced the use of spinal anesthesia at Letterman Army Hospital in 1930–31. His goal was to establish a neurosurgical service in the army.

Sams's second decision was shaped by his early training in research as well as his postgraduate medical training at Walter Reed Army Medical School, where he graduated first in his class in 1931. He credits Dr. Rispler, a German-trained scientist at the Monsanto research department in Saint Louis, Missouri, where Sams worked upon returning from military service after World War I, for having taught him "the scientific method, the ethics of scientific integrity, and the great necessity for thoroughness in doing a job, particularly in the fascinating field of research, seeking the truth." At Walter Reed, he not only learned "how to keep people well" but also found a mentor in the field of preventive medicine, then Maj. James S. Simmons.[7]

During his assignment in Panama from 1937 to 1939, Sams was responsible for malaria control at eleven military installations in the Canal Zone. While travelling along jungle trails in the interior of Panama that had been treated for mosquito control, he observed that, contrary to current practice and belief, the mosquito larvae were able to withstand the army's methods of controlling mosquito breeding. He then devised experiments to study the survival of the larvae under various conditions and developed more effective methods to control their breeding, thereby reducing the rate of new cases of malaria. In recalling this experience, Sams wrote:

> In so many fields in which I have been engaged, I have run into some interesting problems which did not fit the things I had been taught in the textbooks. If one is trained in observation and analysis and evaluation, then you are, in effect, soon continuously engaged in one or more phases of research, and I would like to emphasize that research in medicine is only partially accom-

plished in laboratories. Few of the real problems of health in masses of people, particularly in environmental control, are solved in the laboratory.[8]

His experience with malaria control was formative in convincing him of the importance of preventing infection and disease, rather than treating or suppressing the clinical signs of disease with drugs. It led to his decision to work in the "primitive and neglected" field of preventive medicine rather than pursue neurosurgery:

> The two years of work and research on malaria and in attempting to develop and apply the methods which we learned [at Walter Reed Army Medical School] were most stimulating, and I think it was, perhaps, the experience which finally turned me from my long felt desire to be a neurosurgeon to a quiet satisfaction with a career in trying to keep people well. I found the stimulation of being able to keep people well far greater than that of trying to patch up a few individual cases after they had become ill.[9]

What Sams learned about malaria control in Panama—"that the control should be based on preventing the individual from being bitten by an infected mosquito rather than relying on suppressive drugs"—he applied during the war in the Middle East theater, in 1941–43, to protect U.S. troops.[10] In the Middle East, Sams gained experience with methods of prevention through immunization and environmental controls, which he later applied to the control of smallpox, typhus fever, cholera, diphtheria, typhoid, tuberculosis, and dysenteries in Japan and Korea.

The Theme and Significance of Sams's Recollections

During the early days of the occupation of Japan, the purpose of disease control was to maintain order. The PHW Section of SCAP had been directed to mobilize public health reforms "to prevent widespread disease and unrest."[11] This objective had been ancillary to those of democratizing Japan and disarming its military forces, which the Potsdam Declaration set forth as terms of surrender on 26 July 1945. Yet in the immediate aftermath of the war, the tasks of controlling disease and preventing unrest, themselves technically and administratively complex, became diplomatically precarious; for until communicable diseases were controlled, these remnants of prewar modernization and militant nationalism would cast their shadows on democracy. Yet once initial fears gave way to order, friendly allied officials even found public health reforms "necessary and beneficial."[12] The PHW Section's reforms, which had been ancillary to military objectives, thus became integrated into the occupation's political mission to revive and strengthen democratic tendencies within Japanese society.

The central theme of Sams's recollections is that the control of communicable diseases was the handmaiden of democracy in that it served the aim of demonstrating the value of individual human life to peoples and governments worldwide. Sams memorialized this theme at a meeting of the American Public Health Association in San Francisco in the fall of 1951, shortly after the conclusion of the peace treaty with Japan:

> ... I know of nothing more important in demonstrating to the people of Japan and other nations of the world—particularly those in the Far East—what we mean by the worth of the individual, which we consider to be the essence of democracy, than the literal gift of life which the occupation has brought to some 3,000,000 Japanese who would have died between 1945 and 1951 had these modern programs not been established and had the prewar death rate continued at its normal level.[13]

Sams's trust in public health as a positive feature of democracy not only reflects a highly internalized personal sense of the worth of modern public health programs but also implies that the dynamics of scientific knowledge and political power were no less crucial to the reorganization of public health and scientific medicine during the occupation than they were to their institution in Japan. The association of the control of communicable diseases with a transformation of political goals and governmental institutions in postwar Japan has roots not only in the revolutionary inspirations—both scientific and political—shaping the development of modern public health administration in Europe, but also in modern Japanese history and the founding of modern public health administration in Japan during the Meiji era (1868–1912). In later nineteenth-century Japan, as the Meiji reformers tested the idea that technical weakness could be surmounted by a social and political transformation, scientific medicine based on the European model challenged the social and cultural understanding of disease based on traditional medicine of Chinese origin. Political reform was subsequently decisive for sanctioning and instituting western scientific medicine at the outset of the Meiji period. As Harry Harootunian writes:

> ... The course and character of [political] conflict in Tokugawa Japan ... [was] accompanied by shifts in the structure of knowledge and its relationship to power (what is appropriate and inappropriate).[14]

As we encounter the richness of this theme in relation to the occupation of Japan, as well as its bitterness in relation to the Korean experience, Sams's record reminds us that the organization of health and welfare develops within an historical and cultural setting and that public health and welfare institutions are transformed at the interface of science, law, politics, economics, and culture. His frequent references to friendship, between officers and between nations, also remind us that former enemies from different cultures with different historical orientations can establish a benevolent relationship even after a diplomatic and military collapse.

Acknowledgments

The publication of "Medic" has been a goal that Crawford Sams personally inspired but never solicited. He worked in quiet ways. In writing his memoirs and in making his collection at the Hoover Institution Archives open to anyone who was interested, Dr. Sams desired to provide a source for historical research and understanding.[15] Long afterwards, he continued to grant personal interviews. I am grateful to Dr. Sams for allowing me to visit with him at his home in October 1991.[16] During the course of our meeting, he patiently answered my questions without imposing himself on the line of inquiry, while demonstrating to me the acuity of his memory and the self-possession of his thoughts. He also spoke with high esteem and affection about the people and places pictured in the photographs throughout his home.

Owing to the common interests among scholars, archivists, and publishers, this "forgotten treasure" has been recovered. Among the professors who have guided my interest in this work in subtle and instrumental ways over a period of years and to whom I owe my appreciation are Kim Ha Tai, J. Thomas Rimer, Nathaniel B. Thayer, and Charles S. Pearson. I also wish to thank Elena Danielson and the staff of the Hoover Institution Archives as well as Doug Merwin and Mai Shaikhanuar-Cota of M.E. Sharpe for their courtesies and commitment to this project. Kim Cavallero and Angela Piliouras of M.E. Sharpe also deserve thanks for their efforts on behalf of this book.

In the course of my research and editorial work on this book, I have been rewarded with numerous courtesies extended by individuals who participated in some of the events and organizations that are mentioned in this book. Their courtesies are a tribute to Dr. Sams's mission in the Far East. I thank them and hope the results will be of interest to the readers. I am, of course, especially grateful to Yvonne Johns and Patricia Dwyer for their assistance in answering my questions and for their cordial good wishes and confidence for the publication of their father's autobiography.

—ZZ

Chronology of Sams's Life and Work

1902 April 1	Born East Saint Louis, Illinois
1910	Worked as a groundskeeper at his family's vacation resort in southern Illinois, the first of a series of jobs he held outside of school
1917	Death of his father, Fountain F. Sams, a lawyer and teacher
1918 June	Graduated East Saint Louis High School
1918–1919	Enlisted in the army during World War I
1919 October–1921 December	Laboratory Assistant and Junior Research Chemist, Monsanto Chemical Company, Saint Louis, Missouri
1920 January–1921 December	Studied Chemistry at Washington University, Saint Louis, Missouri
1922 January	Entered University of California at Berkeley
	Enlisted as Private, 159th Infantry, California National Guard
1925 June	Bachelor of Arts in Psychology, University of California
	Promoted to Captain, 143d Field Artillery
	Ordered to active duty
1925 September 2	Married Elva Viola Allen
1925 December	Graduated First in the Battery Commanders Course (for training line officers), Field Artillery School, Fort Sill, Oklahoma

1925 December *(continued)*	Began riding and training horses while learning to play polo at Fort Sill
	Purchased his first car, a Maxwell coupe
	Resigned from military service to attend medical school
1926	Birth of first daughter, Yvonne
1927	Master of Science in Neuroanatomy, Washington University School of Medicine, Saint Louis, Missouri
1929 June	Doctor of Medicine, Washington University School of Medicine
1929 June	Commissioned First Lieutenant, U.S. Army Medical Corps
1929 July–1931 July	Intern and Staff Physician, Letterman General Hospital, San Francisco
	Demonstrated the use of spinal anesthesia and encephalography; hoped to start a neurosurgical service
1930	Birth of second daughter, Patricia Ann
1931 July	First experiences with native people outside of the United States, and with tropical diseases in Nicaragua and Panama, while on his way to Washington, D.C., via army transport with his family
1931 December	Honor Graduate, Walter Reed Army Medical Postgraduate School, Washington, D.C.
1932 May	Promoted to Captain
1932 June	Honor Graduate, Medical Field Service School (for training doctors as medical officers, especially for war-related functions), Carlisle Barracks, Pennsylvania
1932 June–1933 June	Commanding Officer, First Ambulance Company (a mule-drawn ambulance company), First Medical Regiment, Carlisle Barracks, Pennsylvania

1932 June–1933 June *(continued)*	As a mounted officer, bought and broke his first horse, Xanthippe, a four-year-old thoroughbred mare
1933 August–1934 July	Advanced Company Officers Course, Infantry School, Fort Benning, Georgia
1934 July–1936 July	Instructor and Director, Department of Military Art (Tactics, Techniques, and Logistics), Medical Field Service School, Carlisle Barracks, Pennsylvania
1936 August–1937 June	Command and General Staff School, Fort Leavenworth, Kansas
1937 July–1939 July	Assistant and Acting Department Surgeon, Panama Canal Department (an unprecedented assignment for an officer of the rank of Captain)
	Responsible for malaria control, his first broad-scale public health challenge
1939 August–1941 August	Medical Instructor, Infantry School, Fort Benning, Georgia.
	Became the first army medical officer to be trained as a parachutist; organized the medical service for injured or wounded paratroopers
1941 February	Promoted to Major
1941 September–1942 May	Surgeon and Acting Chief-of-staff, U.S. Military Mission in North Africa, headquartered in Cairo (then a secret mission to establish the Middle East theater)
1942 February	Promoted to Lieutenant Colonel
1942 May–1943 September	Theater Surgeon, U.S. Army Forces in the Middle East, headquartered in Cairo
1942 August	Promoted to Colonel
1943 September–1944 December	Director, Department of Military Art, Medical Field Service School, Carlisle Barracks, Pennsylvania
1944 January	Chief, Program Branch, Logistics Division, U.S. War Department, Washington, D.C.

1944 December–1945 February	Toured the European theater to assess needs for medical personnel and equipment to treat soldiers, displaced persons, and prisoners-of-war
1945 February	Chief, Planning Branch, Logistics Division, U.S. War Department, Washington, D.C.
1945 July–1945 October	Chief, Health, Education, and Welfare Division, Military Government Section, U.S. Army Forces, Pacific, the Philippines
1945 August 26–30	Moved from the Philippines to Japan with the advanced echelon of the theater headquarters
1945 October 2–1951 June	Chief, Public Health and Welfare Section, General Headquarters, Supreme Commander for the Allied Powers, Japan
1945–1948	Advisor for Health and Welfare to the U.S. Army Forces in South Korea
1947 January	Arrival of his wife and younger daughter for residence in Japan
1948 April 26	Promoted to Brigadier General
1950 June–1951 June	Chief, Health and Welfare, United Nations Command, Republic of Korea
1950 September–1951 June	Special mission for military operations in Korea
1950 November	Loss of his son-in-law, Capt. Charles M. Struthers, in North Korea
1950 December	Departure of his wife from Japan to resume residence in the United States
1951 March–April	Nominated, selected, and rejected for the position of Surgeon General of the U.S. Army
1951 April–July	Request for retirement from the army denied
1951 July–1953	Assistant Commandant, Medical Field Service School, Fort Sam Houston, Texas
1952 July–1953 January	Resignation from the army denied
1953–1955 July 31	U.S. Army Medical Service, First Army, Governor's Island, New York

1954–1955	Special Board of the U.S. Army Surgeon General for the Study of Korean War Casualties
1955 July 31	Voluntarily retired from the army after thirty-three years of service
1955–1958	Wrote the manuscript, "Medic"
1956 May–1968	Research Physician, University of California, San Francisco Medical Center
1979 September	Granted his personal papers to the Hoover Institution Archives, Stanford University
1988 November 20	Death of his wife, Elva
1993 March 3	Married Tuli Kalau Fifita
1994 December 2	Died Stanford, California
1994 December 9	Buried at Arlington National Cemetery, Arlington, Virginia

—ZZ

"Medic"

This book is dedicated to a young doctor who had all the attributes for a distinguished career as an army medic. His all too brief career was cut short when he was killed in action defending his patients as a battalion surgeon of the First Battalion, Ninth Infantry of the Second Infantry Division, near Kunuri, North Korea, on 27 November 1950. He was Capt. Charles M. Struthers, Medical Corps, United States Army. This young officer represented all that I could have desired in a son of my own: he was my older daughter's husband.

The old saying that a good horse master must first learn to master himself is equally applicable to the commander of men. The man who would successfully command others must first learn to control and command himself. When the army lost its horses it lost not only a means of transportation but also a means of training leaders and commanders and trainers of men.

—***Crawford F. Sams***, "Medic"

Preface

Over the years between 1948 and 1955, I was approached by a number of highly competent writers who desired to collaborate on, or to undertake the authorship of, a book recording my experiences as an army medic in many parts of the world.[1] At that time there was considerable interest in the results of our work in the Far East. A number of authors favorably mentioned aspects of my work in their publications.[2] My friends in and out of the service repeatedly urged me to write a book that would be of general interest so that what they called a unique experience could be made a matter of record. Gen. James S. Simmons, a lifelong friend and one of my most respected mentors, who was then Dean of the Harvard School of Public Health, was particularly insistent, as he felt that a book of this kind had not been written in recent years.[3] He felt it would be of interest not only to those in the medical field but also to the public as a whole.

I deferred writing the book until now for a number of reasons.[4] Many of the historic events in which I participated were a matter of controversy, and many of the programs on which I worked required the passage of time to determine whether they had been effective. Many of the events, which at the moment seemed of great importance, have fallen into their proper place in the scheme of things. Sufficient time has now elapsed to obtain a reasonable perspective of what was important and what was comparatively unimportant.

Some of the historical events in which I participated, and which I discuss in this book, have been written about by many other participants. I have attempted to give one man's version of what happened, as I saw it. This version, when added to those of others, because none of us see events in the same way, may serve a useful purpose in arriving at a conclusion as to what really happened. I have made no attempt through footnotes or bibliography to provide the references and documentation that are part of an historical document or official report. This book is a narrative of my own experiences and my own views; however, all of the factual statements included in it can be documented from my own files or from other sources. The interpretation of events is my own and is, therefore, biased by my own background, my own experience, and my professional interests.

In discussing the medical problems in which, of course, I was basically interested, I have tried to present them in a nontechnical manner. I have discussed only those that I feel might be of interest to the average reader.

I have from time to time mentioned the names of numerous individuals with whom I worked on various large-scale programs. To those whom I have mentioned and to the several hundred individuals whose names I have not mentioned for lack of space, I acknowledge a debt of gratitude and appreciation, because to them belongs the credit for such success as some of our programs may have attained. Without the support of my superiors and without the wholehearted loyalty and hard work of my subordinates, none of these accomplishments could have been achieved.

Crawford F. Sams
Atherton, California
1958

The Move

Just before dawn on the thirtieth day of August 1945, the alarm bells sounded. An announcement over the speakers directed all crew members to take battle stations and all passengers to report to boat stations with steel helmets and the ever present life jackets. All watertight doors in bulkheads were to be closed following the movement topside. This announcement was our first predawn "stand to" since the navy command ship Sturgeon had been plowing steadily northward under destroyer escort from Manila.[1] A predawn "stand to" was routine in the combat area or when the radar had picked up approaching unidentified aircraft, submarines, or surface craft. But the war was supposed to be over: At least, a surrender ceremony was scheduled to take place in Tokyo Bay on the second of September.

Conjectures spread in whispers among the passengers at the boat stations. The Japanese Imperial Government had publicly announced that they had accepted, with certain modifications, the terms of surrender, which had been formulated and announced at Potsdam. A Japanese delegation that had been brought to Manila on 19 August had received from the commander-in-chief of armed forces in the Pacific detailed instructions on preparations to be made by the Japanese for receiving allied troops in Japan.—What had happened to General MacArthur and the handful of officers who were scheduled to arrive by air at Atsugi Air Field near Yokohama this afternoon?—The Japanese had been informed of the Sturgeon's arrival.

Our conversation was not the idle gossip of uninformed men, for the Sturgeon's passenger list read like a *Who's Who* of the army, navy, and army air force of the Pacific war.[2] Aboard were the senior officers of General Headquarters, as well as the senior officers of the Sixth Army, commanded by Gen. Walter Krueger, which had fought its way from Australia; the Eighth Army, commanded by General Eichelberger; and the Tenth Army, commanded by General Stillwell. Gen. Courtney Hodges and his senior officers of the First Army, which was being redeployed from Europe to the Philippines, were also aboard. The British, the Australians, the Dutch, and even the Russians, who had so recently entered the Pacific war, had their senior representatives on the Sturgeon.

All of these officers had been engaged in preparing for the greatest air and amphibious operation of all time: the invasion of the island of Kyushu on the Japanese homeland. This invasion had been scheduled for November 1945, with a subsequent landing in the Kanto Plain on Honshu island in March 1946. Divisions in the Philippines and on Okinawa were being re-equipped and retrained.

6 THE MOVE

Supplies were being stockpiled, major construction of bases was under way, and shipping was being assembled. The redeployment of troops from Europe had begun when negotiations for surrender were initiated by the Japanese; but upon surrender, instructions had been given to plan the movement of troops to Japan for the occupation of that nation for the first time in its long history.

Was this "stand to" preliminary to an attempt on the part of the Japanese to sink the Sturgeon? Had there been a drastic change of plans? Was the war to be renewed as a result of one more act of treachery on the part of the Japanese? What a prize the Sturgeon and its passengers would be for the Japanese if she were sunk. Of course, no one was indispensable in war, and any or all of the senior officers could be replaced in time. But what of the delay, the temporary uncertainty on the part of the troops if all of their senior leaders were removed at once? What about the time necessary for new leaders to learn to work together with that smooth teamwork that time alone can bring about, so that each can anticipate the actions of the others in a given situation? Time was all important, for only two months remained to prepare for the invasion in November. If the war was to be resumed, would there be time enough with new staffs and leaders? Many of these officers had been the victims of Japanese treachery and deceit in the Philippines in 1941, and at Pearl Harbor, and during the many operations on the long hard road up from Australia or across the mid-Pacific.

As I stood with one of the groups at my lifeboat station as the first light began to glow above the horizon, not one word was uttered about the personal safety of these men who were dedicated to the ultimate defeat of the common enemy, Japan. Our concern was for the course of the war. Was the goal for which we had striven for almost four years, and which had seemed so close, to be withdrawn in one final attempt on the part of the Japanese to seize victory from defeat, as the Germans had tried at the Battle of the Bulge in December 1944? It was known that there were approximately seventeen Japanese divisions in the Kanto Plain, that midget submarines were still available to the Japanese, and that several thousand kamikaze pilots and planes were in the homeland as we were approaching.

Only a handful of American troops of the Eleventh Airborne Division were at Atsugi Air Field. Other divisions were loading in the Philippines; some were en route. Were the peace negotiations a giant hoax to draw us into a trap?

We quietly discussed these and many other thoughts as the sun came up over the horizon to starboard. On the port side, we could see the rugged cliffs and hills of Japan surmounted by the profile of Mount Fuji, in all of its perfect grandeur as it reflected the light of the rising sun, hinting at the meaning of the symbol on the Japanese flag. For almost all of us it was our first glimpse of Japan.

The "all clear" sounded, but over the speakers came the warning for no one to go below decks unless required by duty until the ship was docked. Then came the explanation for the "stand to": There had been trouble in Japan. Although the emperor's message announcing the surrender had been broadcast, certain diehard elements of the Japanese armed forces had refused to accept defeat, and there had been some fighting in the streets of Tokyo. As a result of damaged communications, the Japanese Imperial General Headquarters had been unable to reach all of their units to announce the cessation of fighting. Some of the units that had been reached refused to believe the message of defeat was authentic. It had been feared that some Kamikaze pilot or some returning submarine might make one last desperate effort to die in glory for the emperor by attacking the Sturgeon as she approached the sacred homeland.

Mines constituted an additional hazard. Although a path had been swept up the channel, there was always the possibility that a mine had broken loose into the channel we were negotiating; hence, with due prudence, the skipper had ordered the "stand to" as a precautionary measure: There were too many valuable eggs in his basket to run the risk of losing them through accident or otherwise.

As we proceeded slowly up Tokyo Bay, we could see Japanese anti-aircraft guns on the hills. Yokosuka, the great Japanese naval base, was protected by coastal defense guns protruding from what appeared to be fortifications tunneled into the cliffs. Two burned-out Japanese destroyers beached on a small island in the bay were our introduction to the terrible destruction that we were to encounter throughout Japan. Ahead we approached the fleet of the U.S. Navy, including the U.S.S. *Missouri*, on which the ceremony of surrender was to take place. With flights of aircraft from the carriers on constant patrol overhead, the seaworn grey of the ships lying at anchor off the port of Yokohama was a most reassuring sign that there had been no change in plans. The great might of the United States, which had almost singlehandedly brought Japan to her knees, had indeed reached the Japanese homeland; the war was finally over.

A small Japanese harbor craft approached the Sturgeon and a Japanese pilot came aboard. He took the Sturgeon into the dock adjacent to the customhouse. It was the first American ship to dock in Japan since the United States declared war with Japan on 7 December 1941.

So began the greatest experiment in human relations in history.

JAPAN

1

The Perimeter

As the Sturgeon lay tied to the dock, I stood at her rail with a member of the theater engineer's staff wondering what extent of destruction awaited us in this great port and industrial city of Yokohama. With a population of over one million people, Yokohama had been one of the primary targets of our army air force raids. In 1941, Gen. Elmer Adler and other senior officers of the army air corps had predicted that if our bombers could only reach and destroy the industrial centers of the Ruhr in Germany, the Ploesti oil fields in Rumania, and the Yokohama-Tokyo area in Japan, then Germany and Japan would immediately collapse and the war would end. I had seen firsthand the destruction wrought by such bombing raids at targets in North Africa and the Middle East, in Europe, and in the Philippines. Somehow the predictions had not worked out.

As an island empire, Japan was supposed to be vulnerable to such strategy. Some held that if her ships could be sunk, her ports destroyed, and her industrial centers laid waste, there was no need to defeat her armies. Her cities were particularly vulnerable to fire because ninety-eight percent of her buildings were built of wood; by destroying these, her labor force, at least, would be dispersed, even if the factories were not knocked out. Subsequently, according to press reports we had received from home, the bombings of Hiroshima and Nagasaki were credited as ending the Pacific war. Such reports were to be taken as proof of this theory, at least so far as Japan was concerned.

Months later, through study of Japanese records, interviews with top civilian and military leaders of Japan, and firsthand study and evaluation of damage and destruction and her remaining resources, a truer picture began to emerge. Once again the theory and popular wishful thinking turned out somehow to be in error. Japan had recognized her defeat when her armies were annihilated on Okinawa and in the Philippines, and had made overtures for peace through Russia, a neutral at that time, in May 1945, three months before the atomic bombs were dropped.

Man has been seeking an ultimate weapon with which to defeat his adversary without great risk to himself since the first primitive heaved a rock at his barehanded enemy before the fingers of that enemy could close around his throat. The first cutting edge of steel, gunpowder, high explosives, bombs, and now the unleashed power of the atom, have all been hailed, in turn throughout history, as the ultimate weapon for defeating an enemy without too great risk to self; yet, history records that the final decision for victory in every war, even in Korea in 1953, is determined by men struggling in the dust or the mire for some piece of ground, no matter how worthless that ground may appear to be at the time. Perhaps it is justified politically as a deterrent against war to play up the destructive power of each new ultimate weapon, as it has been done throughout history, is being done in the present controversy, and will be done in the future until the end of time, provided, of course, you do not frighten yourself and your own people more than you do your potential enemies. For those charged with the responsibility for the conduct of war or for provision of defense forces, however, to believe one's own propaganda or to fail to study the lessons of history is another and very dangerous matter.

I had spent much of my career studying the history and causes of human casualties, both civilian and military, and the relative effectiveness of their agents, whether disease or weapons of war. I had studied the means through organized medical efforts necessary for minimizing casualties and, particularly, deaths. I had directed such efforts in other parts of the world. Now that the war had suddenly ended without an invasion, that part of our plans for taking care of our military casualties from such an invastion had come to a close. But what of the enemy casualties, both civilian and military, which we would find in this land? That was to be my responsibility as chief of the Health, Education, and Welfare Division of the Military Government Section of General Headquarters, U.S. Army Forces, Pacific.

How accurate were our estimates of those casualties in the homeland from our air attacks, naval shelling, and the atomic bombs? How many military casualties were in hospitals? We had thought that very few had been evacuated from the Pacific Islands to Japan. What about epidemics? What medical facilities, personnel, and supplies remained in Japan?

I had learned through experience to make some correlation between physical destruction in cities and human casualties among the population. As soon as I could go ashore in Yokohama, I hoped to find some indication of the problems with which I would be faced. I had to re-evaluate our plans as quickly as possible in order to modify our requirements for medical supplies and relief supplies of food, clothing, blankets, and other items. Messages would have to be sent to the War Department so that only such quantities as would be required were shipped and the procurement of the sizeable quantities of such supplies that had been programmed were cancelled. All of these thoughts were running through my mind as I stood at the rail of the Sturgeon studying the scene around me.

As we surveyed the waterfront, the docks and warehouses appeared to be undamaged, although far to the north a Japanese aircraft carrier lay canted in a shipyard. No other ships could be seen. To the south, the New Grand Hotel facing the promenade along the waterfront also appeared to be intact. Just beyond the New Grand, the bluffs rose sharply along the shore, and we could see a number of fine homes that were also undamaged. These were the homes of the prewar foreign national colony, which subsequently were to serve as quarters for senior officers of the Eighth Army headquarters. On the skyline to the west we could see a church that had apparently been gutted by fire.

Directly opposite our ship was the customhouse. It was undamaged. We were especially interested in that building because it was to be the location of advanced General Headquarters of which I was a part. The building of reinforced concrete was painted black. We were to learn that all of the important buildings, governmental or private, including hospitals, had been painted black by the Japanese in an effort to make them more difficult to see during our night bombing attacks.

Something about this building appeared to be odd. It was constructed with several setbacks and a signal tower with numerous outside concrete stairs. My engineer companion called my attention to the fact that all of the steel railings and supports of the stairways had been removed. The steps for the stanchions were set in the concrete, but no other metal was apparent. We were to find throughout Japan that all metal had been removed from structures of all kinds. Even the steam radiators had been taken out of the buildings and piled in vacant lots preparatory to being moved to the steel furnaces as scrap.

Here, then, was the first indication of one of the causes of Japan's defeat. Although in 1931 she had begun the development of an industrial empire in Manchuria, where there were tremendous natural resources, including iron ore and coal, and had for some years before the war been stockpiling scrap steel from all over the world, particularly from the United States, Japan had virtually exhausted her supplies of scrap. She had resorted to stripping every available pound of metal that could be gotten from her buildings, bridges, and factories.[1]

Shortly after the gangplank had been lowered, we were called below for a staff conference and orientation. A perimeter would be established around Yokohama when sufficient troops arrived. In the meantime, we would not leave the perimeter area. We could go ashore but must always go in pairs. Side arms were to be worn at all times. We were to avoid any incidents with Japanese we might encounter. Those who so desired could move into the New Grand Hotel, but the Sturgeon would remain at dockside to serve as billets for an indefinite period. We would proceed to set up General Headquarters in the customhouse using field tables, chairs and other field equipment as soon as it could be unloaded from the ship. It would be days before vehicle transportation would be unloaded from ships en route from the Philippines, so we would be on foot until that time.

The Customhouse

Brig. Gen. William Crist, chief of the Military Government Section, and I debarked and started the short walk to the customhouse. As we left the dock, we encountered two Japanese national policemen with their helmets and short swords and one American soldier of the Eleventh Airborne Division, who were guarding the entrance to the dock. They were the only living beings we could see in what appeared to be the remains of a dead city.

The prefecture building, a large brick building painted black and set in a block-square park, was intact. A few other brick or concrete buildings to the south were intact. These included a large department store, which we would later use as a military hospital. To the west we could see a few isolated concrete buildings obviously gutted by fire. The rest of the scene was one of desolation. I had become accustomed to destroyed or damaged cities in other parts of the world and to the sight of huge piles of rubble of brick or stone from well-supported buildings that had collapsed under bombing, shelling, and demolition. Here there was no such picture—only ashes—literally miles of ashes interspersed with tall, isolated brick chimneys and steel safes. Later I learned that the chimneys were the remains of public bath buildings, which had dotted every Japanese town and city.

The steel safes were the result of lessons learned in the 1923 earthquake and fire. After that disaster in this land of major disasters, great difficulty had been encountered in settling insurance claims as records and policies had been burned. When the Tokyo-Yokohama area had been rebuilt, a campaign had been undertaken to sell steel safes to all who could afford to buy them. The campaign had evidently been a success for I had never seen so many safes. Although the people had lost their homes and their possessions, this time, at least, they had their safes and policies and records.

The streets were passable but for an occasional burned-out streetcar, truck, or fire truck that had been engulfed by the fire storms. No passenger cars could be seen burned or abandoned in the streets. Broken trolley wires and power lines dangled across streets and walks, serving to menace the unwary passerby in the night in a city without lights. Thousands of burned bicycles lay in the ashes or along the streets in mute testimony of the speed with which the flames had swept the city. To the north, we could see the twisted skeletons of burned factories and mills. The heat had been so intense that massive steel girders and pillars looked like a writhing mass of reptiles flung to the ground by the hand of a giant.

But what of the people in this great ghost of a city? Nothing moved, there was no sign of life. There was a deathly silence. Had they all been consumed in the holocaust? Because my concern is primarily with people, I wondered as to the fate of those caught in the storm of fire.

Fire storms of such magnitude have never been seen in Europe or America, where our cities of different construction and design do not provide the tinder of a Japanese city. It was not until I had witnessed the second burning of Aomori in northern Honshu a year later that I could visualize what had happened in Yokohama. The endless blocks of closely packed, frequently interconnected frame buildings serve as a powder train through which the flames sweep with ever increasing speed and intensity, creating their own winds of cyclonic force. So strong are they that one can hardly stand upright. The flames fed by these winds increase to such intensity that buildings are consumed with the force of an explosion.

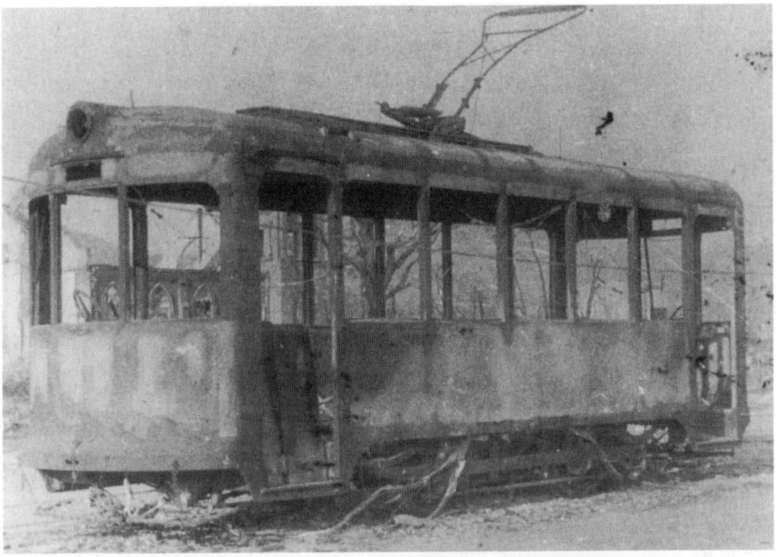

Figure 1. An occasional burned-out streetcar such as this one was part of the desolate scene that occupation forces encountered in Japanese cities that had been engulfed in fire storms during the war. Occupation of Japan, circa September 1945. (Courtesy of the Hoover Institution Archives, Stanford University.)

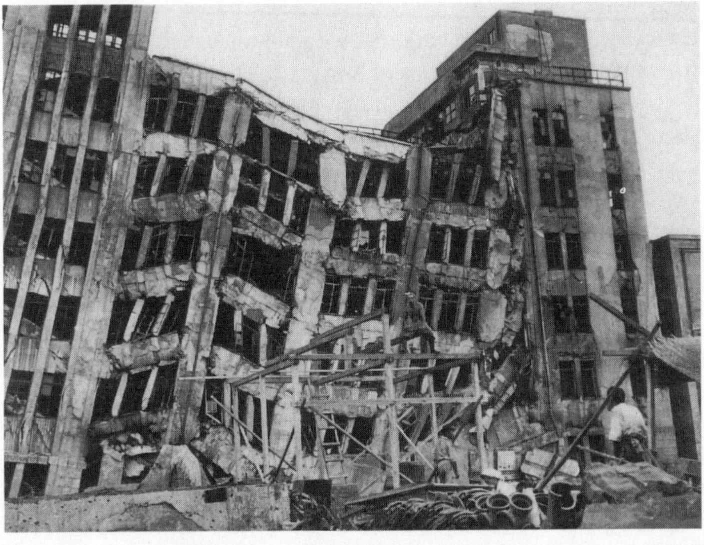

Figure 2. The Yamato Department Store, once an imposing seven-story building, was reduced to a mass of twisted steel and concrete by the intense heat of fire bombs during the war. Occupation of Japan, circa September 1945. (Courtesy of the Hoover Institution Archives, Stanford University.)

At frequent intervals between the curbs and the sidewalks were slit trenches in which people evidently sought refuge when an air raid alert sounded. They offered protection against bomb fragments and flying debris, but, as I was to learn, throughout Japan many people were found dead in these shallow trenches, which had become their coffins. There was no mark upon them, for the cyclonic winds of the fire storm literally sucked the air from these trenches as the fire swept past, and the people died for lack of oxygen. It was something to remember for the future.

The tall steel structure of the Tokyo and Yokohama elevated electric line appeared to be undamaged. At the railroad yards near the station, the tracks had been repaired. A few four-wheeled freight cars, characteristic of European and Japanese railroads, were in the yards. Some were burned. The few modern, double-trucked passenger cars in the yards looked like sieves from machine gun bullet holes of strafing raids. These raids must have been carried out by carrier based aircraft, as army fields for tactical aircraft used in low-level strafing were too far away for such attacks when the war ended.

As we entered the customhouse, we saw a picture that was to become all too familiar throughout Japan. The fine floors were covered with a scum of wax and dirt of several years' accumulation. The walls were grimy with soot; they had obviously not been repainted during the war. The windows were almost opaque from the grime. The radiators had been removed as had all railings. Small single light bulbs hung suspended from cords in the ceiling. Blackout curtains were fixed to all windows.

After walking through the building, we finally located the room on the ground floor to which our staff section was assigned. There were a few old desks and chairs in the room, and I sat down at one that had a knee well. That was my first mistake in Japan, although far from my last. In only a matter of seconds, my ankles were on fire. They were covered with a swarm of culex mosquitoes, who had been resting in the cool shadowed recesses of the knee well. They were obviously starved for some fresh blood. They were not adverse to taking it from an enemy of Japan, and they were not willing to wait until the usual biting time at dusk. This was a bright sunny midmorning.

I had hoped to find some indication of the nutritional status of the Japanese people, for one of my responsibilities was to make such determinations and recommend importation of food for relief purposes, if necessary. Yet my first contact with living creatures in Japan was with insects, who from their actions appeared to be starving. The Japanese had never attempted modern methods of insect control and had no such thing as DDT, which had been so effective in malaria and fly control throughout the world during later years of the war; thus, one of my first tasks would be to obtain DDT and sprayers from my friends in the navy. All buildings to be occupied by our people would have to be given a thorough spraying before we could use them.

The Police Hospital

As our field equipment for the office had not yet been unloaded from the ship and there was nothing yet to be done in the customhouse, I set out on foot with a Nisei interpreter on a reconnaissance of the city. I hoped to locate a hospital in order to form some idea of the medical situation and the work ahead. I had a prewar map of the city, but the widespread destruction made it difficult to identify landmarks. The map, however, showed a small police hospital located near the New Grand Hotel. There were a number of undamaged buildings in that area, including the Helm House apartments, so we proceeded in that direction.

As my interpreter and I walked down the street, we located a painted brick building, which from its location and color should have been the hospital. We entered the lobby, and my interpreter called out in Japanese to learn if anyone was present. Silence greeted us. We then began a tour. It was even more filthy than the customhouse. In the laboratory, drawers were half open; broken equipment was strewn about the floor and tables. In the X-ray room, we found a machine of Japanese manufacture patterned after German machines I had seen in captured German military hospitals in North Africa and Europe. The machine appeared workable, but there was no electricity and no standby electric power generator such as we routinely have in our hospitals. I was interested in the quality of technical work done by the Japanese, which could be judged by an examination of films. To my surprise there was no film. X-rays had been taken on photographic paper, which had a coarse emulsion, so the films were fuzzy and difficult to read. Later I learned that no Japanese hospital had X-ray film during the last three years of the war.

In the operating room, there were only paper bandages and a few cotton bandages on the shelves of the cabinets. The cotton bandages were old; although they had been washed, they were stained from much reuse. In the wards there were no beds, only tatami on the floor on which the patients would lay. But there were no patients in this hospital.

As we worked our way through the second floor, we came to a hall that was lined with sliding doors, probably the quarters for nurses or other hospital staff. We slid back the various doors. The rooms were empty with the exception of one. In this room we encountered three men sitting on the tatami drinking tea. As we entered the room they were obviously frightened. Here was my first opportunity to talk to a Japanese in his homeland.

Through my interpreter, I received one of the real shocks of my life. I had been trained in my profession of medicine and in the military medical service in accordance with occidental standards to provide medical care equally to anyone regardless of race, creed, or color; to friend or enemy. In accordance with the Geneva Conventions, if it endangered the lives of our wounded to move them, it was safe under the Conventions to permit them to fall into the hands of the enemy, leaving medical supplies and even medical personnel behind with them if need be. We were trained to provide medical care for enemy sick and wounded, whether military or civilian, who might fall into our hands. We provided for such care in all of our planning.[2]

On the whole, this code has been observed in the great majority of battles in which our forces have participated. It is true, however, this gentlemen's code has been violated many times in the past, even in the gentlemen's wars of Europe, and I suspect it will be violated many times in the future. I had seen captured Japanese hospitals in the Philippines in which many of the patients had committed suicide rather than fall into our hands. I had listened to harrowing stories from our medical personnel released at Santo Tomas and Baguio of wounded and sick prisoners who had been bayonetted because they could not keep up with the column on the infamous death march from Bataan. Our medical aid men and litter bearers had discarded their Red Cross brassards and went armed into battle because they found the brassards only made them better targets for the enemy.

These violations of our code of conduct and moral standards had been in the heat of battle, or at least had been carried out in the belief that they would contribute to winning the war. They were the result of the brutalities of war when the thin veneer of civilization is stripped away and the raw emotions of self-preservation and hate become dominant. It is the uncontrolled rage that causes a murderer to continue to fire into the body or to continue to slash the body of his victim long after that victim has entered the throes of death. It is the ferocity of a cornered wild animal seeking to preserve its life.

In this filthy room, I was to learn the first of a number of bitter lessons. The war was over. Surrender had been arranged. Fighting had ceased. Yet through my interpreter I was informed that these three Japanese men crouching on the straw mat in this hospital were waiting for us to execute them. They had decided to stay behind as a last gesture of defiance. All of the patients had been evacuated to the country with the nurses and other staff because it was expected that when the barbaric Americans arrived they all would be killed. The hospital looked as though it had been looted because in the haste of evacuation all movable supplies that could be taken had been sent away with the patients, lest they fall into our hands. They expected us to seize all medical supplies for our own use. The city had been evacuated of those who had survived the bombings, as it was expected that we would loot and pillage the remaining buildings and homes, rape the women, and slaughter the men and children.

Through my interpreter, I informed the three doctors that we had come to this hospital to see the patients and to find out the status of medical supplies; not to seize them for our own use, but to find out if they were adequate and to help them, if possible. They were free to go or to remain as they chose. In either case they would be unharmed. The war was over. It was not in accordance with our standard of conduct to go through the country raping and slaughtering the unarmed civilian population.

To be suspected of a code of conduct so alien to all that in which one has been trained and in which one has believed was a shock. But I shall never forget the look of disbelief that replaced the expressions of despair on their faces when my words were translated to them.

Since my return to this country, I have thought over that statement. In the light of present planning, I am not so sure that I was correct in my interpretation of our present code of conduct. Perhaps without realizing it, we have changed our standards of moral values. Certainly with the advent of weapons of mass destruction from the air, we have engaged in wholesale slaughter of unarmed civilian men, women, and children in the bombing of the cities of Europe and Japan. Of course, we can rationalize that the Germans started it all in the senseless destruction of Rotterdam and the bombings of London and that we were merely retaliating; however, I am reasonably sure that we will not initiate such action in a future war. If someone else starts it, perhaps retaliation in kind is justified.

But on that day in August 1945, I was certain that we had no intention of lining up the people in the streets and mowing them down with machine guns. Certainly, we were not going through their hospitals slitting the throats of the patients to get rid of them so that we could use the buildings for our own sick and injured as these three pathetic figures had anticipated.

As there was nothing further we could learn there, we left the hospital. We then crossed the street and entered an undamaged apartment building. I had never seen a Japanese apartment building. This one would become the symbol of a controversy: Inside we found a few Japanese girls who, according to my interpreter, were prostitutes waiting to serve the occupation troops.

En route to the bluff where I hoped to determine the status of a small hospital which before the war had been built and operated by and for the foreign national colony, we passed the New Grand Hotel. We stopped to watch the cavalcade of cars arriving from Atsugi bearing General MacArthur and his party. These were the first passenger automobiles we had seen in Japan. They were American cars that were five- to ten-years-old. I was to learn that there were only about forty thousand trucks and cars in all of Japan before the war, which explained the absence of burned out cars in the streets and ashes of the devastated cities.

The Bluff Hospital

As we reached the top of the bluff, we had a bird's-eye view of Yokohama. Along the hills to the west and north, we could see numerous groups of houses that had escaped the flames. With the exception of the few concrete or brick buildings near the waterfront, the rest of the city had been destroyed. The bluff hospital, painted black as were the others, was a beautiful modern concrete building. Like the police hospital, it was stripped of movable equipment and devoid of patients and staff. This hospital was soon to be one of the first problems with which we had to deal.

The next morning an irate Frenchman entered the office that we were establishing in the customhouse and demanded that I re-equip the bluff hospital and turn it over to him forthwith. Here was a small issue that necessitated a determination of broad policy concerning property ownership. Subsequent investigation showed that a group of foreign nationals had formed a corporation prior to the war to build and operate this hospital for the foreign national colony. The Japanese had replaced the foreign nationals on the board of trustees when war became imminent. The Japanese board had turned over the hospital to the Japanese Medical Treatment Corporation, a quasi-governmental corporation established by the Japanese Government to acquire and operate all nongovernmental hospitals for the duration of the war. This corporation had turned this particular hospital over to the imperial Japanese navy to operate as a naval hospital throughout the war.

Who were the real owners? The original board had been comprised of Germans, Italians, French, Swiss, British, and Americans. Some of these nationals were now enemy nationals and some allied. If all were enemy nationals, the precedent was quite clear as to the disposition of the property. If all were allies, our instructions were clear as to restoring property to allied nationals which had been seized by the Japanese. If title had actually passed to the imperial Japanese navy, the rules of land warfare were quite clear. We, as the occupying power, had a clear right to seize such enemy military property as war booty. Again, as the occupying power, we could requisition either governmental or private property of the Japanese for our own use, but we did not intend to use this hospital for our own troops.

One of my responsibilities was to provide for the health and welfare of foreign nationals who were in Japan at the termination of the war. Unilateral instructions prepared by the State, War, and Navy Coordinating Committee (SWNCC), with which I had become familiar before leaving Washington, D.C., for the Far East, gave detailed procedures for these foreign nationals. They were divided into three groups: former enemy (Nazi Germans, Fascist Italians); friendly nationals (anti-Nazi Germans, anti-Fascist Italians, British, French, Dutch, Chinese, Canadians, and all other nationals who had been on the allied side during the war); and liberated people, particularly Koreans. There were several thousand occidental foreign nationals in Japan and 1.7 million Koreans who, it was alleged, were slave labor brought to Japan during the war to work in the coal mines, steel factories, and other industries.

All foreign nationals were to be given the choice of repatriation to their homeland, except for the Nazi Germans and the Fascist Italians, who were to be repatriated whether they liked it or not. Individuals classed as friendly foreign nationals who were held in concentration camps by the Japanese were to be immediately freed. Because they had been on a semi-starvation diet during the entire war, they were to be given special rations, clothing, and medical care according to occidental standards.

There were several solutions to the problem of medical care for the foreign nationals. One, of course, would be to provide medical care for them in our own military hospitals; however, because the war was over, the plan of the military theater surgeon was to move only those hospitals to Japan in sufficient numbers to provide for our own military people. To provide for the care of foreign nationals, especially Koreans of formidable numbers, would have been a tremendous additional load. By agreement, this was my problem to solve. It was my intention, therefore, to re-equip and staff with foreign national doctors and Japanese doctors those hospitals that we knew had been used for occidental foreign nationals before the war and to use Japanese hospitals for the Koreans.[3] Because the repatriation of such large numbers of people would take many months, and actually extended over several years, and because we could not accurately determine how many would desire to remain, it was necessary to provide facilities for a long-term program; hence, my decision to use civilian hospitals.

Because the bluff hospital had been used for foreign nationals before the war, it was one I had selected in my planning to re-equip and reopen. The answer to the Frenchman and the dilemma of who owned the place was solved temporarily by deciding that the hospital would be taken over and operated under the direction of the Supreme Commander for the Allied Powers (SCAP). Several years later, a succession of legal advisors finally untangled the ownership and title of the property, and it was restored to a new corporation of foreign nationals, businessmen, and others who came to Japan to join those friendly nationals who had elected to remain.

First Instructions

During the first days of the occupation after we had established our headquarters in the customhouse and the Eighth Army had established theirs in the ballroom of the New Grand Hotel, we were concerned primarily with working out a method of operations for dealing with the Japanese. As happens frequently, precedent was established in the field of health and welfare.

Shortly after establishing our headquarters, two members of the International Red Cross Committee (IRCC), Dr. Juno and Marguerita Strahler, came to my office to report a situation that required immediate action. Russia had refused permission for members of the IRCC to cross Russia via the trans-Siberian railroad to Japan in accordance with the Geneva Conventions until shortly before the war ended. The members had arrived in Japan only a couple of weeks before we did. The situation concerned the thousands of injured at Hiroshima, the target of our first atomic bomb. They reported that only two small hospitals had survived the bomb and subsequent fire and that medical supplies for the care of the injured were exhausted.

Gen. Thomas F. Farrell of the Manhattan Project had come to Japan with a number of his scientists aboard the Sturgeon and was most eager to move his scientists into Hiroshima to begin studies of residual radiation and other effects of the bomb. There were no American troops ashore in the Hiroshima-Kure area, and none were scheduled to arrive there for several weeks. The problem was twofold: to take action on the request of the IRCC; and to try to move American scientists into Hiroshima.

I, therefore, decided to send seven plane loads of medical supplies by troop carrier plane to the airfield at Hiroshima and to introduce General Farrell's people into the area under the guise of assisting in distributing the medical supplies.[4] We did not know just what the reaction of the Japanese in Hiroshima would be to the first Americans to enter that city. Frequently, the reaction of civilian populations to bombing is to be so enraged that they will kill any aircraft personnel who may be shot down and parachute into the target area. In view of the reports that I had received from Dr. Juno, it was obvious from his description of signs and symptoms of some of survivors that many were suffering from the effects of radiation. Far more were suffering from flash burns. In either case, the picture was not a pretty one, and the situation was hardly conducive to accepting with open arms the perpetrators of such injuries. It was inadvisable to send an armed escort with the scientific personnel, as that would further aggravate the problem, if a mob action resulted from their entry into Hiroshima; hence, I decided to place on the Japanese themselves the responsibility for the safety of the Americans sent into the area.

Then began the task of setting the precedent for how this was to be done. Should we deal with the Japanese army or civilian authorities? If civilian authorities, at what level? Should we deal directly with local city authorities, prefecture authorities, or the civilian national government? If so, with what agency of that government? Would it be still capable of functioning? What should be the form of the instructions?—An order? A request?—Who should sign such instructions on behalf of our then military headquarters? Such apparent minutia, which can become so frustrating in attempting to accomplish a simple task such as the one I was attempting to do, frequently establish important principles. It became my problem to find the answers to the questions through a process of trial and error in order to send the medical supplies and General Farrell's personnel into Hiroshima.

After several days of conferences with the various staff sections of the headquarters, it was finally decided that I would prepare a letter of instruction, subsequently called "SCAPIN" (Supreme Commander for the Allied Powers Instructions), addressed to the imperial Japanese Government. The letter informed the government that we intended to move in by air medical supplies and personnel for their distribution to Hiroshima, and directed the imperial Japanese Government to provide for their security. Because we desired that there should be no doubt in the minds of the Japanese and no doubt subsequently as to the legality, the first instructions were to be signed by the Supreme Commander, himself. So the pattern was set. After General Headquarters, SCAP, was established, some subsequent modification permitted signature by staff section chiefs or the adjutant general of that separated headquarters on behalf of the Supreme Commander.

The Lessons of *Ikiri*

A few days after the establishment of our headquarters, liaison officers from the imperial General Headquarters of the Japanese army, which was still in operation in Tokyo, were assigned to the various staff sections. Colonel Harada, an officer of the medical section of the imperial General Headquarters, was assigned to my section. He was an outstanding officer and later was to become one of my good friends among the Japanese. His samurai battle sword, which is a family heirloom handed down in Japanese families for many generations, and his dress cap, which he also sent to me, are among my treasured mementos of Japan.

Among the voluminous information that I required Colonel Harada to obtain were data on the incidence of diseases throughout Japan. I was particularly interested in the incidence or presence of various epidemic diseases in the Tokyo area, where we expected to move in a short time.[5]

He reported the presence of *ikiri* in Tokyo. In English, ikiri means cholera. Cholera is one of the formerly dreaded epidemic scourges of the world that has killed literally millions of people, particularly in the Orient, although it has invaded Europe and even the United States in the past. It is a disease acquired through water or food contaminated with the cholera vibrio passed out in the stools of carriers or other cases. It is one of the wildfire diseases which sweep through an area of low sanitary standards like a forest fire. It is a dramatic disease in that people walking along the street may fall and die before your eyes. Frequently death occurs in a few hours after the beginning of symptoms. The dehydration is so intense that one of the characteristic signs of cholera occurs after death. It is a weird sight to see rows of bodies of cholera victims awaiting cremation, for long after death the muscles will contract so that the arms and legs move. I have seen dead men sit up during such contractions.

I had seen cholera in India, when I was en route to the Middle East in 1941, and had seen an outbreak in Meshed, Iran. Our troops had been inoculated against cholera. I inquired of Colonel Harada if the Japanese civilian population had been inoculated against cholera. The answer was negative. I believed that with water systems broken by bombing and low sanitary standards in handling food in Japan that we were faced with a serious situation if a real cholera epidemic was raging in Tokyo. It was therefore necessary for me to see these cases at firsthand and find out the number of cases with which we would have to deal.

This report led me into two mistakes and taught me lessons as a result. One of the mistakes is common among the medical profession; I had made it before in the Middle East. I might add that it is not limited to the medical profession. The mistake is to think that a foreign word translated into English necessarily means the same thing in both languages.

In the Middle East, I had received a report of a number of typhus cases in an Italian military hospital in Eritrea. To us the diagnosis of typhus means a louse- or flea-borne disease with certain signs and symptoms. To the European-trained medical man, the diagnosis of typhus may mean either what is typhoid fever to American-trained physicians or typhus. I had, therefore, made it a practice to inquire of European-trained physicians whether a case they reported as typhus was really louse- or flea-borne typhus or abdominal typhus, which to us is typhoid fever, a distinctly different disease caused by an entirely different organism. Their control, prevention, and treatment are quite different.

To the Japanese, ikiri meant either cholera, as we understood it, or an entirely different disease: a disease of children who acquired a diarrhea, went into convulsions, and frequently died in a few hours. The ambiguity stems from the early days of medicine when, clinically, the two diseases could not be distinguished from each other. To find out what ikiri really was it took a special research mission, which I requested from the United States a year later; however, the lesson is there. In dealing with people of different languages and cultural backgrounds, take a little time to study them. I am firmly convinced as a result of many years of dealing with people of other lands that many of our differences and misunderstandings are due to our own impatience and failure to find out really what words mean to them, as distinguished from our own interpretation of the translated words.

Our inability to communicate ideas in terms that, because of language and cultural differences, are understandable to others is one of the great handicaps of the world. Perhaps one of the most important lessons I have learned through experience is to acquire patience and attempt to have a sympathetic understanding and tolerance of peoples of other lands. Perhaps at the same time I have unfortunately acquired a bit of intolerance with some of my fellow Americans, particularly that small group who is unwilling to concede that anything developed in another country can in any sense equal, and certainly cannot be superior to, ideas or things made in America, or that small group who may spend a week on a whirlwind tourist trip or attend a conference in some foreign land and then return to pontificate as an authority on the attributes or lack of them of the people visited.

I obtained permission to leave the perimeter and go with Colonel Harada in a Japanese army car to Tokyo to determine whether cholera was epidemic in that great metropolis. The slow trip over the twenty miles between the center of Yokohama and Tokyo was a journey through devastation, for the main road or rather what passed for a main road ran through the industrial center of the country. We could go about only five miles an hour without breaking a spring in the car due to the holes in the road. Much of the road was unpaved.

Although a few hundred Japanese men had begun to return to Yokohama to work as labor for the occupation troops, as we entered Tokyo we saw fairly large numbers of people on the streets, including women and children. The women all wore a sort of mechanic's coverall called a *mampe*, which Colonel Harada told me had become the national costume for women during the war. Many thousands of women were working in the war factories, on the railroads, and at other jobs for which the traditional long-sleeved kimono was unsuitable; so the coverall had been decreed.

Tokyo was, of course, much larger than Yokohama. The prewar population of the Tokyo metropolitan area was over nine million people. There were far more fine brick or concrete buildings standing in Tokyo. Some had been gutted by fire, others were apparently untouched. One of the peculiar evidences of the vagaries of fire storms was also evident. Small islands of frame dwellings usually on a hilltop were seen throughout the city. They remained untouched by the flames.

As we drove past the imperial palace, the driver stopped the car on the plaza. Both Colonel Harada and the Japanese soldier-driver got out of the car and bowed low toward the palace as a sign of their great respect for the emperor.

We visited a contagious disease hospital at which some ikiri cases could be found. This hospital was the large Komi-go Hospital, which, unlike the police hospital in Yokohama, was filled with patients. It did not take long to realize that the ikiri of the Japanese was not the classic cholera with which we were concerned. So the mistake was made and the lesson was learned.

Then I proceeded to make a second and more serious error. My second mistake was to lose face or prestige, that fine distinction between the ruler and the ruled. It is a distinction that is alien to our American way of thinking and living but is essential to successful relations with peoples of other lands where prestige is so important, particularly when in the position in which we found ourselves as an occupying power. In my service, particularly in the Middle East, and in my short time in Malaya, Singapore, and India, I had had the opportunity to learn much from our British friends about the art of governing large numbers of people with a minimum of force and a handful of British military and civil servants. For several hundred years, this small island of people had stabilized a large portion of the population of the world. In my study of political science and history, I had wondered how they did it, and I had learned above all the necessity for maintaining face, as it is known in the Far East.

I should have known better from my past experience. But in my desire to obtain at firsthand necessary information concerning the health and welfare and education problems with which I would be faced, I visited the Education Ministry and Ministry of Health and Welfare in company with Colonel Harada. At the Ministry of Health and Welfare, in particular, I was received by the minister and vice minister and his bureau chiefs in a conference room. After the usual ceremonial introductions and the inevitable round of tea, I obtained some of the information I wanted and made arrangements for the ministry to compile additional data. Being quite satisfied with the information I had obtained and particularly happy to learn that we were not faced with an epidemic of cholera, Colonel

Harada and I returned to Yokohama, where I made my report on the trip to General Crist.

Not until I read a copy of the English-language version of the *Nippon Times* the next morning did I realize the magnitude of my error. There for all the world to see in large print was an article concerning the fact that one of the senior officers of General MacArthur's headquarters had journeyed to Tokyo to pay his respects to the Minister of Health and Welfare of the imperial Japanese Government. I had stepped over the fine line. Apparently, I had completely hurled myself over it.

The timing of my action was particularly unfortunate, for much was being written by the American press about General MacArthur's kid-glove handling of the Japanese. General MacArthur, in his personal conduct throughout the occupation, demonstrated innate knowledge of the proper relationship that I have attempted to describe. He maintained an aloofness and isolation in his dealings with the Japanese that was perfectly suited to their psychology, which gained their respect and admiration. He dealt only with the emperor or the prime minister, which fit into their concept of stratification of classes and ranks.

For the sake of future historians, let me parenthetically state that the files of the *Nippon Times* for September 1945, until censorship was established on the Japanese press, will be rich source material for an analysis of Japanese attitudes during the immediate post-surrender period. Although we interpreted the surrender as an unconditional surrender, the Japanese interpreted the surrender as a negotiated agreement. Had they not, in their view, obtained concessions by the allied powers from the original Potsdam Declaration of surrender before they had agreed to surrender? They were, therefore, preparing to negotiate from their side with our side, as they termed it, on every issue, whether it involved acceptance of currency, the issuance of a surrender proclamation, or the processing of logs into lumber.

For many weeks after the occupation began, large numbers of undemobilized Japanese divisions remained throughout Japan and in the Kanto Plain area, in which we were located, while we had only a handful of American troops available to enforce any of our demands if the Japanese flatly refused to accept them. In such a delicate situation, I had made a mistake of etiquette. It was improper for the conqueror to call upon the conquered at that time. As a result, I learned a lesson for my own personal conduct in relation to the Japanese with whom I worked throughout the occupation, which I believe later gained their respect and cooperation.

2

Tokyo

On the tenth of September 1945, the advanced General Headquarters moved to Tokyo from the customhouse in Yokohama. The customhouse was turned over to the Eighth Army for use as their headquarters. The Dai Ichi building, a beautiful multi-storied building owned by the Dai Ichi Insurance Company and located directly across the moat from the imperial palace, was requisitioned as the principle building for our headquarters. Additional buildings nearby, such as the Forestry building and the Meiji building, were requisitioned for the overflow. As the headquarters grew during the course of the occupation, additional space was required; by the end of the occupation, the headquarters occupied many buildings in the city.

Initially, the Military Government Section of General Headquarters, U.S. Army Forces, Pacific was assigned to the Forestry building. On the organization of General Headquarters, Supreme Commander for the Allied Powers (SCAP), as a separate headquarters for the conduct of the occupation, I was assigned as chief of the Health and Welfare Section of General Headquarters, SCAP, to the first floor of the Dai Ichi building.

Here again one of the small things that become so important in human relationships was brought to my attention. In the reorganization, I was elevated from the position of chief of a division within a staff section to the position of chief of a staff section; yet, in the eyes of the Japanese with whom I was dealing, I was moved from the fourth floor to the first floor, which in their literal interpretation of place on the totem pole meant a demotion in prestige. Immediately, my Japanese liaison officer raised the question whether I had been demoted in position and function. As he pointed out to me, the most important individual should be located at the top of the building and least important people were on the first floor. The buildings were designed with the most luxurious offices on the top floors and the large undivided spaces on the bottom floors for the working people. Of such small things one must learn in dealing with people of cultures and standards of values different from one's own.

The Imperial Hotel

As one of the senior officers of the headquarters, I was assigned billets in the Imperial Hotel, the world famous hotel designed by the American architect

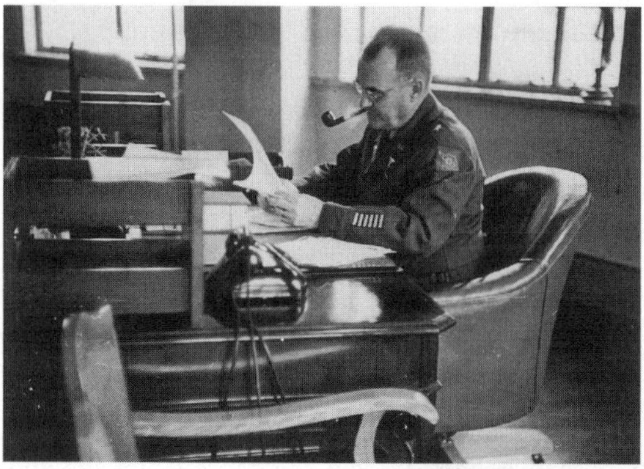

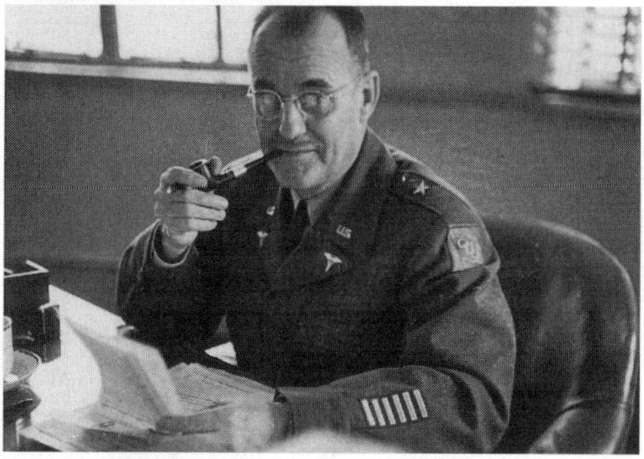

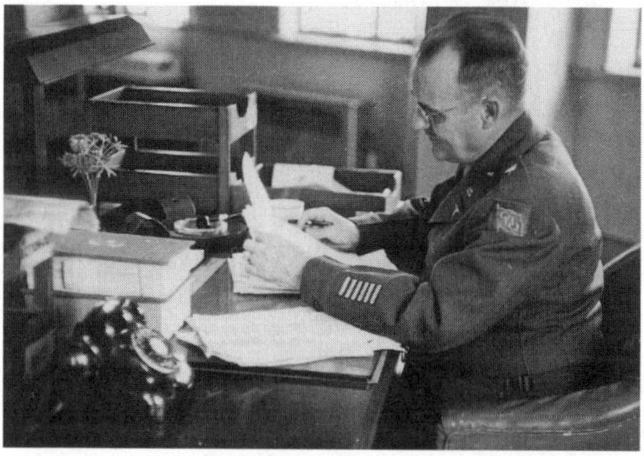

26 JAPAN

Figures 3, 4, 5. Col. C.F. Sams at his desk, General Headquarters, Supreme Commander for the Allied Powers, Tokyo, circa October 1945. Sams served as Chief of the Public Health and Welfare Section of SCAP from October 1945 to June 1951. He considered his peacetime work in Japan to be his greatest professional challenge and most important accomplishment. (Courtesy of the Hoover Institution Archives, Stanford University.)

Frank Lloyd Wright. The rambling three-story building of yellow brick had successfully withstood the earthquake and fire of 1923, but had not escaped unscathed the second burning of Tokyo in 1945. One wing, the ballroom, and the theater within the building had been gutted by fire. In the opinion of some of our engineers, that portion of the building should have been torn down and rebuilt; but to a people whose sense of values is so different from ours and who are used to accomplishing so much with so little, such a course of action was wasteful and unthinkable. The Japanese succeeded in obtaining permission to rehabilitate the gutted portion of the building without tearing down the remaining structure so that within a comparatively short time the ballroom and second wing were ready for use. This patient patching of buildings was used throughout Japan in the case of brick or concrete buildings gutted by fire or partially damaged by high explosive bombs; thus, the cities were literally rebuilt.

The Imperial Hotel was far from a pleasant place to live at that time. The fine furnishings of prewar days had been removed, even the rugs. Straw mats constituted the floor covering of the main lobby and the hallways. The rooms were lit by the inevitable single light bulb of low wattage, which fatigued the eyes by its constant flickering due to low-cycle alternating current. There was no heat. Room radiators had been removed and hot water did not flow from the tap. The metal tubes had been removed from the boilers in the scrap metal drive. At night, life was made miserable by the hundreds of rats that used the ventilating ducts as runways in their constant search for food. Their scratching and squealing and fighting made sleep most difficult. Finally, we initiated a rat-catching campaign and ended that nuisance.

Tests showed that the damaged city water system could produce only contaminated water unfit for human consumption, so drinking water was initially obtained from army lister bags in which the water was chlorinated. They were located in the lobby, hallways, and dining room.

Our meals were prepared by a Japanese chef trained in Paris who could do wonders with American C rations. They were to be our fare for many months until reefer ships became available in sufficient numbers to bring frozen meat and fresh vegetables from the States.

Japanese waitresses, many of whom had been employees of the hotel for years before the war, returned to serve in the dining room in their mompe. It was not long until each received an American nickname. "The Tiger" was one of the most beautiful girls, in spite of the mompe. It was several months before the girls appeared in beautiful *kimono*, characteristic of the beauty of Japan.

How different was this picture from the picture of the Imperial Hotel presented to our dependents a year later when they were first permitted to join us in Japan. By then the hotel had been completely refurnished and rehabilitated, and the service worthy of a world-renowned hotel had been re-established.

A Survey of Hospitals

I moved to Tokyo on Saturday. The next day, accompanied by Colonel Harada and Dr. Manabe Mitsuta, an additional liaison officer assigned to me by the Japanese Ministry of Health and Welfare, I set out on a reconnaissance of the medical facilities of Tokyo, primarily to determine which Japanese hospitals or other buildings should be requisitioned for U.S. Army hospitals to be moved from the Philippines. Out of 4,000 hospitals in the country, 1,027 had been destroyed by fire bombs and high explosives. It would be my responsibility to recommend such hospitals that could be spared from the remainder for requisition. We required three hospitals in Tokyo alone. Aerial photographs showed that several hospitals were apparently in areas that had been destroyed; the civilian population which they had previously served obviously had been moved elsewhere. The buildings therefore would no longer be required for those areas for some time, at least until the areas had been rebuilt and the population returned.

We proceeded first to St. Luke's, a fine modern hospital built with American funds by Episcopal missionaries. It was one of the most modern in design, with spacious sundecks and a beautiful chapel with balconies from the second and third floors of the hospital extending into the chapel so that patients either in wheel chairs or in beds could attend church services. Like all buildings at the time, it was dirty and run down. It would require extensive repainting and some internal rearrangement to expand the capacity to meet the needs of the military hospital scheduled to occupy it.

We next proceeded to the Tsukiji Hospital, which was occupied by the Japanese naval medical school and staff. The hospital had no patients except for about thirty men and women gathered in one ward. The operating room had been moved to the basement for protection during bombing attacks and was heated by a charcoal brazier. We aroused the Japanese admiral in command of the school and asked him to accompany us on an inspection tour of the naval medical school building adjacent to the hospital to determine whether it could be adapted for additional ward capacity. He was extremely arrogant and flatly stated that we could not take over this hospital as the imperial Japanese navy required it. Unfortunately, he had not been informed that the imperial Japanese navy was to be literally abolished under surrender terms and, therefore, would have no further need of the place. Because it was not needed for the civilian population, if it were suitable for our needs, we would requisition it under the Geneva Conventions.

He reluctantly started a march down the halls. I was more interested in the rooms, laboratories, and other facilities than simply marching through the halls, so I requested that we visit each room. He was not eager for us to do this.

Here, again, was a lesson in conduct. In dealing with some of the arrogant Nazi German officers in the Middle East and in Europe, I had learned that the only way to gain their respect was to adopt an even more arrogant attitude toward them. To act with the ordinary courtesy with which we normally deal with each other in this country is only a sign of weakness to such individuals. In this instance, it became necessary to outdo the arrogant vice admiral. I forcefully directed him personally to open each door and then stand aside while I entered the room I desired to inspect. It took only a short time to convince him that cooperation was better than defiance. Soon he was freely explaining in response to my questions the information I desired as to the layout, equipment, and function of the various facilities.

Next we visited the Doai Hospital situated on the banks of a river on the north side of the city. It was located adjacent to the Doai Shrine. The surrounding area had been destroyed by fire, and no requirement existed at this time for its use for the civilian population. This hospital illustrates an interesting point. It was built with American funds donated for the relief of the Japanese people following the great earthquake of 1923. By the time the American people had put on a campaign for funds, which were transmitted through the American Red Cross, there was no real need for the money for direct relief of the destitute people. It had been decided to use the money to build a shrine as a memorial to those killed in the earthquake and fire and to include a modern hospital in the plan. The old pattern of waiting for a disaster to occur and then putting on a fund drive afterward for direct relief usually fails in its purpose. One of the cardinal points of a successful disaster relief organization is to have funds earmarked for direct relief before disasters occur.

We then visited the Seibo Hospital, a fine little hospital in western Tokyo, which we knew had been used by foreign nationals before the war, like the bluff hospital in Yokohama. It was undamaged. The head of the hospital was a British nun who was also a doctor of medicine, and an exceedingly competent one. I decided to re-equip this hospital and, using the foreign national staff who had been released from concentration camps, use it again for care of foreign nationals in the Tokyo area.[1]

The First Imperial Japanese Army Hospital, one of 469 Japanese army and navy hospitals and the largest hospital in Tokyo, was filled with battle casualties. Later, I was to place all of these former military hospitals under the control of the Ministry of Health and Welfare as national civilian hospitals.[2] After rehabilitation, the "First National Hospital" was to be used as the first model of a modern hospital and as the site of the first school for hospital directors in Japan.[3]

I decided to recommend the St. Luke's, Doai, and Skiji Hospitals in the Tokyo area for requisition for the U.S. Army military hospitals. This I could conscientiously do after studying the requirements for the civilian population in the area, because the population had been reduced from 9 million to 3 million people by evacuation before the fire. So far as I know, the three hospitals were still used by our army ten years later.

Uyeno Station

On our return, we went through Uyeno Park, a beautiful park containing a fine museum and drives lined with cherry trees. I was to visit the park many times in the future at cherry blossom time. On one edge of the park was Uyeno Station, which my liaison people wanted me to see.

Tokyo is unique among the large modern cities of the world in having a fine elevated train system, a subway system as fine as the metro in Paris, and a surface street car system to handle the daily movement of its teeming millions. Uyeno Station was one of the points at which all three systems met to discharge and take on passengers to and from the steam railroads, which served the northern part of the island of Honshu and the island of Hokkaido. The Central Station, not far from the Dai Ichi building, served a similar purpose for trains running to the south of Japan. Although the Central Station had been largely destroyed by bombing, for railroad stations seem to be aiming points for aerial bombs, the Uyeno Station was undamaged.

Here at Uyeno Station was my first contact with what was to become one of our major problems: the control of population movement. I saw thousands of people milling about. My liaison people told me that many of these poorly dressed people, all of whom seemed to have all of their belongings on their backs, were either trying to return to the destroyed city from the country, to which they had been evacuated before the bombings, or they were city people who had remained and were going to the country in search of food. The ration distribution system had ceased to function. In addition, there were several thousand homeless people, including many orphans, living in the passageways to the subway system, which had been used as air raid shelters during the war. Many of these refugees were supposedly dying of starvation. It was one of the more horrible sights I have seen in a lifetime to enter the underground passages, dark, damp, with foul air and the stench of thousands of unwashed humans lying in rows on the cold concrete. The ventilation systems had long since ceased to function due to lack of electric power to drive the fans.

In picking our way over and through the rows of men, women, and children lying in the tunnels, it was evident on even a cursory examination of some of them that they were not dying from starvation, but smallpox, typhoid, and typhus fever. We found many cases of these diseases among them. I was told that this picture was typical of the situation I would find in Osaka, Fukui, Sendai, Shimonoseki, and other transportation centers and cities.

A Problem of First Magnitude

The population was in a ferment. Like millions of ants, people were moving all over the country. Koreans by the hundreds of thousands were trying to return to Korea. Demobilized soldiers, sailors, and airmen were trying to go home or to locate their families who had either been evacuated before the bombings or killed in the attacks. People from the country were trying to return to the ashes of their homes in the cities, and the remaining city people were on the move to the country in search of food. Obviously, we had a problem of first magnitude.

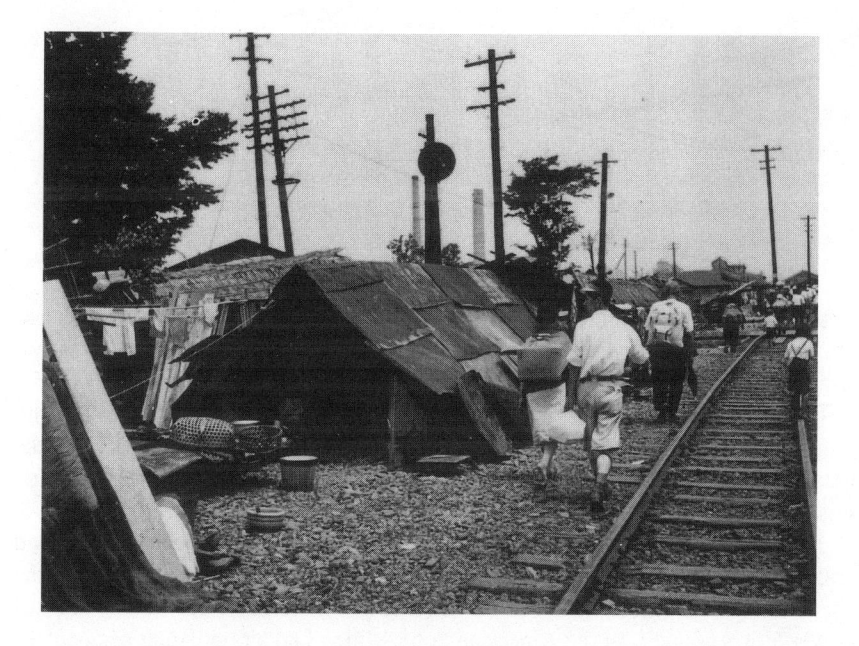

Figure 6. Lean-tos built along the roadbeds of railroads provided temporary shelter for people left homeless by the war. Occupation of Japan, circa September 1945. (Courtesy of the Hoover Institution Archives, Stanford University.)

It was estimated that the homes of 8.5 million people had been destroyed in the cities of Japan, and 6.5 million Japanese were to be repatriated from countries outside of Japan and relocated in Japan. Some of the people who had already returned to the ashes of their homes had erected lean-tos of any material they could find undestroyed, such as sheets of galvanized iron from their former roofs. They were without jobs, and most of them were destitute.

The problem of controlling the epidemics of smallpox, typhoid, dysentery, typhus, and other wildfire diseases from spreading throughout the country by this mass movement and the provision of direct relief in the form of food, clothing, bedding, and some form of shelter, until people could be re-established on their own feet, would be my responsibility and that of the Ministry of Health and Welfare, with whose operation I would be most directly concerned. How these problems were solved is one of the stories of this book. It was a challenge in mere magnitude of numbers and lack of means for meeting the problem that I had not seen equalled in Europe or anywhere else in the world where I had lived and worked.

3

The Decision: SCAP

It was not until the second of October 1945 that the final decision was made, and the necessary orders were published, as to the type of organization to be established for the occupation and government of Japan. This organization was quite different from that established for the occupation of Germany. For those who may be faced with similar problems in the future, the basic differences and the reasons for the differences are worth noting, as they were the source of many misunderstandings and some unfounded criticisms.

In Germany, the country was divided into four zones, each occupied by and under the absolute control of the military forces of a different country, with the exception of the isolated city of Berlin, which was to be governed by a four-power allied council. In the American zone, which had a population of about 15 million people, the commander was responsible only to the U.S. Government. In the British zone, the British commander was responsible to his government; likewise with the French and the Russian zones. In the American zone, we used an American form of local and state government, and the German people could be indoctrinated with the American way of doing things. In the Russian zone, the communist form of local and state government and the communist way of doing things became the order of the day. The success or failure of that method of conducting the occupation of a country is a matter of record and of judgment for future historians.

In Japan, by terms of the surrender, the former empire of Japan was limited to the four main islands of Japan: Hokkaido; Honshu; Shikoku; and Kyushu. General MacArthur, by terms of his designation as Supreme Commander for the Allied Powers in East Asia (SCAP), represented not only the U.S. Government, but also was technically responsible to an allied group, later established by intergovernmental agreement, known as the Far East Commission. As such, he was limited in his authority, so far as the Japanese were concerned and in the conduct of the occupation, to the four main islands of Japan. Although the initial directives to him for the conduct of the occupation were unilateral directives prepared by the State, War, and Navy Coordinating Committee (SWNCC) of the United States, these directives were later reviewed and, with some modifications, adopted by the Far East Commission as their directives to General MacArthur, who was their executive representative. Gen. Frank McCoy, one of our most able diplomats, was the American representative on that commission.

At the same time, General MacArthur, as commander-in-chief of the U.S. Far East Command, the separate military general headquarters, was responsible only to the U.S. Government. Under this other hat, he was responsible for the command and control of all U.S. military forces in Japan, the Philippines, Guam and the Marianas, the Ryukyus, and Korea.

In Germany, Gen. Dwight D. Eisenhower was initially in command of the military components. His deputy, General Clay, was in charge of the military government section. In Japan, General MacArthur had separate staffs for the military command and for the military government; both were responsible to General MacArthur.

On the second of October 1945, General Headquarters, SCAP, was established and organized to cover the extensive functions of normal civil government, with the addition of several staff sections for special functions, such as Civil Property Custodian and Civil Reparations. These functions are peculiar to occupations of enemy nations. The staff sections that made up this organization were responsible directly to the Supreme Commander through a deputy chief-of-staff for SCAP and the chief-of-staff.

The Public Health and Welfare Section

The various staff sections of SCAP were organized to parallel the functions of the various ministries (or departments) of the national government of Japan. In some instances, the functions of one SCAP section dealt with more than one ministry. As the chief of the Health, Education, and Welfare Division of the Military Government Section of General Headquarters, U.S. Army, Pacific, I would have been concerned with both the Ministry of Health and Welfare and the Ministry of Education; however, in studying the problems in these fields with which we were faced upon our arrival in Japan in the light of our directives and missions, I had come to the conclusion that the task of reorganizing a totalitarian national system of education, including all elementary and middle (high) schools, universities, and technical schools, into a decentralized reasonably democratic system would require the full time and effort of a most capable chief. Likewise, the task in the fields of health and welfare, which included the major fields of preventive medicine, medical care, welfare, and social security, was so tremendous that it would also require the best efforts of a single chief.[1] Following the sound principle of grouping like or closely related functions together, I had found it organizationally most unwise to group general information and education with the rather specialized and unrelated fields of health and welfare.

I had, therefore, prepared a memorandum outlining my views and recommended that in the reorganization which was to result in the establishment of staff sections of SCAP, Information and Education should be divorced from Health and Welfare and established as a separate staff section. This recommendation was favorably considered and acted upon by the chief-of-staff when the organization was set up. The first chief of this new Information and Education Section was Gen. Ken Dykes, who was succeeded a year later by Col. Don Nugent, a marine officer of wide educational experience. By agreement with the section chief of Information and Education, I, as chief of the Public Health and Welfare Section (PHW), was to retain the principle interest in the field of professional education and training of those engaged in the health and welfare fields, such as medicine, dentistry, pharmacy, veterinary medicine, nursing, nutrition, and social work. Likewise in the field of industry, which was the primary responsibility of the Economics and Scientific Section, Colonel Kramer and the subsequent chief, Maj. Gen. Bill Marquat, and I agreed that I was to retain primary interest in the pharmaceutical and medical supply industries.

In any well-organized and smoothly functioning organization, such informal agreements and close coordination among the various major subdivisions of the organization are required if needless bickering and feuding over internal jurisdiction are to be avoided. Although at some time or another during the course of the occupation of Japan various problems required close coordination with every SCAP staff section, PHW had almost daily contacts with the following staff sections:

The Civil Information and Education Section in the reorganization of professional schools in the fields I have already mentioned; in the school health programs for elementary and middle schools; in health education for the entire lay population; and in the establishment and operation of a school lunch program.

The Natural Resources Section, whose able chief was a former Stanford University professor, Col. Hugh (Hubert G.) Schenk, in the fields of food production, particularly the types of foods needed to provide a balanced nutritional diet for the Japanese; in food processing as it pertained to the establishment of modern sanitary standards; and in animal husbandry with which PHW veterinarians were primarily concerned.

The Economics Section, headed by Gen. Bill Marquat, in the fields of pharmaceutical and medical supply industries; in requirements for allocation of raw materials or the importation of either raw materials or finished pharmaceuticals and supplies; in licensing for production under foreign patents; in relation to nutritional requirements in the types and quantities of foods required for importation; in control of the Japanese budgets as they pertained to the Ministry of Health and Welfare; and in scientific research as it pertained to the fields of medicine and the allied sciences.

The Government Section, whose chief was Gen. Courtney Whitney, particularly in establishing a nationwide health and welfare governmental organization; and in the preparation and passage through the Diet of all legislation pertaining to the fields of health and welfare.

The Professional Teams

It was the intention of SCAP to deal only with the national level of the Japanese Government in giving them instructions to be carried out at all levels of government down to the local level. After much discussion prior to the establishment of SCAP, it was decided to use the structure of the Japanese Government for accomplishing the mission of the occupation, gradually reorganizing that Japanese structure as needed, rather than having American military government teams take over entirely the actual functions of government at local and prefectural levels.[2]

For the first several months, it was thought that no surveillance would be required below the national level of government, and the personnel of the military government teams who had been shipped to the Far East and organized into companies and groups were kept in Manila. Later they were moved to Japan and Korea and attached to the various army, corps, and division headquarters, as those units moved to occupy the entire country; but for some months they were held without any function other than obtaining local Japanese labor and supplies to support occupation troops. As a result, many individuals who were highly trained in the specialized functions of civil government, and who were brought into the service during the war and trained in military government schools in the United States, were lost. Many of these individuals were reassigned to military units or, when the army began to disintegrate in late 1945 and early 1946, they returned to civilian life rather than stay on in assignments which they felt were boring or at least not fitting for the training which they had received. I had health officers, welfare officers, and sanitary engineers on each of the teams.

But by the time it was realized that these teams would be required to exercise surveillance at the prefectural and metropolitan city levels, the experienced personnel were gone. As replacements, I had medical officers from deactivated military medical units who were older doctors, usually already committed to surgery, roentgenology, or some other medical specialty, and who had neither the training nor the inclination to learn anything about the many problems involved in organizing and administering the many-faceted field of health and medical care from a governmental standpoint. Furthermore, most of them had served in military hospitals throughout at least a portion of the war and justifiably were most interested in going home.

By the spring of 1946, I was faced with a decision of continuing to receive that type of replacement or to accept approximately 150 recent graduates of medical schools who had been inducted into the military service after the war had ended. I decided to accept the young men, for at least they were sufficiently mobile in their thinking that they could be trained on the job by frequent seminars and could be a real asset. Unfortunately, the turnover of personnel was so rapid during the year of 1946, and the military medical manpower so short, that on a trip to the United States in the summer of 1946, I was informed by the personnel officer of the office of the Surgeon General of the Army that no more replacements would be furnished for my program in Japan.

It, therefore, became necessary for me to recruit civilian doctors, nurses, sanitary engineers, and welfare and other personnel directly by contacting professional organizations in the United States and by placing advertisements in professional journals at my own expense. The efforts were successful in spite of dire predictions in Washington, D.C., that it could not be done. The response was so gratifying that we were able to fill completely the requirements for professional personnel on my own staff, which I purposely kept small, never exceeding 150 people, but also the requirements for professional personnel on the military government teams at the prefectural and local levels.

Over the years, there were frequently gaps for months at a time in certain specific positions because we could not recruit replacements until vacancies actually occurred, and there was a time lag for security clearance, processing, and so forth, after I had submitted names of applicants to the civilian personnel office of the secretary of war. But on the whole, we were able to maintain a highly competent corps of professional and administrative people in the health and welfare organization over the years of the occupation. I am very proud of these people and their superior accomplishments. Over the years, several thousand people came and went through our organization. Many, particularly the younger medical men whose first contact with the manifold and broad problems of public health was in Japan or Korea, became sufficiently interested to make a career of that most important field of medicine following their return to the United States.

Over the years we were able to replace the less desirable and to retain the most desirable personnel so that by the time the occupation neared the end, I can, I believe, state that the organization and its professional personnel had few peers and no superiors in any part of the world with which I am familiar for the development, organization, and supervision of a nationwide, integrated health and welfare program. This group, together with the various missions or individual experts whom I invited to review or study special problems from time to time, accomplished a task in the fields of health and welfare that has not been equalled to date in the history of medicine, even in our United States.

The Method of Operation

The initial plan was for SCAP to issue orders to the national government, which in turn issued ordinances implementing these orders through the governors to the local government officials who were to execute them.[3] At the same time, copies of these orders and copies of the Japanese ordinances were sent through military government or civil affairs channels to the prefectural and local military government teams so they, through surveillance, could ensure that SCAP instructions were being carried out throughout the nation. Initially, such civil affairs channels were cumbersome and involved long delays in transmitting instructions because the areas occupied by military units with their attached military government teams did not in any way correspond geographically to the prefectures or metropolitan areas of the Japanese civil government.

Because General Headquarters did not want to become involved in the housekeeping responsibilities of military personnel of the civil affairs teams located throughout Japan, Sixth Army and Eighth Army headquarters were given this responsibility. Military government sections were established in each of these headquarters and their respective corps and division headquarters. By January 1946, Sixth Army was deactivated, leaving the Eighth Army as the only remaining army headquarters in Japan. Although the commanding general Eighth Army did not have the authority to issue instructions to the Japanese Government, he was charged by SCAP with ensuring through the military government teams compliance with SCAP's instructions at the local levels. Technical supervision of the various specialists, such as health officers, sanitary engineers, public health nurses, veterinary officers, welfare officers, and others engaged in the health and welfare fields and assigned to these teams, was exercised, for instance, by my own health and welfare staff section at SCAP.

As I began my staff visits throughout all of the prefectures, the difficulties of this system soon became evident. Frequently, the Japanese officials at the prefectural and even local levels had received their instructions through the Japanese Government to comply with some instructions we had given the national government weeks before my health officers on the local teams had received the corresponding instructions. As an example, instructions were issued to the Japanese on certain mass immunization programs. The corresponding instructions were issued to Eighth Army, whose military government section in Yokohama, in accordance with accepted military procedures, copied them and republished them as Eighth Army instructions to the I Corps in Kyoto and the IX Corps in Sendai, who in turn republished them. It often took weeks to get instructions through such channels to a health officer in Tokyo, who was located a few blocks from my own office.

Again as so often happens, because PHW was the first staff section engaged in programs that required action at all levels of government, as our programs affected the entire population, it was "P, H and W," as it became known throughout Japan, that had to prepare, at General Chamberlain's direction, the first standing operating instructions for military government teams in their conduct of surveillance. After many weeks of conferences and coordination with other staff sections and final approval by the chief-of-staff, they were finally published as the pattern pertaining to all fields involving nationwide compliance.

It took some time to iron out the wrinkles. One of the first steps to prevent the embarrassment of having local Japanese officials receive instructions before the American civil affairs officers of the teams who were supposed to enforce the instructions knew about them was to obtain permission to publish a weekly bulletin prepared by PHW, which was distributed directly to all American health and welfare officers. This bulletin served two purposes. It enabled the local civil affairs officers to obtain a picture of what was being done on a nationwide basis in these fields and served as a medium of exchange of ideas. It also served as a means of placing in the hands of the civil affairs health and welfare officers on the local level advance copies of instructions from SCAP, which had been approved and were in channels on the way to them. Copies of Japanese Ministry of Health and Welfare instructions to the local Japanese officials were also sent in this way, enabling our officers to keep ahead of the Japanese officials they were supposed to lead.

As the years passed, the teams were deactivated as military table of organization units and were reorganized as table of distribution units, which permitted the replacement of military officers by qualified civilian specialists. The teams were finally placed directly under Eighth Army headquarters as successive military headquarters, including the two corps headquarters, were eliminated from the channels. Finally, in 1950, the military government civil affairs section of Eighth Army was moved to Tokyo under Maj. Gen. Whitfield Shepard and placed directly under SCAP.

There was, as could be expected, some disagreement among those most concerned as to how rapidly this evolution of five years should take place. Those of us most concerned with fundamental programs directly involving the daily lives of all of the people were most eager to speed up the evolution in order that the progress of the programs could be expedited. On the other hand, there were many good reasons why Eighth Army headquarters should have been kept in the picture as long as it was, particularly because it was directly concerned with the destruction of war material formerly belonging to the imperial Japanese army, navy, and air force, which had been abolished. The matter of military security of our own forces spread throughout Japan was another factor in keeping Eighth Army headquarters in the picture.

Any organization can be made to work, no matter how faulty it is in concept, if there is the will to make it work on the part of those staffing the organization. Certainly in the military government or civil affairs organization in Japan, there was a universal desire on the part of all those concerned to make it work, and it did. There were occasional disagreements on matters of jurisdiction or some other aspect, but they were usually quickly resolved and a method was found to keep things humming, because of the high type of men who were in the key spots throughout the entire organization.

Much credit for the comparatively smooth functions of the organization is owed not only to the outstanding men who headed up the various SCAP staff sections but also the chiefs-of-staff who succeeded Lieutenant General Sutherland, such as Maj. Gen. Paul Miller, Maj. Gen. Steve Chamberlain, Lt. Gen. Ned Almond, and Lt. Gen. Tom Hickey. The first deputy chief-of-staff for SCAP, Gen. Steve Chamberlain, who did so much in the initial development of the organization, was succeeded by Lt. Gen. Pat Fox. He remained in that position from 1946 until the end of the occupation. It had been my privilege to serve with him, as with some of the other officers, in various assignments before the beginning of World War II in 1941. His common sense, quick grasp of the essentials of any problem in the multitude of programs involving the entire civil government of Japan, and his ability to arbitrate any disagreements which might arise, contributed as much to the success of the occupation as that of any other individual, in my own opinion.

A Student of Organization

By virtue of necessity, I, like many others, have had to become a student of organization over the years and have been assigned to some that were "beauts." They were so involved with overlapping or duplicating areas of responsibility and authority in some fields on the one hand, and the consequent complete lack of responsibility on the part of anyone for other fundamental aspects of the mission, that ninety percent of the time of the staff was involved in trying to find ways to overcome the organizational difficulties in order to accomplish anything pertaining to the basic mission or reason for existence of the organization in the first place. Personally, I have found that the smaller and simpler an organization is in its concept, the more efficient it is in accomplishing something worthwhile.

I lack one of the requisites of a successful bureaucrat. I am not an empire builder in its usually accepted definition of trying to create a large complicated organization of some sort which I can head and point to with pride as an indication of my own prestige and power. Nor do I enjoy the favorite pastime of so many bureaucrats of trying to take over functions and personnel of colleagues in order to build up my own importance.

During the fall of 1945, there was considerable uncertainty as to the location and place of the General Headquarters, Far East Command, as the old military headquarters had been renamed. Except for the general staff, the signal officer, and engineer officer, the remainder of that headquarters had stayed in Manila. The theater surgeon, Maj. Gen. Guy Denit, had maintained a liaison officer in Japan with the advanced echelon of the General Headquarters with whom I dealt on matters of mutual interest. It was not until January 1946 that the rest of General Headquarters moved from Manila to Japan.

During this period, in November 1945, Maj. Gen. Raymond Bliss, the Deputy Surgeon General of the Army, and a party visited Japan for the purpose of inspecting the military medical service there as part of the entire Far East military medical service. In the many discussions which occurred during his visit, he proposed that all army medical facilities in the Far East be placed under a separate medical command and did me the honor of proposing that I should wear two hats: That is, in addition to being the chief of the Public Health and Welfare Section of General Headquarters, SCAP, I should take over the assignment of theater surgeon from Major General Denit, who was due to return to the States. This dual assignment would mean an immediate personal promotion for me.

I had been an assistant department surgeon and acting department surgeon in

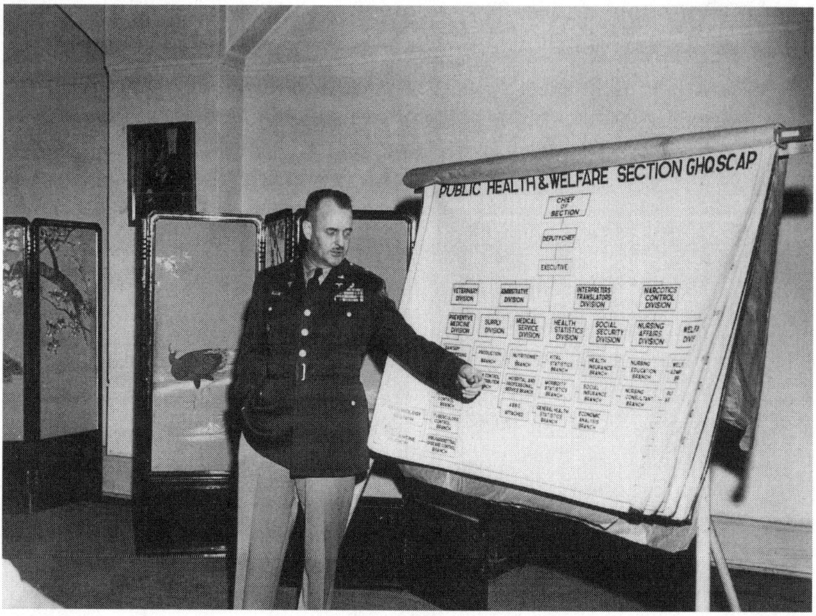

Figure 7. C.F. Sams was a student of organization and an experienced teacher. Here, Brig. Gen. C.F. Sams is shown reviewing an organizational chart of the Public Health and Welfare Section of SCAP with members of the Reserve Officers Association at a meeting held at the American Club, Tokyo, 11 January 1949. Photocredit: U.S. Army, Photographer Turnbull. (Courtesy of the Hoover Institution Archives, Stanford University.)

Panama (the name given to overseas commands before they were called theaters of operation when World War II began), and had been the theater surgeon of the U.S. Army Forces in the Middle East until 1943, so I had some idea from past experience of the importance of the assignment and the magnitude of the work in the adjustment from the wartime forces to a semi-permanent peacetime basis. I also had been in Japan long enough to obtain some idea of the magnitude of the problem in establishing or re-establishing a nationwide health and welfare program for that devastated nation of 72 million (later to be 83 million) people.[4]

The fundamental dissimilarity and magnitude of the two programs, which in reality overlapped in only a few small areas, as in the case of the education program versus the health and welfare program within the civil government, caused me to believe that they should not be placed under one head, in justice to both programs. In such a situation, one or the other of the programs would suffer. If I devoted my primary interests to the military medical program, then the civil health and welfare program would inevitably suffer or vice versa. I, therefore, could not concur in his proposal.

His official written report did not reach General MacArthur until after General Bliss's return to Washington, D.C., at which time I was called in by General MacArthur and asked for my views on the Bliss report. I restated to General MacArthur the same reasons I had given General Bliss for my nonconcurrence. He agreed with my views, and the report was not favorably acted upon. I asked that I retain only my assignment as chief of Public Health and Welfare Section, General Headquarters, SCAP, as the challenge offered for constructive work in the civil government health and welfare program would require all of the best effort of which I was capable.

I believe that the passage of time and the results accomplished have proven the soundness of the decision. Although I paid a personal penalty by having my own promotion delayed three years as a result of my recommendations, were I faced with the same decision today I would make it again.

Throughout my life I have followed a code of conduct which has placed what I believed to be the best interests of the service or of the position which I was trying to fill above my own normal personal ambitions or welfare. The empire-building and pyramiding of jobs to increase eligibility for personal advancement which has been especially prevalent since the end of World War II, and particularly since the passage of the Officer Personnel Act of 1947, have done more to undermine the morale of the officer corps of the army through the incentive to scramble for personal advancement rather than to work for the good of the service than any single factor. I have been told many times by friends in the service that in the modern day of "dog eat dog," particularly in the military service, my ideas of dedication to the service are obsolete and old-fashioned; however, I think that I shall stick to them for the remaining years of my life. I am satisfied with the peace of mind and sense of accomplishment that are my good fortune to have as a result of that code of conduct.

"The Men Who Sit Behind the Bamboo Screen"

In Japan, as in all other countries including our own, there was a group of individuals of great power and influence who in that country are called "the men who sit behind the bamboo screen." Of these men, none was more powerful than Prince Tokugawa, formerly head of the House of Peers of the prewar Diet, and senior member and head of the Tokugawa Shogunate, the most powerful clan in the feudal days, which was largely responsible for the restoration of the emperor during the Meiji Restoration in 1868. In this country, we would say they are the men who pull the strings that make the elected or appointed government officials dance. They usually do not seek or hold elective or appointive office for themselves, but through their influence they have a most important role in determining who shall be nominated for elective office and who shall be appointed to office; through these individuals, they have a major voice in determining policy and even the passage of laws which determine policy. In our own country, such influence is usually coupled with or measured by financial contributions to political campaigns. Of such are the realities of practical politics and practical political science.

During the course of the occupation, it was my privilege to get to know rather well some of these men and to acquire a liking and respect for them because of their sincere interest in the health and welfare programs for the Japanese people as a whole. During the first winter of the occupation, I was invited for private teas at either the homes of a number of "the men who sit behind the bamboo screen" or at some out-of-the-way teahouse for a private conference. In each instance, I was, in effect, asked what I was up to in initiating the many and various programs to improve the health and welfare of the Japanese people. After outlining the motives and purposes of these programs, I was assured of their support.

As the occupation progressed, it was General MacArthur's decision that all of the directives given to the Japanese Government and implemented by imperial or governmental ordinances should be reviewed and, where applicable, embodied into Japanese law by 1 July 1949. Over a period of several years, new laws were drawn up, either by the Japanese who brought them to us for approval or by my own people working with the Japanese in the Ministry of Health and Welfare, and presented to the Diet for passage. I am sure in my own mind that the relative facility with which all of these laws were passed was a result not only of the general acceptance of the basic programs of health and welfare by the Japanese people as a whole but also the strong support of "the men who sit behind the bamboo screen." This was equally true of the budget of the Ministry of Health and Welfare. I might add at this time that in the six years since the end of the occupation, Japan has had a code of health and welfare laws as modern as any in the world.

It was from one of these powerful men that I learned a most important fact later on in the occupation. At one of our meetings, I asked why, on the whole, the Japanese people had cooperated with us in carrying out our mission when they were a conquered people and could be expected to resent and attempt to sabotage our work rather than assist us in carrying it out. In response, he pointed out that at the beginning of the modern era of Japan, they had sent their people throughout the world to observe particularly the European nations and our own nation and to bring back to Japan those ideas and material things that were the best in each nation and adaptable to the Japanese. Modern railroads, electrification, manufacturing processes, and other important contributions had been made to Japan's rapid development into a modern power in the world prior to World War II. Of all the nations of the world, Japan had looked upon Germany as the *ichibon* (first) nation from which they desired to copy.

The United States had defeated not only Japan, and had, thereby, demonstrated its superiority over Japan, but also Germany. Had we not defeated Germany, there would have always been a doubt in the Japanese mind as to our ultimate superiority. Now there was none. We were now the ichibon nation of the world, and they desired to learn from us all that could be adapted to Japan.

In accordance with oriental thinking, the people always are on the side of the winner and quickly lose respect for those who are no longer winners. This statement should give all those who are concerned with our relationships with non-European nations throughout the world much basis for thought. If we continue to follow the course of appeasement, and by repeated acts continue to demonstrate weakness to nations which have given us their respect and allegiance, we should not be too surprised if we find our former friends in Asia, the Middle East, and Africa quietly turning toward the opposite side in the present cold war.

4

First Reconnaissance of Japan

As part of my concept of my responsibilities in any position I have held, I have felt it necessary to find out at firsthand by frequent visits how the programs for which I was responsible were being carried out by subordinates at lower or more distant echelons. Such visits not only give me firsthand information in order that I might evaluate the progress being made or the correctness of having initiated the program in the first place, but also serve other useful purposes in that they give the subordinate who often is isolated and frequently develops the idea that he is "the forgotten man" a sense that I have a personal interest in him and appreciation for his work and his particular problems. Therefore, it was my plan, which I carried out throughout the years, to visit or revisit a number of prefectures each month. This plan was particularly important early in the occupation when the extent of the problems and their many facets could not be adequately grasped by reading reports or studying long columns of statistics.

During the course of the occupation, through this plan I was privileged to meet and to get to know many thousands of Japanese and to visit every part of the country. It is indeed one of the most beautiful countries in the world.

Utsunomiya

My first visit beyond the Tokyo-Yokohama area was a trip to Nikko, the location of the famous Tokugawa Shrine, as well as many other Shinto shrines and Buddhist temples. I had been informed that this lovely community with its many fine hotels was a site to which many of the children from Tokyo had been evacuated to escape the bombing. These children included those of the Peers School, a school to which the children of the nobility were sent before the occupation. The report indicated that these children were very much undernourished and that illness was prevalent among them. Although I had already taken steps to tackle the problem of the several thousand orphans inhabiting the ruins of the cities, I had not up to this time had an opportunity to see at firsthand the status of the great majority of children who had been evacuated to the country for the duration of the war and who were still there.

Accompanied by Gen. Dale Ridgely, Colonel at that time, who was chief of the Dental Division, and Dr. Manabe, the liaison officer at that time from the Ministry of Health and Welfare, we set out by rail from Uyeno Station for our first ride in a Japanese train. The railroads are owned and operated by the government as in most European countries.[1] Because this trip was made before special cars had been put on the various trains for occupation personnel, we were introduced intimately to the Japanese people on this train. Because of the mass movement of people which was occurring at the time, all of the trains were overcrowded; the people entered not only through the doors but also climbed through the windows in the mad scramble for even standing room. When we finally left the station, the train looked as if it were inhabited by a colony of bees: People were not only completely filling the cars but also clinging to the steps and riding on the roofs and on the couplings between the cars. The particular car in which we rode had been the victim of a strafing attack; the numerous machine gun bullet holes served not only to increase the ventilation with fresh air, which was badly needed in the overcrowded car, but also to fill the car with smoke from the low-grade brown coal used as fuel by the locomotives of Japan. The smoke filled the car whenever we passed through a tunnel, and there are many hundred tunnels on Japanese railroads.

At Utsunomiya, a junction where we had a short wait before boarding a branch line train for the remainder of the ride into the mountains, we were invited to rest in the station master's office and reception room. Utsunomiya had been badly destroyed by bombing because its status as a rail junction with appropriate marshalling yards made it a legitimate military target.

The station master in Japan is a government official and is a man of importance in his community. One of his functions appeared to be that of official greeter for the community whenever visitors of so-called importance stopped at his station. Dressed in his uniform, with white gloves as part of the equipment, he not only escorted and looked after the comfort of the visitors but also, on their departure, took his post outside of the car in which the visitor departed and rendered a smart military salute. During our wait, there occurred one of the small incidents that serve to enlighten one about people of different backgrounds and cultures.

Several hundred Japanese children had detrained at the station and were patiently waiting with their escorts for the arrival of another train. They were quiet and orderly. I was interested in observing their physical appearance for signs of malnutrition of which there were many and asked that we join a group on the platform. General Ridgely, who was largely responsible later on for the remodeling of the profession of dentistry in Japan, has a particularly friendly way with children. Soon peals of laughter and shouts were coming from the children in response to his antics.

On our return to the station master's reception room, the station master, his assistants, and Dr. Manabe began to cry. Although I, like most of my countrymen, had been under the misconception that orientals were stoic and unemotional, I was to learn that the Japanese are a highly emotional people, and for men to break into tears is a common manifestation of joy; however, at the time of this

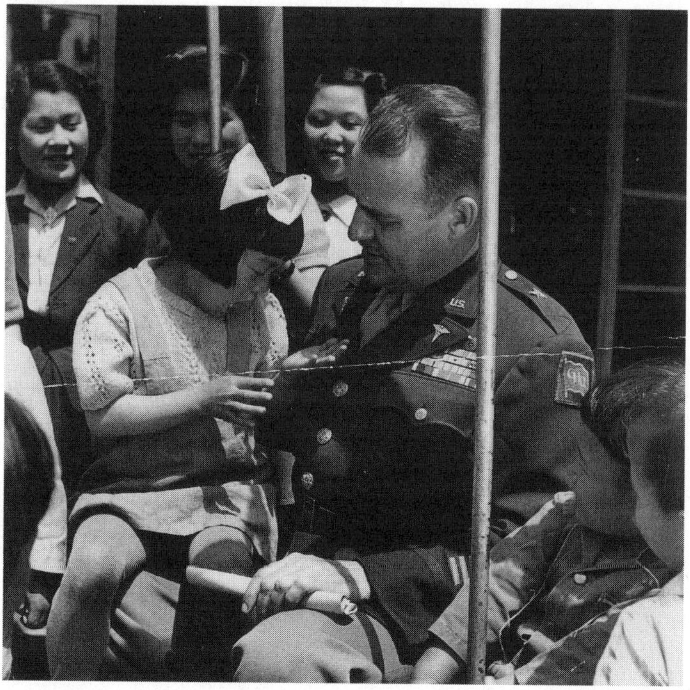

Figure 8. Although it was then contrary to Japanese norms for an army officer to show interest in children other than his own, Brig. Gen. C.F. Sams took time to visit with healthy and well-nourished Japanese children. Occupation of Japan, circa 1951. (Courtesy of the Hoover Institution Archives, Stanford University.)

incident, I had not yet learned this fact and was concerned that in some way we had offended the Japanese officials and that the tears were either of sorrow or anger, which is the usual cause for an American to weep, if he is ever going to do so.

It took considerable time to learn what it was all about. Finally, Dr. Manabe told us that he and the others were crying with joy because two senior American army officers had not only shown a real interest in the Japanese children but also had won the hearts of that particular group. This interest was quite contrary to Japanese custom, for it was unheard-of for an officer of the imperial Japanese army even to pay attention to children other than his own, let alone to amuse them. And, as he said, it indicated that we had "hearts."

Nikko

After our arrival at Nikko, we went to one of the fine European-type hotels in which some of the children were staying. We had brought our own military K rations, as our policy was to provide our own food owing to the actual food

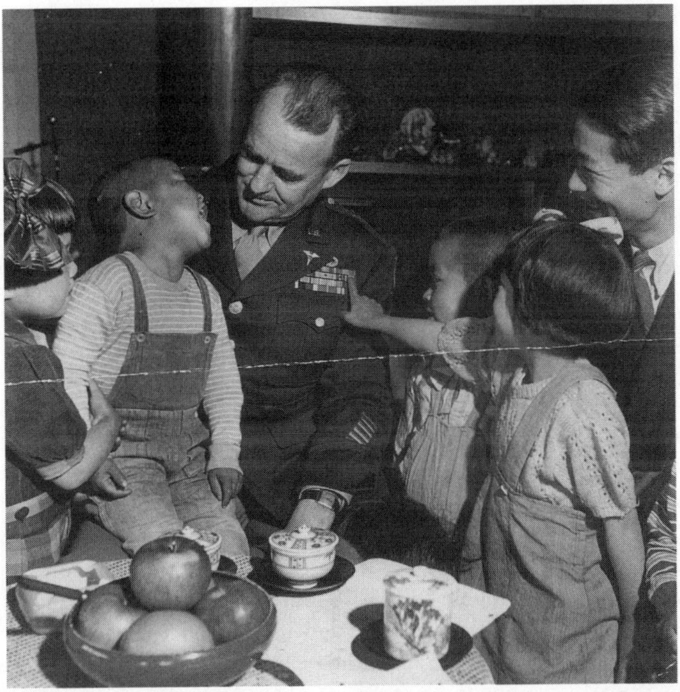

Figure 9. Curious Japanese children crowd around Brig. Gen. C.F. Sams to get a closer look at his insignia. The man at the right is a Nisei who served as a translator for the PHW Section, SCAP. Occupation of Japan, circa 1951. (Courtesy of the Hoover Institution Archives, Stanford University.)

shortage in Japan at that time. I noted that many of the children were apathetic, were shorter in stature for their ages than previously obtained figures for average growth rates for Japanese children would indicate as normal, and showed other physical signs of nutritional deficiencies, particularly certain vitamin and protein deficiencies. On observing the evening meal served to the children, I found that it consisted mainly of sweet potatoes. I was informed that sweet potatoes had formed the principal item of Japanese meals since May, when the last year's rice crop had been largely consumed. It was obvious that sweet potatoes provided an entirely inadequate diet so far as nutritional balance is concerned, regardless of the quantities consumed as represented by caloric intake.

After spending the night at the hotel, we visited the various temples and shrines for which Nikko is famous. There were many shrines in which the spirits of various animals as well as humans had been deified. The shrine to the cat for which the place was named, the shrine to a horse, and the shrine to the three monkeys who "see no evil, hear no evil, and speak no evil" are examples. The shrine to Tokugawa Ieyasu, the first Tokugawa shogun, is the largest and most beautiful in all of Japan, so far as I can determine.

Although it is not my intention, nor am I qualified, to discuss in detail the religions of Japan, it is useful to learn about the religious beliefs and culture of people with whom one must deal on a daily basis, particularly when they differ radically from our own, in order to develop health and welfare programs adaptable to them. So far as I was able to learn over the years of the occupation through many discussions with numerous Japanese, including Shinto and Buddhist priests and one "living god," all Japanese except for about 100,000 Christians were Shintoists and about 55 million were also Buddhists. In addition to State Shintoism, which was subsequently abolished in accordance with directives by the occupation, there were some thirteen private Shinto sects.[2]

The essence of the Shinto system was an extension of the tight family system into the hereafter. As one learned Japanese explained to me, the Japanese do not really worship their ancestors as we worship our God. They frequently adopt a grown man, if they have no sons, or adopt a younger brother as a son to maintain an unbroken chain of ancestors so that as the elder head of the family passes on there will be a successor to take his place. They enshrine the souls of their ancestors; and when going to the shrine in which his spirit hovers, they attract his attention by clapping their hands three times and then report on important events in their family as well as report on their troubles and ask his assistance in their daily lives. In the case of shrines dedicated to someone other than their own ancestor, who was enshrined because they possessed certain virtues, such as bravery or loyalty or stamina (in the case of animals as well as humans), they ask for the assistance of that spirit in solving their particular problems. In the case of the State Shintoism, the emperor, as the direct descendent of the Sun Goddess, was the "father" of all Japanese, and as a "living god" was therefore entitled to the respect and "worship" of all Japanese.

On a subsequent trip to the seat of a private Shinto sect known as Tenrikyo ("Teaching of the Heavenly Truth") near Nara, I was the guest of another living god who, as the direct descendent of his grandmother (his grandmother having been deified because she had performed some miracles), was, as head of this sect, entitled to be called a living god. He had some twelve hundred shrines throughout Japan and some 5 million followers. In this particular sect, a complete Japanese apartment was maintained at the central shrine in which the spirit of his grandmother resided.

The Buddhist beliefs are, of course, better known throughout the world than are those of Shinto. A succession of reincarnations in which you progress either up or down the scale, depending on your conduct during this life, with the ultimate hope of reaching nirvana, is the essence of the religion, as I understand it. Because the spirit of one of your ancestors may, through reincarnation, not be inhabiting a human body, the eating of animal flesh or the taking of life of any animal, including that of rats, may prove embarrassing to your own advancement up the scale in successive reincarnations. It was this belief that caused us some difficulty in altering the nutritional patterns of the Japanese to provide adequate balance in their diet and in carrying out a rodent control campaign as part of our sanitation program.

Kyoto and Nara

It is possible to go completely around each of three of the four main islands of Japan. Shikoku is the only main island that lacks a complete encircling rail line. It is also possible to go by rail from the northernmost town of Wakkanai on Hokkaido, opposite the Russian-held Sakhalin, to Kagoshima at the southern tip of Kyushu. Such a trip takes about three days and nights and in mileage is equivalent to a trip in this country from San Francisco to Chicago. The trains are transported across the Tsugaru Strait by a seagoing ferry ship between Aomori and Hakodate on the trip between the northern island of Hokkaido and Honshu. The trains pass through an underwater tunnel between Shimonoseki and Moji on the trip between Honshu and the southernmost island of Kyushu. I have found that the trip across the Tsugaru Strait can be exceedingly rough in the blizzards which sweep across that strait during the winter months.

My first overnight trip by rail was to Kyoto and Nara, the old capitals of Japan. Neither city had been damaged by fire or bombing. They were the only major cities spared throughout Japan. The Miyako Hotel in Kyoto is a beautiful place built on the side of a mountain overlooking the city. It is a building of many levels fitted into the side of the mountain.

Nara is one of the oldest cultural centers in Japan and is the site of many beautiful temples and shrines. It was spared from bombing on the assumption that it would not be used by the Japanese for military purposes; however, on my first trip to Nara, I found stacks of artillery shells dispersed throughout the parks and within the temple and shrine grounds, for it was used by the Japanese as an ammunition depot. Our intelligence on that point apparently was not too good.

Osaka and Takarazawa

Nearby Osaka, the second industrial area in Japan, had been badly hit, as had Kobe, the inland seaport for that part of Honshu. It was on my first trip to Osaka that the governor of Osaka took me to Takarazawa, a resort town and the home of the all-girl opera troupes. I believe that the all-girl opera troupes are unique. Certainly they are in the Orient, where it is the custom for men to take all parts on the stage, impersonating the female, particularly in the ancient dramatic theater, the Kabuki. There are numerous Takarazawa troupes, the Snow Troupe and the Frost Troupe being, I think, outstanding. It was my privilege to witness *The Mikado* and *Madame Butterfly*, and although I have seen both numerous times in other countries, I have never seen more beautiful performances than were put on by these troupes. The costuming could not be equalled, and the voices of these girls, many of whom I was told were Eurasians, were outstanding.

It was also at Takarazawa that I witnessed a most unusual puppet show. I am not sure that technically it would be classed as a puppet show. The figures were not manipulated by strings from overhead, but each figure was manipulated by the fingers of a player who held the puppet and who himself was completely covered by a black cloth. The various voices came from a group of men seated on the floor of a raised platform at one side of the stage. Amazingly, the black clad figures moving about the stage, which at first were so obvious, eventually seemed to disappear; they were no longer noticed as attention became more concentrated on the little figures they were holding and manipulating. Backstage, the senior puppeteer presented me with the figure of a samurai warrior. Because raising and lowering of the eyebrows appears to be essential to the fierce expressions desired by samurai warriors, even these eyebrows move when a short string is pulled by one of the fingers inserted into the body. I have not seen such a type of puppet show any other place. It has no similarity to our ventriloquists and their dummies.

Tenrikyo

While at Osaka, Dr. Manabe suggested that we accept the invitation of the living god to visit Tenrikyo. As a tuberculosis sanitarium was located there as one of his institutions, we accepted, making the trip in a fifteen-year-old Packard which he had sent over for us. Several thousand of his followers inhabited this small community, and I was told that each year new followers made a pilgrimage to the central shrine and worked there for a year as part of their service to this private Shinto seat. It was my first experience as an overnight guest at a Japanese home, and it was here that I learned why the Japanese class Americans as "barbarians."

It appears to be a custom in Japan when one makes a visit that theoretically you are tired and the first procedure is to take a bath, which in that country at least can become quite a social event. Because I was eager to learn all that I could about the customs of the people, we were to have dinner and entertainment in the Japanese house and subsequently to spend the night in a European-type guest house. After stripping, we were presented with a small wooden tub about a foot in diameter, filled with hot water, and a bar of Japanese soap with which we washed ourselves while squatting on the tile floor of the bath. Then several Japanese girls entered and began to pour small tubfuls of hot water over our heads as a sort of rinse. Now we were prepared to enter the large tub of almost boiling water where, besides being slightly parboiled, you also engage in conversation with others sitting in the hot water up to your chin. In the more modern communities at least, the old custom of community bathing as a means of relaxation and gossip was still prevalent. The Japanese girls kept pointing at my companion, General Ridgely, and me, and were giggling and talking among themselves. The word *Ainu* frequently occurred in their conversation. I inquired of Dr. Manabe what the amusement was all about. He told me that this was the first time these girls had seen a barbarian or hairy Ainu. Both General Ridgely and I had considerable body hair on our chests. This hair is the mark of a barbarian in Japan, because the Ainu, the original inhabitants of the islands of Japan, were considered barbarians.

The Ainu, who are now concentrated in a small area of the northern island of Hokkaido, were later to be the subject of one of our numerous research projects. A considerable body of anthropological knowledge had already been acquired by the Japanese anthropologists at Hokkaido University in Sapporo. The Ainu are apparently Caucasians who thousands of years ago migrated by way of Siberia and Sakhalin to Hokkaido. They have none of the characteristics of the oriental. Their features, their eyes, their hair, including heavy beards and body hair, are like our own. They are important to the anthropologist because the path followed during the spread of the human race to our own western hemisphere is still a matter of controversy. We found that there are only about one hundred fifty pure-blooded Ainu left.

Because the Ainu are primitive in their culture and still hunt bears, large numbers of which inhabit the mountains of Hokkaido, they are looked upon as barbarians by the oriental Japanese. To an oriental, a minimum of body hair and a sparse beard is a mark of civilization and high culture. So it was in a bath in a Japanese home that I learned it was by my physical appearance rather than my conduct that I was labeled as a barbarian.

After a suitable period of boiling and conversation, we were given hot wet towels to dry ourselves. There are certain advantages to using a wet rather than a dry towel, and it is worth trying. We were slightly nonplussed on re-entering the dressing room to find our clothes missing. They had disappeared and we were not to see then again until the next day, when we found them neatly pressed and hanging in a closet in the European-style guest house. Instead, there were men's kimonos, *obi*, and *tabi*. [The obi is a long broadsash worn on the outside of the Kimono.—Ed.] (The tabi is a split sock in which the big toe is inserted in a separate compartment like a mitten so that the thong of a *geta* [a type of shoe or clog] can be passed between the big toe and the other toes.)

A Japanese meal, particularly if it is a formal dinner served to guests, is worth describing; this was such a dinner. Only one dish of food is brought in at a time. After a round of *sake*, the rice wine for which Japan is noted, soup is served in individual covered bowls. This soup may be fish-head soup, complete with fish head and eyes, or *miso* (broth of fermented bean paste). Raw fish dipped in a dish of *shoyu* (soy sauce) flavored with ground *wasabi* (a radish of potent odor and flavor) is a favorite dish. *Tye*, a deep sea fish served raw, is perfectly safe to eat so far as fish tapeworm is concerned. Other species are not, however, to be eaten raw without some trepidation. Then there may be several kinds of tempura, which may be almost anything from a small piece of sweet potato to a shrimp or piece of fish dipped in batter and fried in boiling oil; then sukiyaki, the oriental version of a beef stew; and finally *gohan* (cooked rice). The host watches very carefully how you eat your final gohan, because if you eat all of it to the last grain, then he feels badly because he has not fed you well enough. If you do not eat all but a few grains then you have not liked his meal or you are wasteful. As a matter of politeness, I learned to eat all of this last dish except for a few grains of rice to be left in the bottom.

I have never been able to figure out the Japanese custom of consuming alcoholic beverages. I had been raised in the tradition of using caution in the consumption of beer, wine, and whiskey at one time, but I learned in Japan that the indiscriminate mixing of these three throughout the course of a dinner is not too hazardous if moderation in quantity is practiced.

It has been my privilege subsequently to be invited to many Japanese homes, some belonging to the nobility, and to have the hostess prepare sukiyaki on a little hibachi or charcoal burner for me as the guest of honor. Usually, except for the Japanese who have had previous contact with occidentals either in Japan or Europe or America, it is the custom for the husbands to attend dinners outside of their homes unattended by their wives.

As at this dinner, each guest is assigned a *geisha* for the evening. Because geisha are much misunderstood and often maligned by occidentals, it might be well to describe their place in Japanese society and culture. Geisha are primarily entertainers who look after the serving of food to the guest and keep the sake cup filled. They may sing, dance, or play the *samisen* during the course of the evening. They are not always young or exceptionally beautiful by any means; but they are ususally highly intelligent and can carry on a conservation on other than household affairs. At several subsequent dinners in Tokyo, I was honored by having the ichiban (number one) geisha of Tokyo assigned as my companion. She was a charming and brilliant lady in her seventies. When the evening's entertainment is over, the first-class geisha returns to her home. She is not about to spend the rest of the night as a companion. If that sort of companionship is desired, then a *jo-ru* is obtained, but not a first-class geisha, who may be the mistress of some wealthy patron or the "second wife," but who is not a promiscuous harlot, as is so often charged.[3]

At this particular dinner, our host inquired if there was anything we desired which had not appeared, apparently to show his alleged magical power as a living god. We were urged to suggest something, and as sort of a test we asked for a particular brand of scotch whiskey produced only in Scotland. A bottle appeared. We were again urged to ask for something. Because Japan had been cut off from American imports for five years, we decided to make a real test and asked for an old brand of American bourbon. This bottle also appeared. Out of curiosity I examined the label. It was a bottle bearing the mark of the U.S. Army Medical Department and had been bonded in 1915. I was later told that this was part of a shipment of relief medical supplies sent to Japan by the American relief group following the 1923 earthquake and had come into the hands of the living god many years before World War II. I had never before, nor have I since, had the privilege of drinking thirty-year-old whiskey.

On our departure the next day for our return to Osaka, I was introduced to the Japanese custom of exchanging gifts, it seems to me, at every occasion possible. I am convinced that each Japanese home must have hidden someplace a store of gifts received from others which, in turn, are passed on to someone else on appropriate occasions. The custom of exchanging gifts was always a source of embarrassment to me, particularly in the early years of the occupation, because we were not permitted then to give or sell anything American to the Japanese. Even had I violated such an order, it might have proved embarrassing to the Japanese recipient, who, if found with anything in his possession produced in America since the war, was subject to prosecution for black marketing if he could not prove that he had received the item as part of relief supplies.

We had been authorized to accept gifts of small value from the Japanese which could not be considered any form of bribe for special favors. We were encouraged to accept such gifts on social occasions, so as not to offend the Japanese, with the clear understanding that we could not, in turn, give them an American gift.

On this occasion, I was presented a small wooden figure of a Japanese samurai warrior which represented to me at least a new form of art. I was told that this was a one-stroke carving: The artist must make each cut with one stroke of the knife. If an error is made he is honor bound to start all over again on a new piece of wood. I do not believe that anyone other than a Japanese would have the patience to acquire such skill.

For our return trip to Osaka, we rode in a beautifully kept Straight Eight Gardner touring car, the like of which I had not seen for twenty-five years. As additional evidence of the supernatural powers of my host, it was propelled with gasoline, an exceedingly scarce commodity in Japan at the time. All of the other cars, trucks, and buses which had appeared on the streets shortly after the occupation began were propelled by some form of charcoal burner fixed either on the rear or the side of the vehicle.

5

Food Relief and Nutrition

Not long after our arrival the clamor began about mass starvation. Each day, laid on my desk were translations from the Japanese press concerning health and welfare matters, including stories of hundreds dying of starvation. There were almost daily reports of deaths from starvation among the refugees living in the tunnels at Uyeno Station. Each story was investigated. One story indicated that truckloads of bodies of those dying from starvation were being hauled out of Shiba Park, across the street from the Imperial Hotel where I was living. That one I investigated myself. I found that an elderly man had been found dead in the park. The autopsy showed that he had died of cancer. This lone individual had been multiplied by several hundred in the press and the imaginary deaths were attributed to starvation.

We were never able to verify that anyone died in Japan at any time during the occupation from starvation; but, the alarming reports resulted initially in some confusion. In some areas occupied by our troops, truckloads of American rations were being given by the local military commanders to the Japanese, while in other adjacent areas any Japanese found even with an American candy bar was prosecuted for black marketing. It took a directive from SCAP to end the confusion. No relief supplies were to be turned over to the Japanese people without SCAP authorization.

The Rice Culture

So far as I could determine through study and from such information as I could obtain from the many Japanese I consulted, the Japanese had made a fundamental decision concerning nutrition: to rely on grain crops as the principle source of food, rather than a combination of grain and domestic livestock. This decision was made centuries ago when very little was known scientifically about human nutrition, and the reasons to base the Japanese economy on a grain, particularly rice, were many, one of which was religious. This decision was to lay the basis for a quantitative food deficit as the population subsequently increased.[1] More important, it was to be the basis for many other problems, particularly in the health field through the creation of faulty nutritional patterns, which not only contributed to the exceptionally high beriberi and tuberculosis incidence in prewar Japan, but also contributed to the steady decrease in height and stamina of the people.

Japan has become an industrial nation basically to produce manufactured goods for export and sale to food-producing countries in order that she might obtain through exchange the additional food necessary to feed her own people. In fact, there are many among the Japanese who explain their actions in China in 1931 and the initiation of World War II in the Pacific in terms of food shortage. Their perhaps over-simplified explanation is that, as they had to become industrialized in order to import sufficient food for their expanding population as a result of their initially unfortunate decision to base their economy so many years ago on a rice economy, they found it necessary to seize control of other areas for three aims: first, to ensure access to raw materials, which could be imported and converted into manufactured articles; second, to ensure control of the market for the sale of their manufactured products; and third, to control the sources of their food imports. This was the pattern followed by European nations that led to the creation of the great colonial empires of the past; thus, some Japanese leaders maintained that if Japan had not been denied access to the sources of food, raw materials, and markets for her manufactured products, she would not have entered World War II.

There is, however, another partial solution to this food deficit problem. A principal facet of the solution is to change the nutritional pattern of the Japanese and concurrently to change land utilization. Another principal facet is to stabilize population growth. Both of these major changes were initiated during the occupation and are continuing at present. If they are properly continued into the future, they will help to maintain peace in the Pacific, as far as the Japanese are concerned.

The Nutritional Pattern

One of my responsibilities was to determine the nutritional status of the Japanese people. To determine the facts as accurately as possible, we initiated the largest nutritional survey that has ever been scientifically undertaken in Japan. We studied a cross section of 150,000 people of all age groups, all economic groups, and all geographic areas. They were given physical examinations every three months in order to record the signs and symptoms of nutritional deficiency, including height and weight. In addition, their homes were visited, and their food consumption was determined quantitatively and qualitatively.

These surveys were continued throughout the years of the occupation. Certain refinements in survey techniques were added in 1948, but on the whole the data were comparable throughout the six years of the occupation. The surveys not only revealed new knowledge of scientific value but also upset the traditional concepts of methods for determining food requirements in mass feeding programs.

The Japanese nutritional pattern as revealed in the surveys was an exceedingly high carbohydrate, inadequate protein, inadequate calcium, and inadequate vitamin diet. The rural population with comparatively ready access to grain foods had a higher quantitative consumption, as was expected. It must be emphasized that an individual or group of people can be less well nourished on 3,000 calories per day than on 2,000 calories, if qualitatively certain essential elements are lacking, particularly proteins, minerals, and vitamins. This important scientific fact created one of our most difficult problems in obtaining food imports.

At the beginning of the occupation, the Japanese were consuming only about seven grams of protein of animal origin per day in the rural areas and about sixteen grams in the cities, against a minimum normal requirement of twenty grams per day for the normal consumer, that fictitious individual who is a composite of all age groups and all economic groups in the nation. There were many reasons for this pattern of consumption.

Although among meat substitutes fish most nearly approach a complete protein, the Japanese were not the great fish eaters we had thought. The lack of household refrigeration and inadequate transportation facilities made it most difficult to distribute fresh meat or fish without spoilage to the rural population; hence, most of the fish and such products of animal origin as are consumed were largely consumed by the urban populations, which are usually located near or on the coast. So far as domestic livestock were concerned, the inevitable pig and a few chickens or other poultry, which are found in most households in other oriental countries such as China or the Philippines, and which furnish some of the protein requirements of those countries, were lacking in Japan, although work cows of a small size and limited milk-producing capability and a few Holsteins in the dairies of Hokkaido and Chiba Prefecture were slaughtered for food when too old or incapacitated for work.

Our studies indicated that for an average Japanese adult, the basal metabolic requirement was 1,250 calories, as contrasted to 1,500 for an average 150–pound occidental adult. The basal metabolic requirement for a human represents the energy requirements expressed in calories when converted to heat to simply exist; that is, to lie quietly without even providing additional energy for the digestion of food. To perform any type of work, of course, requires energy above the basal metabolic requirement. When an individual falls below his basal metabolic requirement for energy, by limiting his food intake, he then literally consumes his own body and converts his own stored body fat, carbohydrates, and proteins into energy to keep his body alive, to simply breathe, and to circulate the blood through his body. When this debilitating process is occurring, he has little resistance to any infection and may die from some infection before he literally starves to death. To state that individuals have been living for months or years on as little as 80 calories per day is fantastic and inconsistent with either reality or scientific or mathematical fact, although such claims were frequently made for propaganda purposes.

Our nutritional surveys indicated not only an inadequate qualitative nutritional pattern in Japan, but also indicated that the period from May to July 1946 would be a critical time. May, June, and July were the critical months because the greatest quantitative shortage occurs after the staple food, rice from the preceding November harvest, has been consumed and the wheat crop and sweet potato crop are not yet ready for harvesting: The rice crop is planted in July and is harvested in November. Then the wheat crop is planted on the same land in December and is harvested in June. The Japanese could not afford to let the land rest in their never-ending struggle to produce enough grain.

Such a critical period did develop. Scheduled imports of food, which had been developed and requested during the winter of 1945–46, had not yet been received in Japan, so we were much concerned about the possibility of rice riots during that period.[2]

Competing for Food Resources

We had to compete with other nations for a fair share of worldwide food resources, which were allocated by the Food and Agriculture Organization. Obtaining these resources was a difficult problem and involved two areas.

First, we were dealing with laymen who were thinking in terms of scientific information that was twenty years old; that is, they were thinking only in terms of calories or quantities rather than qualitative nutritional requirements. To try to sell the idea to such individuals that it would be better in terms of balanced nutrition to provide imports of items such as powdered skim milk, a cheap source of protein of animal origin which could be utilized and distributed in Japan to make up the marked deficiency in protein intake, than to ship large quantities of additional carbohydrate in the form of wheat, grain, or corn, was like talking to someone in another language. They were prone to take a slide rule and multiply tons of grain by the number of calories per ton and divide this total by the number of persons to be fed, then to point out that this provided adequate food. It did quantitatively, but it completely ignored the simple scientific facts of nutrition that I have tried to emphasize: The kinds of food expressed in terms of proteins, carbohydrates, and fats, as well as mineral and vitamin content—in other words, food in qualitative terms—was even more important than quantity.

It took a long time, in fact a number of years, to sell this now obvious and simple fact. Herbert Hoover and Maurice Pate, who visited Japan in early 1946, and Tracy Voorhies, assistant secretary and later undersecretary of war, are due much credit in assisting us in ultimately selling these simple facts to the people with whom we were dealing back home. It finally became well recognized in Europe when individuals who had been on semi-starvation diets, particularly in concentration camps, failed to respond to large quantities of food in the form of carbohydrates. It was not until adequate quantities of protein and, in some cases, intravenous feeding of proteins in the form of essential amino acids was begun that these people began to recover. Today it is almost routine in serious postoperative cases to give intravenous feeding of protein to hasten repair of damaged tissue in addition to the intravenous use of carbohydrates in the form of glucose, which was routine twenty years ago.

Second, as one of many claimant nations for the limited food supplies available worldwide, we were having our difficulties because we were perhaps too honest. In our surveys, we were actually determining the total food consumption of the people by weighing and measuring the food found in their homes. The people were most cooperative in this work. They also were perhaps too honest because they were reporting the sources from which they obtained each item and relative quantities of food, whether it was received through the ration or not. Non-rationed food came from home gardens, black markets, or other sources. We found to our amazement that people can be really ingenious when the chips are down and that almost fifty percent of the food actually consumed came from non-rationed sources.

Unfortunately for us, we were reporting total food consumed. As we found out later through private correspondence and conferences with those concerned, other claimant nations, particularly occupied nations such as Germany, were reporting as food consumed only that which was rationed. Consequently, when the propaganda drives about potential mass starvation increased in intensity in each area, in order to put pressure on the food allocation organization for a larger share of the available food supplies, we were at a disadvantage. When the authorities in Germany were wailing that the German people were approaching the starvation level, they were speaking in terms of only the rationed component of the food consumed. We were speaking in terms of total food consumed. I have since verified from sources actually engaged in nutrition work in Germany at the time the truth of these statements. Like the Japanese, the Germans were actually consuming approximately twice the amount of food they were alleged to be receiving. Only the rationed food was publicly acknowledged.

At one time, we were urged to present evidence supporting our food requirements in the form of photographs of individuals dead or dying from starvation and to show that our tuberculosis death rate was climbing, as it was in Europe at the time. We could, of course, have prepared such photographs by using individuals emaciated from the ravages of cancer or tuberculosis and alleged that they were dead from starvation, as some of the other claimants for food allocations were not averse to doing, we were informed. As for our tuberculosis death rate, it was dropping rapidly instead of increasing in the face of all of the adverse known factors which should have caused that death rate to climb rapidly, because we had begun an effective tuberculosis control program. I, therefore, recommended to General MacArthur that "we stick to our guns" and present only the facts as accurately as we could, hoping that eventually honesty would still be the best policy. He wholeheartedly backed this recommendation, knowing the full implications of what the results might be. It took several years before our position was accepted.

The solution for the future is obvious. In the event of any future occurrence of food shortage, such as existed after World War II, in which numerous nations or areas are claimants for allocations of available food supplies, they should be required by the allocating authorities, whether they be a temporary body such as existed immediately after the war or the United Nations, to conduct accurate and complete nutrition surveys including total food consumption, rather than present data on only the rationed component, which fails by far to give an accurate picture of the real situation. The second element of a successful solution is to incorporate in such an allocating body individuals who are abreast of modern scientific knowledge on nutritional requirements in terms of quality as well as quantity.

The Critical Time

In the meantime we were in difficulty. Our May and August 1946 surveys showed that the urban people in the major cities of Japan were near the danger point of mass starvation as their total quantitative food consumption had dropped to 1,570 calories, of which only 760 were being received from rationed foods. It was during this most critical period that I was thankful that General MacArthur had authorized the retention of the 100,000 tons of wheat from the initially planned relief supply of food which had been shipped to Japan and stored.[3] This relief supply was finally released on my recommendation and did barely tide us over until the programmed food imports that had been developed and requested by SCAP during the winter of 1945–46 actually arrived in the fall of 1946. It was not until 1949, four years after the occupation began that the rationed component of the total food consumed by the urban population reached the 1,250 calories considered essential for even basic metabolic requirements of the normal consumer in Japan.

New Foods

In addition to trying to change the nutritional pattern to provide a more properly balanced diet as a means of improving health and resistance to disease, we had the problem of teaching the Japanese how to use new foods with which they were unfamiliar, such as wheat, corn, flour, butter, and some meat products, but which could be obtained through imports.[4] These particular types of foods were available for worldwide redistribution. This situation required a nationwide nutrition education campaign, which went on continuously, but especially during the first four years of the occupation.

The first shipments of corn to Japan caused some concern. The Japanese normally did not bake or have ovens in their homes for baking any sort of bread, whether it be from cornmeal or wheat flour, with the exception of a few westernized areas in a few of the large cities. They normally cooked all foods over a small charcoal burner called an hibachi. To bring in these new foods was to create a problem in teaching the Japanese people methods of preparation which could be carried out with the simple cooking utensils available to the average home.

In addition, corn is not used for human food in many places outside of the western hemisphere. Instead, it may be used exclusively for livestock feed. A mission made up of experts in corn utilization in the United States visited us during this period to assist us in our educational campaign, which was carried on through the nutritionists in our health centers, the schools, the press, and the radio to induce the Japanese to use corn products. Although we had some temporary success, the stigma that they were eating stock feed still remained in the Japanese mind. I doubt that many Japanese today are eating corn in any recognizable form as part of their daily diet.

Food Relief and Propaganda

We worked with Natural Resources Section people, who were concerned with food production, and with Economics Section people, who were concerned with imports, to determine the quantities and types of food to be imported into the country by SCAP using U.S. funds appropriated for Government and Relief in Occupied Areas (GARIOA). Nonetheless, the failure of some individuals to think of nutrition in terms of factors other than a mathematical calculation of calories consumed resulted in some major headaches. One such incident was the shipment of several hundred thousand tons of sugar to Japan, in lieu of a grain requirement. In terms of calories, it was the quantitative equivalent of the food requested, but try sometime to live for a couple of weeks on a bucket of sugar as the principal staple food.

The carbohydrate diarrheas which developed particularly among the children gave the communists a propaganda opportunity they were looking for. In their constant efforts to undermine the confidence of the Japanese people in the intentions of the occupation, they immediately seized on this incident to start a whispering campaign, which later spread to the Japanese press, that the Americans were only shipping food to Japan to get rid of surpluses and that this shipment of sugar instead of grain was proof. It was alleged that there was a surplus of sugar in the United States and that sugar was sent to keep up the price of sugar in the United States. Moreover, this sugar had come from Cuba, which was evident from the markings on the bags, and had supposedly been contaminated by the organism that causes leprosy, which was the disease from which their children were suffering.

Unfortunately, there was some small truth in their propaganda about the sugar being surplus. This element of truth made such fantastic tales difficult to combat with counter-propaganda. It was not until the arrival of other food, which permitted substitution of grain for any further sugar as the principal staple food component of the ration, and the resulting disappearance of the illness, principally diarrhea, from the thousands of children, that this wave of communist attack could be stopped.

Another incident which unfortunately played into the hands of the commu-

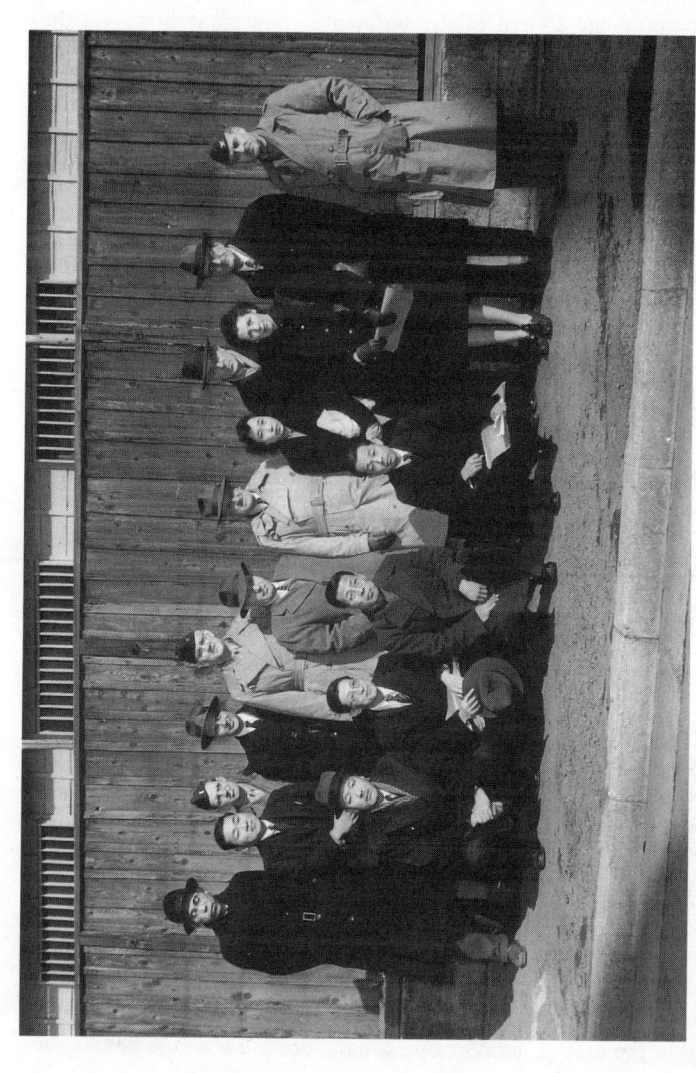

Figure 10. Members of the United States Food Mission, who were sent to Japan by the U.S. State, War, and Agriculture Departments to study the food and fertilizer situation, gathered for a photo with officials of Japan's Ministry of Health and Social Affairs and representatives of the PHW Section, SCAP, in front of the Central Health Center, Tokyo, 6 February 1947. Standing, from left: unidentified, unidentified, unidentified, Ross H. Whitman (State), Col. J.W. Scobey (War), Nathan Koenig (Agriculture), Col. R. Harrison (Agriculture), unidentified, W. Hallam Tuck (War), Agnes O'Donnell (Assistant Nutrition Consultant, PHW, SCAP), Capt. Tracy B. Kittredge (USN) (Navy), Col. C.F. Sams. Kneeling, from left: unidentified, unidentified, unidentified, Nisei translator (PHW, SCAP). Photo credit: U.S. Army Signal Corps, Photographer Dargis. (Courtesy of the Hoover Institution Archives, Stanford University.)

nists was the shipment of soybean flour in bags marked "stock feed." Some of this soybean flour had been contaminated with staphylococcus, and several outbreaks of enteritis resulted. Again the communists were quickly on the job, this time maintaining that the Americans were shipping cattle feed to the Japanese for human consumption and that it had been poisoned. It took a short time to find out the facts concerning the source of the outbreaks of the enteritis, and the remainder of the soybean flour was immediately withdrawn from the ration channels.

Changing Nutritional Patterns: The School Lunch Program

A special study of the average growth of elementary school children in rural and urban schools indicated that since 1937 there had been a steady decrease in height and weight in each age group. In 1946, the average twelve-year-old child in urban schools weighed twenty percent less than the average twelve-year-old child in 1937, the prewar year used as a base year in the study. These children showed all of the manifestations of a high carbohydrate, inadequate protein, and inadequate calcium diet, regardless of economic status.

By the spring of 1946, we had obtained sufficient information on the nutritional status of the people to begin action. In changing nutritional patterns of a nation, precedents had been established in our own country. Within my own lifetime, the nutritional pattern of our own people changed for the better, with the result that each succeeding generation of Americans since the turn of the century has on the average been taller, stronger, and healthier than their parents. The widespread and beneficial use of liquid whole milk has become one of our great nutritional assets in providing part of our protein requirements of animal origin. We have over the years established sanitary standards for handling milk and have made household refrigeration an essential of living.

Such is not the case in most other countries with which I am familiar. Relatively few children in the world consume cow's milk, because through many generations the people have found that to give contaminated and unrefrigerated milk to children has all too often led to their death or illness from typhoid fever or the other enteric diseases. Milk is one of the best media for the incubation of bacteria-producing diseases in humans, and if adequate sanitary standards and refrigeration are not available during the course of its distribution, it can become one means of the spread of disease. Modern methods of processing milk, particularly into powdered skim milk, which contains the essential proteins of animal origin so deficient in the diet of many peoples, have opened a whole new era in nutrition. Powdered skim milk can be distributed and stored until used without the tremendous cost of providing refrigerator cars and household and public eating-place refrigeration.

The point of attack in any such program as in any other major change in a nation is always to begin with the children. In 1929, private social welfare agencies in Japan had initiated a supplementary food program for malnourished children in the form of a school lunch program, which eventually included some 22,000 children. By 1940, this program had been expanded, but during the war it had completely collapsed.

After many conferences, including those with Maurice Pate, who had much experience with Herbert Hoover in large-scale food relief programs in Europe following World War I, I decided to begin our action with the children of Japan by establishing a nationwide school lunch program. This program not only would directly provide the food needed by these malnourished children but also would teach them to acquire a taste for foods, such as powdered skim milk and meat, with which they were unfamiliar but which were essential to provide the proteins of animal origin in which their diets were deficient. We would in the course of many years produce a nation which no longer preferred, to the exclusion of other foods, white rice, the principal source of their nutritional deficiency.

Because this program would require the cooperation of the Ministry of Education as well as the Ministry of Welfare, a joint task force was established of representatives of these ministries and representatives of the Public Health and Welfare and the Civil Information and Education Sections of SCAP. Other interested sections such as the Economics Section were invited to attend because the program would require food imports and financing.

The program began in December 1946. A total of 250,000 children in the selected schools of the Tokyo-Yokohama area were fed a school lunch using powdered skim milk as the basis for the meal. This milk was used in combination with fish to provide a fish soup, which was not too alien to the taste of the children. This program, together with the teaching of simple but fundamental facts about a balanced diet, met with immediate success. Within one year, the children in the demonstration group on an adequate protein intake had surpassed the control groups, that is, those not receiving the high protein food, by over an inch in increased height and a sharp upturn in weight. But it was not without some amusing incidents.

There was much discussion as to whether the children would touch the milk, because Japanese children, once they had been weaned by their mothers, did not drink milk. There was also some discussion, as I have previously mentioned, of the religious training of the children causing them to refuse cow's milk, for as one outstanding Japanese physician assured me, he himself had been taught by his mother that he should never drink milk from a cow because "the cow would cry."

An epidemic of a new "mysterious disease" also appeared among some of the children on the program in one of the schools in Yokohama. The new disease turned out to be simple hives, because the children had become sensitized to protein, a problem with which American mothers are often confronted when they first feed their infants egg or other new proteins for the first few times. In Japan, because the children had not had such protein, they had reached the ages from six- to twelve-years-old before going through the experience American infants do in the first year of life.

Many difficulties had to be solved: financing; obtaining kitchens and kitchen equipment; preparing the meals in the schools; obtaining fuel and, above all, the particular types of food needed. Some canned meat that had been seized as Japanese military food stocks was released, and Licensed Agencies for Relief in Asia (LARA) initially contributed the imported powdered skim milk.

Counterpart funds were used to defray administrative and transportation costs, counterpart funds being that ingenious financial device by which governments of nations receiving financial assistance from this country are required to expend local currency on a comparable basis on U.S. Government-approved programs. The children initially paid three yen per day for the school lunch. Children of destitute families were provided with their yen under the public assistance program, known as the Daily Life Security Law, which we inaugurated, so that there was no discrimination among the children on any economic basis.

As the program expanded, our most important problem was the never-ending fight to obtain sufficient powdered skim milk to meet requirements. Our annual requirements were calculated as 45,000 tons of powdered skim milk. Under U.S. laws, if funds appropriated under Government and Relief in Occupied Areas (GARIOA) were used to purchase this essential food from the Surplus Commodity Corporation, another federal agency, there had to be transfer of funds at the rate of fifteen cents per pound, the price paid by our own government to the dairy industry in removing this surplus from the American market. Our financial experts found that if we used funds from what was termed "the commercial account," we could obtain the same milk at four cents per pound, provided we removed the milk from the U.S. market. The commercial account consisted of American dollars earned by the sale of Japanese products in dollar markets and was under the control of SCAP for the purchase of raw materials or other products for importation to Japan. Finally, after lengthy negotiations, we were able to persuade UNICEF (the United Nations International Children's Emergency Fund) to contribute additional powdered skim milk to Japan, which was of considerable assistance.

I have found throughout the years that I could talk myself "blue in the face" trying to sell a new idea without much success, but if I could demonstrate it—and in this case we did demonstrate what we were trying to sell about the protein deficiency—I could sell an idea. Many Japanese, including the prime minister at that time, were extremely sensitive about their short stature.—The prime minister was about as big around at his equator as he was tall, but he was less than five feet tall.—When we succeeded in proving to him that not only would an adequate protein intake give the Japanese better resistance to disease and more stamina but also would increase, over a period of several generations, their height to equal that of other peoples who had been on an adequate diet for many generations, we had an ardent supporter of our school lunch program. The program was quickly accepted by the people, contrary to some dire predictions, and rapidly spread throughout the nation. At the end of the occupation there were 8 million children in the program.

Imports and Foreign Aid

The inevitable question arises, and was raised particularly by some of the American officials with whom we were dealing, as to the wisdom of initiating a program, such as the school lunch program, on the basis that once the occupation was ended, the Japanese would be unable to continue the program, because it would indefinitely require large-scale importation of powdered skim milk. We had made many studies as to the long-range problems before we initiated the program and continued these studies through the course of the occupation. We found that there were several possible solutions, any one of which would work.

One solution was to continue indefinitely the importation of powdered skim milk from surplus areas, such as the United States. Our economics and financial experts had studied the pattern of Japanese import and export earnings in the prewar years and could predict with reasonable accuracy the postwar pattern. Of the several hundred million dollars earned annually, the question of expenditures was one of priority to be established by the national government, which in such countries rather tightly controls the foreign exchange. The money could be used to import additional quantities of white rice or automobiles or other comparative luxuries, or a small part could be used to import the required powdered skim milk for their children. I had no personal doubt, after having learned a little about the Japanese people and their strong interest and devotion to their children, that among all of the claimants for allocation of dollar exchange, if left to the choice of the Japanese people, their children would not be left out once the benefits of the program had been demonstrated to them.

A second solution was to continue the importation of the powdered skim milk until such time, and it would take many years, as it would be possible through a change in basic policy of land utilization to increase domestic livestock production eventually to produce sufficient milk to meet her own requirements without importation. Japan is a country which, if the land is properly utilized, can increase its own food production, particularly in the types of food in which the diet of her people is most deficient. Although only 16 percent of the land on the four main islands of Japan is arable for grain crops, our studies indicated some 18 million domestic animals could be supported. Much of the heavily vegetated and unutilized slopes of the hills and mountains could be utilized for pasturage for domestic livestock, particularly sheep and goats. Instead of relying solely on grain crops as the base for her agricultural economy as in the past, she is quite capable of combining domestic livestock with grain production as so many other nations have done whose land does not provide sufficient acreage to meet their food requirements through grain crops alone.

A start was made through the work of my veterinarians and the Natural Resources Section, in cooperation with the Ministries of Health and Welfare and the Ministry of Agriculture. Breeding stock of cattle and sheep and goats were imported with the assistance of many agencies, including the Friends Service

Organization, to increase the badly inbred and depleted livestock herds which did exist in Japan. The first problem was to begin an educational program in animal husbandry for the Japanese. On the whole, the Japanese farmer was unfamiliar with the handling of herds of animals as is done other countries that use grazing ranges for feeding. If a Japanese farmer was fortunate enough to have a work cow or a goat, he usually treated it as a member of the family and kept it until it was too old or incapacitated for work and then obtained a new one from some neighbor. The breeding and handling of herds was a new field for him.

I tried for several years to obtain the services of a mission of experts in animal husbandry from the United States to begin such a program, but without success. Our own Department of Agriculture apparently was only interested in disposing of surplus crops of grain. We did, however, receive great assistance in the form of technical help from the International Dairy Company of the United States and its representatives.

In the early days of the occupation, the Quartermaster General of the Army had made a contract with the International Dairy Company for the construction and operation of a milk reconstitution plant, in fact, a number of plants in Japan, in which powdered skim milk and butter were recombined into whole milk for sale to, and consumption by, the occupation forces and their dependents. During the course of many conferences with their representatives as to the status of the very small dairy industry in Japan, our own proposed requirement for milk, and the potential through dietary changes of creating a large and permanent market for dairy products, these farsighted gentlemen designed the plants so that when the time came, they could through expansion produce greater quantities of reconstituted whole milk than would be required by the occupation forces. The question of converting the yen profit to dollars, always one stumbling block for such a project, was eventually solved. In addition to this agreement, the American dairy people from time to time gave most valuable advice and assistance to the Japanese on the problems of expanding their own industry, which was part of our goal, if Japan was to sustain her school lunch program over the long run.

In my last meeting with Prime Minister Yoshida before my return to this country, this basic food and nutrition program with its many ramifications, which I have only touched on in this chapter, was a principal topic of discussion.[5] I was assured that so long as he was in a position of power and influence, this far-reaching and fundamental program for the benefit of the Japanese people would be carried on.

It has apparently become our responsibility whether we like it or not to assume a position of world leadership. So long as our own great country is a farm surplus-producing country and, in this instance in particular, a dairy products surplus-producing country, we should consider as long-term foreign aid for peoples of underdeveloped nations that we are trying to keep on our side those programs for our mutual benefit. The decision must be a top-level one as to just what form of aid will produce the best results at the least costs and, at the same time, directly and beneficially affect the most people. I have found that most underdeveloped countries with which I am familiar are in that state not from choice or lack of capacity for improvement, but they are underdeveloped because most of their populations are chronically ill and malnourished. Whether we export automobiles, trucks, household appliances, and other things that have become necessities to ourselves but which are decidedly luxuries to such nations, or whether we export such simple but effective tools in the cold war as powdered skim milk is the basic question. The financing, the impact on export programs of other food surplus nations, and the eventual possibility of making such nations capable of sustaining such programs, can all be solved, as was done in this instance, if the will to do so is there. We do have men in this country of vision capable of initiating and carrying out such broad programs. These programs can favorably influence other countries in spite of what appears to be an era of shortsightedness, expedience, and quick profits on our part, which has resulted in a rapid loss of former friends throughout this globe.

This story of the food relief and nutrition programs in Japan has been presented simply as one illustration of the fact that it can be done. It is a question of weighing human values in the balance against material values alone.

6

The Reorganization of Health and Welfare

All too many people have stated that either we were operating a dictatorship or we had a simple task in rebuilding Japan, because the people were used to regimentation. The same individuals are most apt to think that there are only two forms of government, either a highly decentralized form of federal government or some form of despotism. They are also apt to express the idea that our form of government should be spread throughout the world. Because we were building a nationwide governmental health and welfare organization, which, of course, must fit into the pattern of governmental structure, it was necessary to have a clear understanding of the overall governmental structure and functions.

The Government of Japan

The structure of the Government of Japan with which we worked and for whose final modifications we were responsible is the most common form of government in the world and is just as democratic or representative as our own in that the people are masters and not the servants of the government.[1] The government is representative and democratic in that the people, by direct vote, elect their representatives to the national Diet: The Diet is the national legislative body in which all residual legislative power resides. The Diet, in turn, may delegate certain legislative powers to prefectural or local legislative bodies.[2] This delegation is the exact reverse of our own federal form of government. The Diet elects the prime minister, who is the actual head of the executive arm of the national government.[3] The emperor, who formerly was the actual head of the government, is now a symbolic head without executive power.

In the past, the governors of the prefectures, which do not have constitutions, were appointed by the prime minister on recommendation of the Minister of Home Affairs. However, under the new Constitution, governors are elected, although they are in fact still an extension of the executive branch of the national government in that they are responsible for execution of the national laws within their respective prefectures. Likewise, mayors of local communities, who formerly were appointed but are now elected, are an extension of the executive branch of the national government in that they are responsible for the execution

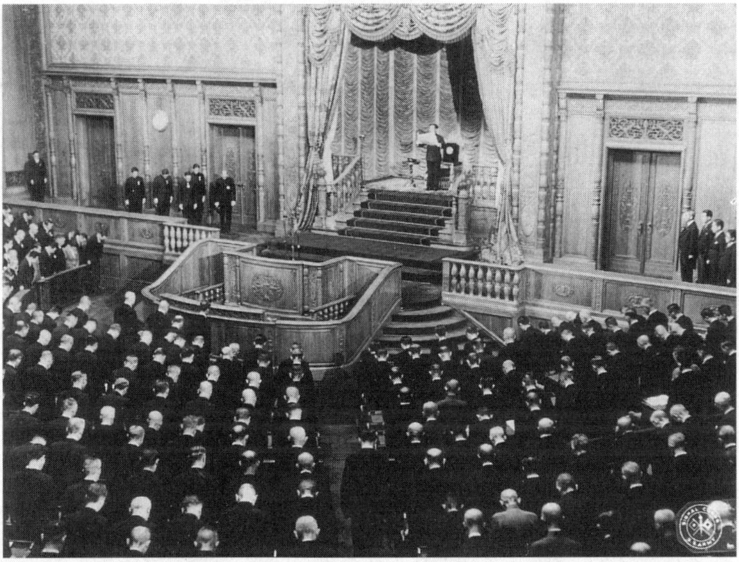

Figure 11. The promulgation of the Japanese Constitution at the House of Peers, Tokyo, 3 May 1947. Photo Credit: U.S. Army Signal Corps. (Courtesy of the Hoover Institution Archives, Stanford University.)

of the national laws under the supervision of the governors within their respective towns and cities. They, like the governors, are additionally responsible for the execution of the laws in the few fields which the Diet has delegated to prefectural or local legislative bodies.[4]

This chain of command is characteristic of a national form of government, which so many Americans failed to understand. Even some of our military government officers at prefectural or local team levels frequently attempted to stimulate prefectural or local legislative bodies to enact some local or prefectural law, which was contrary to the Japanese Constitution. For instance, under Article 25 of the new Japanese Constitution, the national government, rather than prefectural or local governments, is charged with promoting the health, welfare, and social security of the people; this is unlike our own Constitution, which makes no provision whatsoever for our federal government to legislate in the fields of health.[5]

Under a national form of government, almost all tax money is collected by the national government. Because the bulk of such taxes come from that comparatively small segment at the top of the social pyramid which controls the wealth in the country, there is a redistribution of wealth principle involved. The national government, through appropriations to implement its various legislative acts, in fact, reallocates the tax money to prefectural and local governments for their governmental functions in carrying out the national laws.[6]

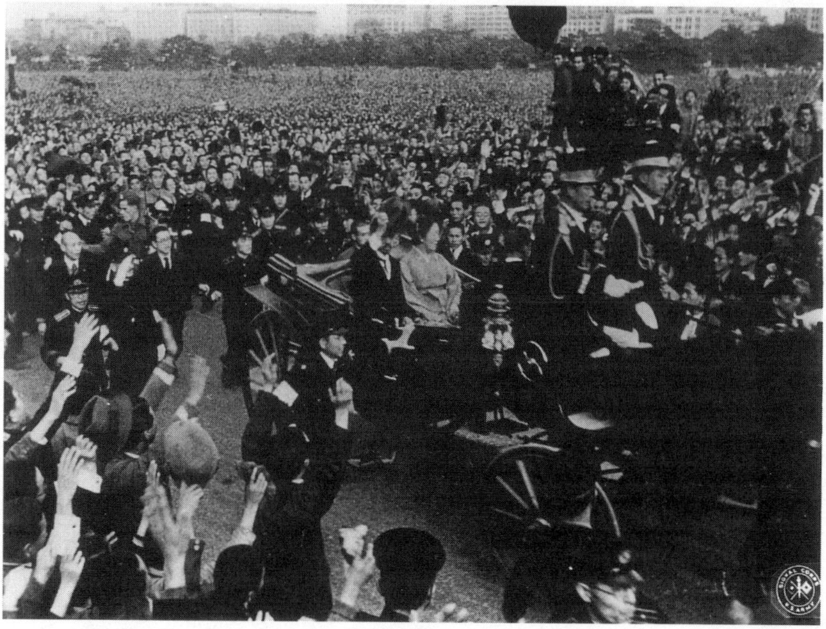

Figure 12. The emperor and empress of Japan at the mass celebration of the promulgation of the Constitution, Tokyo, May 1947. Photo Credit: U.S. Army Signal Corps. (Courtesy of the Hoover Institution Archives, Stanford University.)

There are many facets to the great responsiveness of the executive branch of such a parliamentary system of government to the will of the people. Through their elected representatives in the Diet, they can cause the fall of the prime minister and his cabinet through a no confidence vote at any time, if they believe that his policies and actions are contrary to the best interests of the nation.[7] They do not have to wait four years for a presidential election, as in our own country. Four years is frequently too long a time after the act [sic] to really take corrective action, so it seems. There are also, of course, inherent weaknesses in such a form of government, as are all too evident in some countries in which there are so many splinter political parties that a prime minister cannot obtain an effective majority and, hence, cannot remain in office for any length of time, with the resulting paralysis of governmental functions.

The Ministry of Health and Welfare

Prior to the occupation, the Ministry of Home Affairs carried out, through the national police, activities pertaining to health under the old national laws. In the early 1930s, the Ministry of Home Affairs had established a small number of health guidance centers. In 1937, the Ministry of Health and Social Affairs was established as a planning agency, and the first health center law was enacted.[8] By 1938, fifty health centers had been established in various parts of Japan. As far as we could determine, the primary functions of these health centers were the advancement of health education and the operation of clinics for maternal and child hygiene and for the diagnosis and treatment of tuberculosis.

The health center facilities varied from a few large, well-constructed buildings to small, deteriorated cubby holes located in the poor districts of the cities. Usually, there was a part-time or full-time doctor as director. In some cases, he had a number of assistants. These centers were basically clinics. The director had no idea of the population he was serving or what the health situation was in the area surrounding the health center. This concept of the function of health centers was similar to that held in our own country in the early 1920s.

[With the reorganization of the cabinet in 1947, the new Ministry of Health and Welfare (Kōseishō) (MHW) replaced the prewar "Ministry of Welfare." The MHW's functions now included medical care, disease prevention, social welfare, and social insurance. Labor affairs, which were previously administered by the Ministry of Welfare, were reassigned to a newly created Ministry of Labor, thereby separating labor administration and social insurance functions. With the dismantling of the Ministry of Home Affairs, public sanitation, which had formerly been a police function, became the MHW's responsibility. Administration of vital statistics, formerly a police function of the Ministry of Justice, also came under the MHW's purview. These changes served to reorganize public health and welfare administration as an integral part of postwar democracy on a technical and professional basis removed from police control.—Ed.]

The Health Center System

Even more important than the reorganization of the Ministry of Health and Welfare was the establishment of a nationwide organization for carrying out the national laws pertaining to health at the local level. Over the years in the United States and elsewhere, it had been found that the local political unit of a city, town, village or county is frequently not a suitable unit for carrying out the administration of health laws, which in the United States are based on state or even local ordinances. We, therefore, established health departments and welfare departments in each of the forty-six prefectures and established an echelon of government as an extension of the prefectural government.[9] This new governmental unit was the health center district, which was administered by a district health officer. The district health officer was under the supervision of the chief of the prefectural health department and was responsible for the administration and implementation of the national laws within a given health center district. This responsibility required an administrative organization. In addition, there was, of course, the necessity of providing services, some of which were clinical services.

Health center districts were organized on a nationwide basis with an entirely different philosophy as to their responsibilities and functions. Based on experience in our own and other countries, the principle of the population unit, rather than the geographical area, became the primary determinant in locating a health center district. A population unit of approximately 100,000 was selected as the manageable size to constitute a health center district.

Under the modern concept, a health center district is a governmental administrative organization; it is also responsible for certain basic services. Initially, these services consisted of twelve public health services: public health nursing; maternal and child hygiene; public health statistics; public health laboratory services; dental hygiene; nutritional services; sanitation and hygiene, including meat and food inspection; health education; communicable disease control; medical social service; venereal disease control, including diagnosis and treatment; and tuberculosis control.

After considerable planning, a new Health Center Law was passed by the Diet on the fifth of September 1947, establishing eight hundred health center districts. In the large metropolitan areas in which more than one health center district was located, a city health department was established, which, in turn, supervised the district health officers. The chief of the city or metropolitan health department was then under the technical supervision of the prefectural health department chief. Within each health center district, there was, in addition to the administrative organizations, at least one completely organized and staffed health center that included the clinics and as many branches as might be required.

The staffs of these health center districts were a fundamental part of the nationwide public health organization. Initially, an organization of 109 persons was considered desirable to carry out the twelve basic functions within a district. This number included eight doctors, one dentist, fifteen public health nurses, public health veterinarians, sanitarians, nutritionists, medical social workers, X-ray technicians, and miscellaneous personnel. A Medical Affairs Division was established to integrate the preventive medicine functions of the health center with the medical care facilities within the district by establishing liaison with the local medical associations and medical care facilities. It was also responsible for carrying out the inspection of medical care facilities, as required under a new medical services law which set minimum standards for these facilities. The Division of Medical Social Service acted as a link between preventive medicine functions of the health center and the welfare and social security organizations within the district.

The Model Health Centers

This organization was designed in an attempt to integrate on a population unit basis, at the local level, the four basic functions of a sound health and welfare organization: preventive medicine; medical care; welfare; and social security. It was a tremendous task to implement such a program. After the initial plans and the establishment of the necessary legal basis were completed, the next step was to reconstruct, equip, and staff a model health center in one of the newly established health center districts in Tokyo, as a demonstration. The staff of the model health center were trained by my own staff and a series of demonstrations were carried out.

The first demonstration was for all of the American health officers in the various prefectures in order that they might be thoroughly familiar with the new organization which was to be established within the prefectures. The second series of demonstrations was carried out for all of the new chiefs of the prefectural health departments, who were Japanese, and then the various specialists. When the demonstrations were completed, the prefectures were then directed to establish one such model health center in each of their respective prefectures so that, by the end of 1948, there were forty-six model health centers throughout Japan. These, in turn, became training institutions for the estimated eighty thousand personnel who would eventually staff the newly created or reorganized health centers in each of the health center districts within their respective prefectures.[10]

The construction of health centers, the staffing and training of personnel, and the provision of necessary equipment all took time. A nationwide health education program was undertaken as to the reasons for establishing these health centers and the services which they provided.[11] As the health centers were established over a period of years, the competition among prefectures and metropolitan areas became very keen. In 1948, the health centers provided approximately 3.4 million health consultations. By 1951, that number exceeded 5.6 million. In 1948, there were 382,000 visits by the public health nurses; by 1951, there were over 2.3 million visits. The number of individuals who attended health education courses had increased from 2.9 million to over 21 million by 1951. Food and milk sanitation inspections had increased from 705,000 in 1948 to over 3.1 million in 1951.[12]

Certain modifications were incorporated as the program was carried out. It was found, for instance, that in the rural and semi-rural areas, modifications could be made in the initially established organization of 109 personnel. The health centers were later classified into three types, designated as A, B, and C. By the end of the occupation in 1952, there were 724 health centers, of which 180 were class A centers, each having a staff of 61 persons; 60 class B centers, each having a staff of 54 people; and 484 class C centers, each having a staff of 35 people. The establishment of this nationwide health center organization was one of the accomplishments of which we are most proud.

The Institute of Public Health

There was a great need in Japan for workers trained in modern public health practice. The only qualified public health officials, mostly doctors, were the few who had been educated abroad, principally in the United States, England, and Germany.

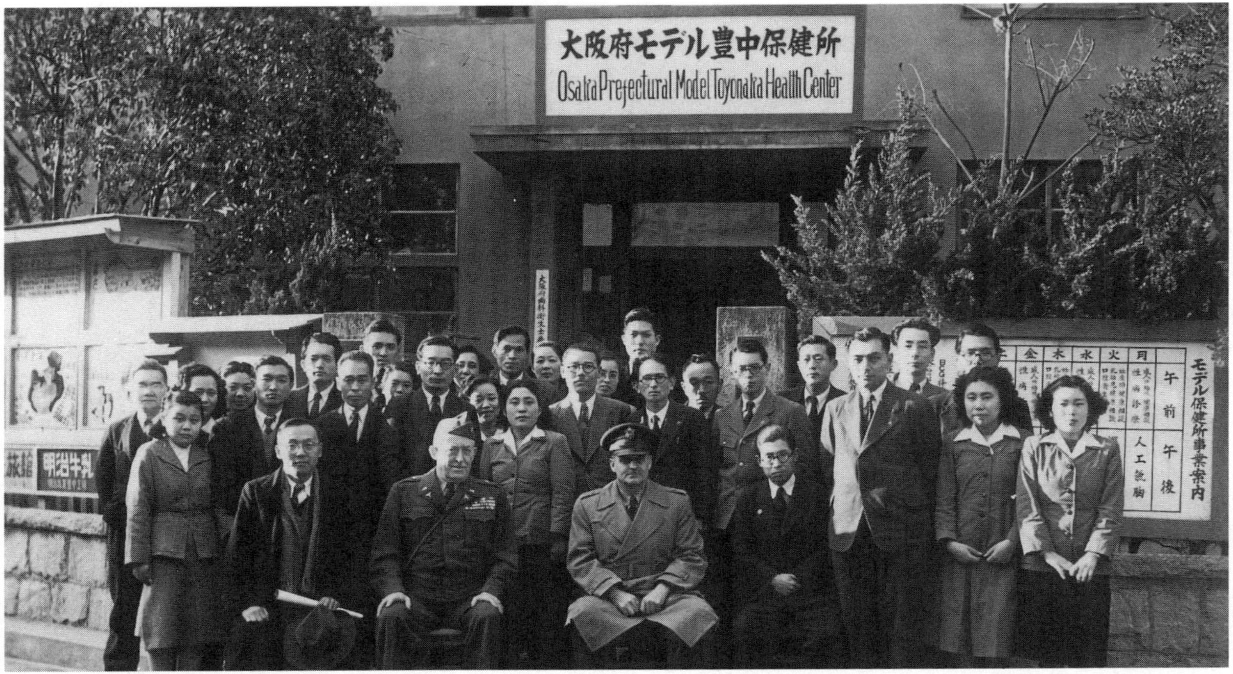

Figure 13. The Toyonaka Health Center was the model health center in Osaka Prefecture. Staff of the Toyonaka Health Center gathered for this photo with Gen. James S. Simmons and Brig. Gen. C.F. Sams on the occasion of receiving a national award for their work in health education. Toyonaka, Japan, 1951. Seated, left to right: Dr. Ito Canada (Director, Division of Preventive Medicine, Osaka Prefectural Health Department), Gen. James S. Simmons, Brig. Gen. C.F. Sams, Dr. Yasuda Kazuo (Director, Toyonaka Health Center). Dr. Hashimoto Masami (Head, Division of Health Extension, Toyonaka Health Center) is standing to the right of Dr. Yasuda; Katayama Tsuneo (Dentist, Toyonaka Health Center) is standing in the back row, second from the right. Photo Credit: Sugimoto of Toyonaka. (Courtesy of the Hoover Institution Archives, Stanford University.)

During the early 1930s, when there were no schools of public health in Japan, the Rockefeller Foundation of the United States became interested in Japan. In 1935, after negotiation with the imperial Japanese Government, they provided the funds for construction and equipment of a modern seven-story building to be known as the Institute of Public Health; however, between 1939, when the building was completed, and 1945, the Institute of Public Health emphasized research activities and accomplished comparatively little in the training of public health workers.[13] All activity of the Institute of Public Health was suspended in 1943, when the Ministry of Welfare occupied the building for the remainder of the war.

Early in 1946, a program was adopted to re-establish the Institute of Public Health as an institution for teaching. Upon its reopening, the initial courses were refresher courses designed for key personnel to be placed in the new prefectural health departments and in the newly created health center system.[14] These initial courses were taught by members of my own staff. As time passed, Japanese instructors took over the task. Dr. Koya Yoshio, who was director of the institute, made a great contribution to the public health field in Japan in carrying out this program of education of key personnel in the various fields of public health: medical officers, nurses, sanitarians, public health veterinarians, nutritionists, public health engineers, and others.

From the time this institute was reorganized as a teaching institute in 1946, until the end of the occupation, 4,786 persons completed its various regular and short courses.[15] Prior to the end of the occupation, the Rockefeller Foundation agreed to permit Dr. Oliver R. McCoy, who was a member of my staff on loan from the foundation, to remain as advisor to the director of the Institute of Public Health. In addition, the foundation provided badly needed funds to subscribe to modern professional journals and to establish a library of modern professional literature at this teaching institute, which to this date is the heart of the public health training program in Japan.[16]

In attempting to improve environmental sanitation, it was necessary for us to establish courses for sanitarians and sanitary engineers in the Institute of Public Health, as there were no courses in sanitary engineering as such in the universities.[17] At the end of the occupation, the sanitary engineers and sanitarians were still being trained primarily in the Institute of Public Health. Great credit is due to the succession of sanitary engineers, headed by Mr. Turner and later Mr. MacLaren and Warren Kaufman and their many compatriots, who served not only on my staff but also on the prefectural civil affairs teams in training sanitarians and sanitary engineers for this nation in which, prior to the occupation, such a profession was unknown.

The National Institute of Health

There was no institute under government supervision in Japan designed to control the assay of biologic products as well as to conduct fundamental research on problems of national importance in the field of public health. The nearest approximations to such an organization was the Institute of Infectious Diseases, which had been established under the Ministry of Home Affairs, but which had been transferred to Tokyo Imperial University in 1933, and was under the control of the Ministry of Education. It, in fact, was a medical research institute for the university.[18] As a secondary function, it acted as an agent for the Ministry of Welfare in matters relating to licensing of biological laboratories and assay of their products. In addition, it became the largest manufacturer of biologic products in the nation and sat in judgment over the products of other commercial manufacturers as well as their own products.

It was the custom for a graduate of a particular medical school to look to that school in future years for his knowledge about advances in medical research. There were no nationwide professional publications. Considerable jealousy existed between the various universities, and nowhere in Japan could be found an institution where graduates of various universities were assembled together to exchange their knowledge and work together on common problems in the medical field.

In May 1947, we were able to establish the National Institute of Health as an official institution of the Ministry of Health and Welfare and to bring together under one roof representatives from the various universities to work together on fundamental research and the assay of biologics. I was warned by many of my Japanese friends that such an undertaking would not be possible. It did work, however. Although there was initially some friction, the staff learned to work together and exchange ideas. This organization has become one of the keystones in the control of biologics and antibiotics and in the medical research program in Japan.

7

Statistics: A Health and Welfare Tool

Numerical information on the occurrence of diseases, known as morbidity statistics, and on the occurrence of deaths, or mortality statistics, as well as births and other vital events, constitutes an important tool, if used properly, to evaluate the overall medical problem in an area or a nation. After evaluating the problem, such statistics are useful in planning programs to control diseases and to reduce deaths and disease. When used in this way, this statistical information can serve as a vast medical intelligence system for channeling information to those responsible for the operation of medical programs; yet, unless these statistics are made available to the proper echelons of the medical service, and unless they are current, they are of no value except for historical interest. Therefore, I established a Statistical Division within the PHW Section, which was headed by Leonard Phelps, to study the vital statistic- and morbidity statistic-reporting system of Japan, and to develop a nationwide reporting system which would furnish the necessary information to the people concerned in time to be of value.[1]

The *Koseki* System

In Japan, since 645 A.D., there had been a reporting system of the family. This system tied in to religious beliefs that required an unbroken line of ancestors in each family. Great care was taken to be sure that births, deaths, and marriages, regardless of whether they occurred in Japan or outside of Japan, were eventually accurately entered into the ancestral records.

Under this system, in the decades prior to the occupation, the vital statistics of births, marriages, stillbirths, and deaths were registered at the ancestral home of the family, known as the *honseki*. The local registration office, the *koseki*, forwarded reports of these events to the Cabinet Bureau of Statistics. Annual and national statistics were published based upon these reports. There were delays of some years before this information was published. None of it was used as a tool to evaluate the medical problems or to plan and execute medical programs for the control of disease.

Such a system was of no value to us as a working tool, except for historical study, and much confusion could result. For example, if a man died of smallpox in Tokyo, his death might well be reported from Hokkaido, because the report was made to the ancestral home. The event was not related to the place at which it actually occurred. There was, therefore, no way in which the distribution of smallpox and deaths from smallpox could be accurately determined.[2]

Rebuilding A Reporting System

We were concerned with where diseases were occurring, quantitatively how much disease there was, and, of course, what the death rates were.[3] In visiting many of the surviving health centers, I found that the health center director had no means of knowing the population in the area which he was serving, the incidence of disease, or the mortality rates from various diseases. In other words, he was blind: He did not have the statistical tools that would enable him to see his problem and plan his work accordingly.

It was, therefore, necessary to build from the ground up a morbidity- and mortality-reporting system, which would channel reports through the nationwide health organization that we were developing, from the national level through the prefectural level down to the health center level, so that a health center chief would know how many people he was serving and what his disease problems were.[4] These reports would, in turn, be sent from each health center to the prefectural health office, where the entire situation within a prefecture could be visualized. They were then sent to the Health and Welfare Ministry, where the national health situation would be compiled and studied.

Publication of the data when it could be useful as a daily operational tool is, of course, a most important element. The immediate publication of this information, in the case of certain acute diseases, even by telegraph, would be channelled downward so any local health officer could know not only what his own problems were but also those of the health districts around him and within his prefecture. He would also know what the national problem or situation was so that he could compare his own situation and the progress he was making.

The attempt to build up such a reporting organization was a tremendous task. As the health center system developed, many thousands of individuals were trained to staff the Health Statistics Divisions, which were established in each health center and in the newly established prefectural health departments. Prior to the occupation, some ten diseases were reported to the Cabinet Bureau of Statistics. Under the new system, the number of reportable diseases was increased to thirty-five.[5] There was also the task of establishing a health and welfare statistics section within the Ministry of Health and Welfare. There was, of course, some difficulty in divorcing the handling of morbidity and vital statistics under the old system from the Cabinet Bureau of Statistics and placing it in the Ministry of Health and Welfare, where the information could be useful; eventually, this reorganization was accomplished.

Using the Data

Many studies were made by the statistics section of the Ministry of Health and Welfare, including studies on the utilization of medical means and the distribution of doctors, nurses, and hospitals, for use in overall planning of the expansion of the hospital system. In addition, welfare statistics, used in implementing the Daily Life Security Law, or public assistance law, which we established, and the Child Welfare Law, were incorporated as a function of this section. Computations made with the ancient abacus and hand tabulations were the means available for handling the tremendous number of transcripts and schedules throughout the nation until the latter part of 1950, when we were able to procure through importation, modern coding, sorting, and tabulating machines for the Ministry of Health and Welfare.

An interesting problem developed in our attempt to analyze past statistics. Under the old system, a child presumably was one year old at birth. Apparently, when this system was established, the normal gestation period of human pregnancy was not known to the Japanese. The first of January was the birthday of all people born the preceding year, at which time another year was added, so that it was possible for a child to be born one minute before midnight on the thirty-first of December and be two years old sixty seconds later. This discrepancy between the age of an individual and ages as determined in most other nations of the world made our study by age groups a little difficult for comparative results, because the average Japanese was a year and a half younger than his occidental or other oriental counterpart. It took some time before this system could be altered so that the reported ages corresponded to those used in other statistical-reporting systems. I might mention that this system in which everyone had a birthday on the first of the year is similar to that used in the United States for the registration of thoroughbred horses.

The Quality of the Data

Completeness of reporting is an important element in evaluating such an organization. From time to time, various consultants were invited to Japan to evaluate this program and to make recommendations and suggestions for improvement. In 1947, Dr. Selwyn T. Collins, head statistician of the U.S. Public Health Service, spent several months evaluating the vital statistics organization.[6] Many tests were made on the completeness of reporting of this essential information. They showed from 95 to 99.8 percent completeness, which is remarkable in any country.

There are many reasons why this level of completeness was attainable.[7] The registration of pregnancies is one example. Under the new system, women were required to register pregnancies at the end of five months at the Maternal and Child Hygiene Division of the nearest health center. This registration then entitled her to receive additional or increased rations, which she could not receive as a pregnant woman unless her pregnancy had been registered.

Today the nation of Japan has one of the most complete, efficient, and modern health and welfare statistic-reporting organizations of any nation in the world.[8] Great credit is due to Leonard Phelps and his staff for the work they accomplished.

8

The Preventive Medicine Program, Part I: Controlling Wildfire Diseases

During the first two years of the occupation, the population was in a state of mass movement. About 6.5 million Japanese who were repatriating from all over the world were being dispersed throughout the country. Another 1.7 million Koreans who had been living in Japan were moving toward the ferry port of Shimonoseki, in southern Honshu, to return to Korea. People who had been dispersed from the cities to the country to escape the bombing during the war were trying to return to their destroyed homes. People who were living in makeshift shelters or the few islands of undestroyed homes in the burned-out cities were making almost daily trips to the country to search for food, because the ration distribution system had ceased to function in urban areas.

With the people in constant movement, Japan was like a huge anthill. Under such conditions, outbreaks of wildfire types of disease could be expected, as the opportunities for multiple contacts with carriers or cases of disease were increased many thousandfold over those in a stable population. By the time we arrived, such epidemics were already spreading rapidly.

Smallpox

Smallpox was one of the most dreaded wildfire diseases. Although Japan had produced smallpox vaccine in the past, the production laboratories, like all other facilities of this kind, had practically ceased to function during the war; vaccination programs had been discontinued. Consequently, over 17,000 cases occurred in the first year of the occupation.[1]

My first problem in controlling the smallpox epidemic was to begin the production of enough potent vaccine to vaccinate the 72 million people who were in Japan at the beginning of the occupation. Our policy was to produce in Japan, whenever possible, all supplies, including biologics, antibiotics, and pharmaceuticals, rather than import them. This policy was designed to place Japan on her own feet and to save American tax dollars, which would have to be expended if these products were imported in finished form.[2]

Smallpox vaccine rapidly weakens and becomes useless without proper refrigeration during storage and distribution. Such refrigeration was unavailable, so it became necessary to establish numerous production facilities throughout the nation. Establishing production facilities involved not only obtaining buildings and personnel but also obtaining calves, which are used in the production of smallpox vaccine, and forage for the calves. The latter was the more difficult part.

The initiation of this program illustrates the detailed instruction and supervision that was required at the beginning of the occupation. I would receive a report that although a building, equipment, and personnel had been obtained and arrangements had been made for procuring the necessary calves from nearby farmers, no vaccine was being produced. On investigation I would find that the officials were sitting in their offices waiting for the calves to be delivered by the transportation officials. Although the transportation officials might be in an office in the same prefecture building, no initiative was shown in contacting them to expedite the movement of the cattle. My own people would have to be the expediters to get things moving and to get production underway.

On the other hand, one of the amusing incidents that frequently compensated for the ever present frustrations involved one of my own health officers. A naval medical officer assigned to the team in Kyushu had obtained the use of some buildings in a former Japanese army barracks in Kumamoto. In his zealousness, he had simply requisitioned cattle and equipment and had selected a competent Japanese to head up the production laboratory. Reports began to reach my office that a certain Japanese man in Kumamoto was becoming wealthy through the sale of smallpox vaccine. I personally investigated this situation and found the reports were true. This man, without expending one yen of his own, had been set up in business, utilizing the buildings, equipment, and cattle which had been requisitioned by the government on our instructions, and had been reaping profits from the sale of the vaccine.

I complimented the young officer on his accomplishment of producing smallpox vaccine, which was the important thing, but pointed out that there were certain methods with which he had to comply if the laboratory was to be run as a private institution for profit. The matter of using government requisitioning powers to obtain equipment and livestock was not quite the proper method, particularly when this equipment was turned over without compensation to a private individual who was acquiring considerable wealth from the profits. On the other hand, if the laboratory was to be a government-operated laboratory, which was the original intent of the instructions, then the use of governmental powers of requisition were in order, but the profits, if any, from the sale of the vaccine belonged to the treasury and could not simply be handed over to a private individual of his own selection. It took about six months for the legal people to untangle this situation. In the meantime, vaccine production continued, which was the essential point.

We promptly began the largest mass immunization program ever undertaken up to that time. The epidemic should have subsided after about 60 million people had been vaccinated. It did not. In my visits to the communicable disease hospitals throughout the country, which might be a one-room building in the small communities—a building which reminded me of the pesthouses that were prevalent in our own country in my boyhood—I found numerous cases of smallpox in individuals whose history showed they had been "vaccinated" only a short time ago. Something was wrong.

We tested the vaccine for potency. It was potent. Not until I began to check the vaccination teams at work did we find the answer. Under an old Japanese law, the individual's arm was swabbed with alcohol, four small superficial cuts were made with a scalpel, and the liquid vaccine was spread over these cuts. Under the conditions of mass immunization, no time was allowed for the alcohol to dry. Because the alcohol killed the vaccine virus on contact, and it was physically impossible to follow up each individual to read the vaccination seventy-two hours later to see if a proper take had occurred, we had not really vaccinated 60 million people: We had only gone through the motions.

It was, therefore, necessary to send out detailed instructions and exercise close supervision to see that no alcohol was used in the future. The whole program had to begin all over again, but it succeeded. The epidemic was stopped.[3]

In public health practice in our own country, it was then presumed that a successful take conferred lifetime immunity. Having had some experience with smallpox epidemics in the Middle East, I had considerable doubts about the generally taught and accepted theories about the duration of immunity from one successful smallpox immunization. In 1945, when we were negotiating with representatives of the various nations from which Japanese repatriates were to be returned, the validity of certificates of successful vaccination against smallpox became a matter of controversy. In most instances, smallpox was then prevalent in these nations, and I insisted that all repatriates be revaccinated if they had not had a successful vaccination within one year before boarding ship. Much pressure was put on me through various channels, including our own State Department, to accept certificates within three years, particularly from British-controlled areas of Southeast Asia. Fortunately, I resisted these pressures.

In the military service, we had found that lifetime immunity was not conferred; revaccination was required every three years. In spite of such an interval, several hundred cases developed among our soldiers. The first cases I saw were in Korea during a staff visit; in Japan, the first cases occurred among enlisted medical personnel at the U.S. Army hospital in Osaka who had been keeping company with some of the Japanese girls who worked at an infectious disease hospital next door where several hundred smallpox cases were hospitalized. Cases also began occurring among soldiers on their way to the United States for demobilization. The disease began to spread among our own people on the west coast. Smallpox cases developed in one trainload of soldiers shortly before reaching Chicago.

The occurrence of an outbreak within three years after immunization of the entire population of Japan confirmed my suspicions about our previous knowledge about the duration of immunity. In March 1949, 124 new cases of smallpox were reported in Fukuoka and Osaka. Investigation showed that smallpox had been reintroduced into Japan from Korea, where an epidemic was in progress. Each of the cases in Japan could be traced to contact with a smuggler who was operating in the Fukuoka and Kobe-Osaka areas.

I directed the revaccination of the entire population. This time, considerable movement of the population had subsided, and it was possible to study the percentage of people who had been successfully vaccinated three years earlier but had lost their immunity. We found that 42 percent of the individuals successfully vaccinated had lost their immunity within less than three years. Following completion of the second nationwide immunization program, only five cases occurred throughout the entire population in 1950. This experience illustrates one of the numerous contributions made to world medical knowledge during the occupation.

Smallpox was reintroduced in 1951, this time by our own people. In the spring of 1951, 86 cases were reported among Japanese people working for the American forces in a cleaning and laundry establishment in Kobe. They were cleaning winter clothing returned from Korea, where our troops were engaged in the Korean War. The troops had been in contact with Korean civilians during a smallpox epidemic. Investigation showed that a long-forgotten fact was the cause of the outbreak in Japan. In the early days of smallpox vaccination, the virus was distributed by shipping the dried scabs from the poxes on calves.

Smallpox virus will remain viable for long periods of time on clothing or other articles which have been in contact with those who may have the disease. Apparently, some of our soldiers had been in rather intimate or, let us say, at least close physical contact with some Koreans, and their winter clothing had been contaminated with the virus. When the clothing was shipped back to Japan for cleaning and storage during the summer, the workers handling the clothing were exposed to the virus. Because some of them had lost their immunity from the previous immunization program, they came down with the disease. Only one locality was involved, so I directed focal reimmunization: Only 13 million reimmunizations were required.

Typhus Fever

Typhus fever has been one of the scourges of war and its aftermath. The humble louse, with its ability to spread this killing disease, has become well known in military medical history. Typhus literally decimated Napoleon's armies during his ill-fated invasion of Russia, and over 10 million deaths were attributed to typhus epidemics in Europe after World War I.

Our intelligence reports showed that typhus had been increasing in Japan during the war, so we had stockpiled DDT and typhus vaccine in the Philippines, preparatory to the planned invasion of Japan. In addition, members of the Typhus Commission had been sent to the Far East to assist in the control of the expected epidemics.[4] When the commission was disbanded shortly after the end of the war, Dr. Speck Wheeler, who was on loan to the military service from the Rockefeller Foundation, stayed on as a permanent member of my staff.

Because the great majority of the cases were reportedly occurring among Korean slave laborers in the coal mines of the northernmost island of Hokkaido, it was my intention to establish delousing and vaccination stations at Hakodate and Aomori, the ferry points across the Tsugaru Strait, and in this way prevent the spread of the epidemic. My plans did not work out.

While the surrender negotiations were being carried out, the Koreans revolted and decided to go home. They proceeded to travel the length of the main island of Honshu to the ferry points of Shimonoseki and Moji, carrying lice and rickettsia and spreading typhus throughout the entire length of Japan, before we even arrived.

Because little was known at the beginning of the occupation as to what violence might occur, priority was given to the movement of guns and ammunition. The movement of DDT, vaccine, and dusting equipment in the quantities required was not completed until November 1945, after a direct appeal to the Supreme Commander.[5] I pointed out that this epidemic was getting out of hand, and serious unrest and other repercussions would occur if thousands of people began dying in the cities of Japan with nothing being done to stop the outbreak.[6] Fortunately, General MacArthur is a man who can quickly grasp the essentials of any situation. He immediately authorized the necessary priorities to enable us to begin controlling this disease, the techniques of which had been developed in the Middle East and proven effective in a small outbreak in Naples, Italy.[7]

Between September 1945 and 1 July 1946, 33,500 cases occurred; 30,000 of these cases occurred between January and July 1946. To bring the epidemic under control, some 48 million people were deloused, and 5.3 million were inoculated with typhus vaccine.[8]

The DDT used in our delousing was authorized for production in Japan by our government, although it was under a Swiss patent. The powder might have only 10 percent active ingredients, the other 90 percent being talc. Therefore, our first step was to continue to import the DDT concentrate, mixing this with Japanese talc and packaging it in Japan, which resulted in a considerable savings in shipping costs. After production of the concentrate was large enough to meet our requirements, we discontinued all importation.[9] Before the end of the occupation, Japan was not only meeting all of her own requirements for DDT products and dusting equipment but also producing sufficient quantities for export for our requirements in Korea.

Dr. Herald R. Cox had succeeded in developing a method of inoculating chicken embryos with rickettsia, so they could multiply in the living tissue of the unhatched chick embryo, thus opening the door for the first time to large-scale

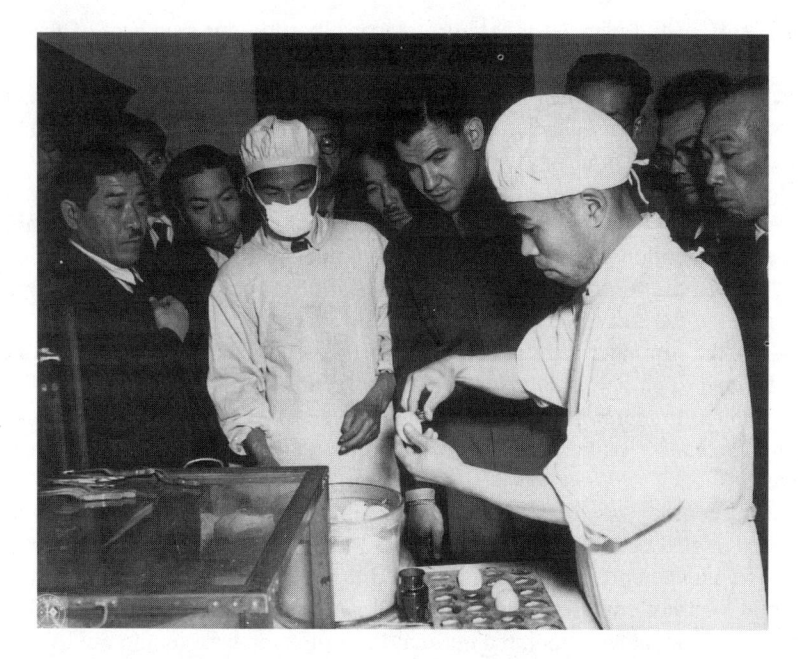

Figure 14. A demonstration of the Cox method of producing typhus vaccine was held at the Institute of Infectious Diseases, Tokyo, 16 April 1947. Here, prefectural laboratory inspectors observe the harvesting of the infected yolk sac membrane. Front, left to right: Dr. Fukuzumi (Chief, Typhus Vaccine Production, Institute), unidentified, Dr. Herbert Volk (Laboratory Consultant to PHW, SCAP), unidentified. Background: prefectural laboratory inspectors. Photo Credit: U.S. Army Signal Corps, Photographer Mularski. (Courtesy of the Hoover Institution Archives, Stanford University.)

production of a successful vaccine for use in prevention of this scourge of war. The Cox method of producing typhus vaccine was introduced in Japan at subsequent savings of many millions of American tax dollars. It also led to one of the amusing but sometimes irritating incidents.

When we decided to introduce the production of typhus vaccine, we had difficulty finding enough fertile eggs for inoculation to produce sufficient quantities of the vaccine to meet our needs. The poultry flocks, which were never very large in Japan, had been badly depleted during the war. Chicken feed, in particular, was almost nonexistent because the people were using all available grains for human consumption. Therefore, one of my requests in the Government and Relief in Occupied Areas (GARIOA) budget was for funds for egg settings and a few hundred tons of chicken feed. This request was greeted with some ridicule in Washington, D.C., particularly by those who said, "We are not approving the use of American tax dollars to feed Japanese chickens." It took considerable, detailed step-by-step explanation to convince the financial people that a few thousand dollars invested in chicken feed at that time would result in a very sound

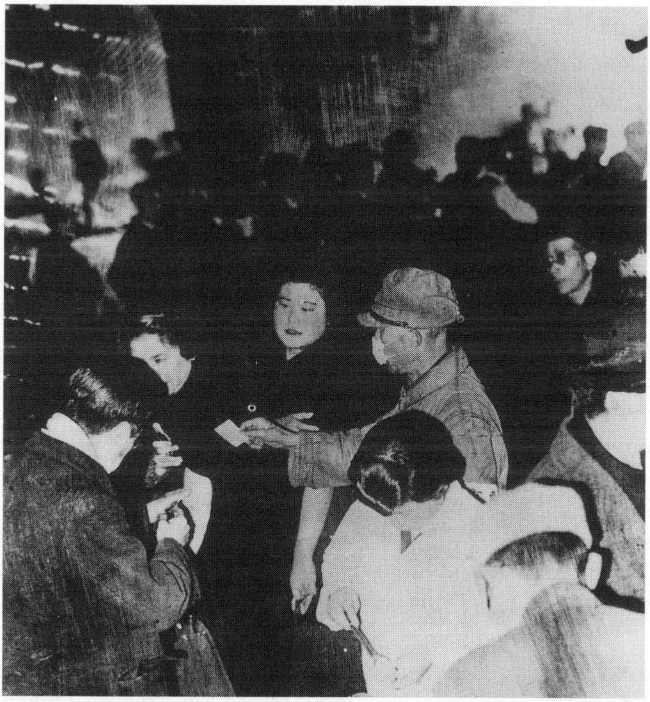

Figure 15. Two women receive typhus vaccinations at Yurakucho Station, Japan, circa May 1947. Although the mass movement of people aided the spread of typhus, this disease was controlled by a combination of case finding, vaccination, dusting with DDT, and health promotion using radio broadcasts, newspapers, posters, and pamphlets. Photo Credit: U.S. Army Signal Corps. (Courtesy of the Hoover Institution Archives, Stanford University.)

investment and a savings of approximately 50 million dollars in taxpayers' money over the period of several years by avoiding the importation of many millions of doses of typhus vaccine.

Typhus was important not only quantitatively but also because we again found that our previously held knowledge of the disease would not explain the epidemiological phenomena with which we were dealing. Typhus is primarily a disease of rats and other members of the rodent family. In the winter when rodents seek shelter in human habitations, they bring their typhus and fleas and mites, which transmit the disease in its various forms from one another to humans. Through this close contact with humans, particularly in time of war when mass movement of people follows mass destruction, the disease known as murine typhus is transmitted by fleas to humans.

As the masses of people, military or civilian, who are brought into close contact during and after war all become lousy, it appears that what was originally a rat disease transmitted as murine typhus to humans through rat fleas gradually, through serial transmission from one person to another by means of a new vector, the human louse, assumes a more virulent character with a comparatively high mortality rate. This disease is then known as epidemic typhus fever.

Although the two diseases, murine typhus and epidemic typhus, have been considered in our textbooks as separate and distinct diseases which could be diagnosed and differentiated by laboratory tests, I had long suspected that our knowledge of these typhus diseases was incomplete and somewhat inaccurate. In the Middle East, I had seen epidemic typhus break out apparently from nowhere in an area where murine typhus was endemic, that is, cases occurred frequently throughout the area each year. Our studies in Japan could not be reconciled with the accepted belief that these were two separate diseases. Our serological studies showed that some 47 percent of the cases were epidemic typhus, some 29 percent were murine typhus, and some 23 percent were of an undetermined type. The peak incidence of typhus was in May, with a lower peak in January, which was not as it should be.

To determine whether we were dealing with a single disease or two separate diseases, we initiated several research projects. We found that we could transmit the rodent disease, murine typhus, by fleas to human volunteers. Serologically, these cases demonstrated murine typhus; however, when lice were fed on these cases and the disease was transmitted serially, that is from one individual to another, for many passages by lice, the disease began to show the clinical and serological picture of epidemic typhus. The serological findings passed from clear murine typhus through the undetermined or transition group to clear epidemic typhus as the rickettsia were passed serially by lice.

Through the important finding that we were really dealing with one disease, we could explain the epidemiological picture in the Middle East as well as in the Far East in terms of the human environment. In Japan, because of the difference in living habits, murine cases acquired from rat fleas, which reached humans in the close contact of winter quarters, constituted the first peak. As the cold weather continued and fuel was negligible for heating water to bathe and the people became lousy, it was possible to have a natural serial passage of the rickettsia by means of lice from one human to another. This passage occurred over a four-month period and resulted in the second peak in May, of which the majority of the cases were epidemic typhus.

There is much more work to be done on this problem. In our naturally human desire to classify and neatly file each scientific fact, particularly in our attempt to create order in the disorderly field of medical knowledge, I believe that we have tended to overclassify into separate diseases what are really different manifestations of a single disease, whose causative organism has been modified through mutations caused by changes in its environment. These changes occur in vectors of intermediate insect or other transmitters of the disease.

Cholera

Cholera, that wildfire killer of the ages, had not been present in Japan since 1920. But the repatriation of 6.5 million Japanese, which began immediately after the war, reintroduced this hazard, as many thousand Japanese were being returned from areas of Asia where cholera was endemic and epidemic.

Because this was the largest overseas population movement ever attempted in such a short period of time, a conference was held with representatives from the Chinese, Southeast Asian, and Russian theaters of operation, where most of the repatriates were located. The shipping was furnished by the United States and manned by Japanese crews. The operational control of ship movement was under SCAP, operating through the Far East Navy Command. G-3 of General Headquarters, SCAP [the staff section in charge of planning and conduct of operations—Ed.] was the agency coordinating the operation of repatriation ports in Japan and the islands under U.S. control as well as the overland movement and dispersion of people within Japan.

In accordance with international custom, an exchange of information about the incidence of diseases in the vicinity of the ports from which repatriates would leave for Japan was established. Certain quarantine procedures were agreed upon. These included delousing and immunization against smallpox, typhoid, and typhus, which were to be carried out at the outbound ports. We were to send the necessary supplies on the ships from Japan, as they were either nonexistent or in short supply in the countries from whence the Japanese were returning.[10]

In the meantime, I was responsible for establishing a quarantine service at each of the repatriation ports to process the returning Japanese and the outgoing foreign nationals, including some 1.2 million Koreans.[11] Japan had had quarantine stations at its ports before the war, which were operated by prefectural or local authorities, but they had been discontinued during the war. We initially established eight quarantine stations and later added six more, each of which was staffed by Japanese who were under the supervision of one of my American health officers. I was particularly fortunate in having received, through the assistance of Tom Parran, the Surgeon General of the U.S. Public Health Service, some twenty-three young American medical officers whom he had especially trained for this task. The chief of my Quarantine Division in my own office was a senior officer the U.S. Public Health Service who was loaned to me for this assignment.[12]

At our stations, all repatriates were redusted, immunized or reimmunized. They received chest X-rays for tuberculosis and examinations of malaria smears.

Our first report of trouble came in April 1946. It was our first knowledge that the repatriation agreement was not being carried out by the other theaters. A convoy of fourteen ships on their way from south Chinese ports reported many of their passengers were sick and dying of cholera. The first ships were due at

Kagoshima, the port at the southern tip of Kyushu, and arrived before they could be diverted. The passengers were held aboard.

All cholera ships were diverted to Uraga, our largest repatriation quarantine station, where I quickly assembled personnel and supplies capable of handling 15,000 stool cultures and examinations per day and immediately visited the first ships on their arrival. We began a real fight, which lasted for many months, to keep this wildfire disease from spreading throughout Japan.

A total of 233,000 persons were held in quarantine at this station after their arrival from what became known as cholera ports. Stool cultures were made on all individuals. Through this means, some five hundred carriers were identified, who, had they been permitted to disperse throughout Japan, would have spread the cholera vibrio in their stools throughout the country. In addition to the carriers, 711 cases of cholera were found among the repatriates. Many of them reported that they had been ill when carried aboard the ship. In addition, 250 cases of typhus and 107 cases of smallpox were picked up and detained. The sick, the carriers, and the dying were removed from the ships to a hospital at the station. The remainder were kept aboard ship until repeated stool examinations were negative and they had passed the incubation period of this disease.

Because the excrement from the ships was dumped into the sea while the ships were at anchor, there was a grave danger that the cholera vibrio in these stools might be carried by the currents into Tokyo Bay, where the shellfish might become infected and, in this way, spread the disease in that metropolitan area where these shellfish were consumed. It became necessary, therefore, to prohibit the procurement of shellfish from Tokyo Bay as a safety measure for some time.

Immunization against cholera was immediately begun at all quarantine stations and gradually spread throughout all port cities. I had a report from Kagoshima that two cases had occurred in that city. I immediately and personally investigated the report and found how easily this dreaded disease can spread.

The investigation showed that the young American health officer at Kagoshima had never seen cholera, and upon learning that the ships at anchor, before being diverted to Uraga, had cholera aboard, he had visited one of the ships to see the cases. In his scientific zeal, he had brought ashore a stool specimen for examination. The young Japanese laboratory technician who handled the stool in making a culture either did not wash his hands before eating his lunch, which he ate in the laboratory, or his lunch had been contaminated by flies who had fed on the stool culture; he became ill. His own stools had been spread with the "night soil" (untreated human excrement) collected from his home and that of neighbors on one of the neighboring gardens. One of the farmers who had handled this night soil had also become ill. I immediately directed a citywide immunization program, and all vegetables normally eaten uncooked from that particular garden were destroyed.

Sporadic cases did occur—1,200 in total—before cholera was completely eradicated from Japan. No cases have since been reported. Two cases of cholera among Korean repatriates from Canton, China, landed at Pusan, Korea; before that epidemic was stopped, 17,000 cases occurred with 11,000 deaths.

I should like to pay tribute to those Americans and Japanese who worked night and day to prevent a greater catastrophe which this dreaded disease might well have caused. As for the American theater surgeon of the China theater who failed to carry out the quarantine processing agreement, I have never forgiven him for his responsibility for this episode and for so many needless deaths.

9

The Preventive Medicine Program, Part II: Environmental Sanitation and Viral Diseases

Standards of sanitation and public health practice in Japan had declined during the war. Public water supply and waste collection facilities had been severely damaged in all areas that had been bombed. Those that had escaped the devastation of war were badly deteriorated through neglect and shortages of materials, labor, and supplies, which had been diverted to sustaining the war effort. By the war's end, the standards in Japan were, in most instances, far below those of the more advanced nations.

Enteric Diseases

Enteric diseases were responsible for the second highest number of deaths in Japan at the beginning of the occupation, exceeded only by tuberculosis, which was the number one killer.[1] This group of diseases is acquired by eating or drinking food and water that has been contaminated by human feces. Human carriers or unrecognized mild cases of these diseases pass the causative organisms out of their intestinal tract in feces. In a land where untreated human excrement called "night soil" is habitually used on the land for fertilizer, the causative organisms are spread on the fields and then spread to uninfected persons through vegetables or other foods that are grown on the ground and normally eaten uncooked. They are also spread to all of the surface streams and shallow wells when rains wash the fertilizer into these streams or wells.

The dysenteries, typhoid and paratyphoid fevers, and poliomyelitis in subclinical form were all prevalent and were particularly hard to combat because of the poor environmental standards of the country, which were aggravated by the widespread destruction of the war. Only a few of the major Japanese cities had modern water supply systems. These systems, which had been damaged by the bombing, supplied only a part of the population of these cities. Most of the people obtained their drinking water from heavily contaminated streams or shallow wells.[2]

Flies are another means of carrying these organisms from feces to food. Flies normally breed and lay their eggs in decaying organic matter. The adults have the nasty habit of feeding on human feces, which may contain the causative organisms of the enteric diseases. At their next meal, which may be the food in the kitchen or in a bowl, they will pass out of their intestinal tracts their own feces containing the organisms they ingested in their previous meal. The Japanese had never attempted large-scale fly, mosquito, or rodent control programs. In fact, there was an old Japanese saying that the better the cook the more flies she attracted to her kitchen.

An effective vaccine for typhoid and paratyphoid fevers had been developed in 1910 in the United States, which was widely used in the military services beginning with World War I. But no successful vaccine had been developed for the large group of dysenteries. The only approach, therefore, to the problem of controlling these diseases for which we had no immunizing agents was to undertake a program of improving the sanitary standards of the entire nation. I had had considerable experience with the use of sanitary teams for the control of insect-borne diseases and the general sanitary environment in Panama and in the Middle East. But to use such methods on the scale which would be required for a nation of 84 million people had never before been attempted.

Long before the war, Japan had organized neighborhood sanitary societies called *Eisei Kumai* that carried on a twice-a-year clean up campaign under the supervision of the national police, which remind me of the spring clean up campaigns of my own town during my youth. During the war, the *Eisei Kumai* had been incorporated into the *Tonarigumi* (Block Associations), which had become the local agencies for controlling all activities of the people, including so-called "thought control." Complete dossiers were maintained on each individual covering all of his activities, including when he left his home or who visited him during the day or night. Such an instrument of tyranny was quite properly abolished by the occupation forces as part of the program to establish individual freedom and democracy in Japan.[3]

At the beginning of the occupation, we could find only two sanitary engineers in all of Japan. They had been trained in the United States, but neither was engaged in practicing his profession of sanitary engineering as applied to environmental sanitation. As in most of our programs, it was, therefore, necessary to begin a large-scale training program. Training courses were first held in Kyoto, and later in Tokyo and Sendai. These were expanded to the nine regions of Japan and eventually to all forty-six prefectures. During the course of the occupation, approximately 160 sanitary engineers and 870 sanitarians were trained in the courses established and carried out under the supervision of SCAP personnel in this field.[4] In addition, some 360,000 men were eventually trained as members of the sanitary teams, which we organized throughout the nation beginning in the spring of 1946.

The initial plan was to have one team for each 2,000 population, which made weekly visits to all human habitations in an assigned area. The first hastily organized delousing teams used in the typhus control program in the winter of 1945–46 were retrained and incorporated into the permanent sanitary teams. By the end of 1946, only 9,000 sanitary teams of six men each, or 54,000 men, had been trained and were carrying out a house-to-house sanitary program. These teams were trained and equipped to carry out insect control measures, including the spraying of fly-breeding places with DDT and the killing of adult flies. They also accomplished much in the field of sanitary education by teaching the householders the basics of simple personal hygiene in handling food and protecting water supplies, including home chlorination of wells with calcium hypochlorite. In the devastated areas in which few people were still living, much of the work of removing insect and rodent breeding places was carried out by these men. In the summer, first priority was given to the control of flies and mosquitos and to environmental sanitation, with emphasis on the enteric diseases. In the winter months, they emphasized rodent control and dusting with DDT for lice.[5]

As time passed, and the initial health center system was established, these sanitary teams were incorporated into that organization.[6] Trained sanitarians headed up each team on a permanent basis; the labor component of each team was increased in the summer and decreased in the winter. By 1948, the teams were reduced to one for every 15,000 population. At the end of the occupation, there were only 2,039 trained sanitarians as inspectors and 7,000 trained assistant inspectors in the permanent organization.[7]

So far as the dysenteries are concerned, the program bore worthwhile results. Dysentery, which had an annual incidence of 138 per 100,000 population in 1945, with a peak of 480 in the months of August and September of 1945, was reduced to 18.3 in 1948.[8] This rate was approximately half of that in the United States that year.

Beginning in 1948, the first steps were taken to stabilize the economy of Japan by Joseph Dodge, which included halting a runaway inflation that had inflated the currency ninety times its initial postwar value. As the first step in halting inflation is to balance the national government budget and curtail excessive spending, our budget for sanitary teams was drastically reduced as part of the overall reduction in yen expenditures. As a result, the dysentery incidence began a steady return to its prewar rate, which was reached by 1951 and exceeded in 1952.[9] There were many other factors which entered into the picture, such as drug resistance to sulfanilamides used in treatment and DDT resistance in flies. The primary importance of the entire program, however, was to demonstrate conclusively that it is possible through proper organization and administration to carry out a nationwide program to improve environmental standards and control the enteric diseases in an underdeveloped country, if the will and the necessary expenditure of effort and funds are there.

The control of the typhoid fevers was important for two reasons. The program settled a scientific controversy which had been going on in the medical profession throughout the world since 1910. It also gave us an insight into a grave danger that can develop among scientists in any country. Japanese scientists, like others throughout the world, had tried the production of typhoid vaccine when news of its development was published. Unfortunately, there had been some difficulty in producing a potent vaccine, for the controlled inoculation experiment among a group of Japanese failed to demonstrate that the vaccine would protect against this disease. They had, therefore, turned their backs on typhoid vaccine as a means of protecting their people against a hazard that, before the war, caused 40,000 to 50,000 cases per year and 6,000 to 12,000 needless deaths per year.

I was informed by some of the leading Japanese doctors and scientists that Japanese typhoid must be different from the typhoid fevers of other parts of the world and that our vaccine would not protect against Japanese typhoid; however, the cases I saw were exactly like those I had seen in our own country, in Central America, and in the Middle East, and laboratory studies failed to show any difference in the causative organisms. I, therefore, decided to begin the production of typhoid and paratyphoid vaccine using methods that we had found satisfactory in our own country.

In spite of the dire predictions of the respected and learned medical men of Japan that typhoid vaccine would not protect the Japanese people against this disease, because they themselves had failed to produce a potent vaccine in past years, we did succeed in protecting the people. Some 60 million persons from 3 to 60 years of age were immunized by the end of 1948; the incidence of the disease promptly dropped to 11.9 cases per 100,000 population, from the 1945 rate of 80 per 100,000 population.[10] This caused the Japanese scientists to lose face in the eyes of their own people and the Americans who were responsible for the introduction and success of the program to gain the confidence of the people as a whole.

Because this drop paralleled the drop in the dysenteries, the old scientifically controversial question was raised as to whether the drop in incidence was due to improved environmental sanitation or to the vaccine. This question had been repeatedly raised in our military service, as many claimed that it was the careful supervision of environmental sanitation by the army medical service that had been responsible for the virtual elimination of typhoid fever as a major cause of disease among our troops, rather than the effectiveness of the vaccine we had used throughout the years.

The answer to this important question was found in the next three years, for as the dysenteries began their rise after the low point of 1948, due to the necessity of curtailing our sanitary team program, the typhoid fever incidence did not rise, but continued to drop steadily.[11] In 1953, it reached the low of 2.9 per 100,000 population, a reduction of 97 percent of the 1945 rate. This steady drop in the face of deteriorating sanitary standards proved once and for all that while improved environmental sanitation, of course, does play a part in controlling this disease, as it does in the dysenteries and other enteric diseases, typhoid vaccine will protect in spite of poor sanitary standards.

The second, and to me more important, lesson we learned from this program is the great danger that scientists of a nation, being only human, may assume, as did the Japanese scientists in this case, that only that scientific knowledge which they themselves have developed is worthwhile and that the rest of the world is wrong. This closed-minded attitude stemming from extreme nationalism led to the loss of scientific leadership in medicine which Germany held for so many years until the advent of Hitler. I am sorry that in my own beloved country there is a tendency in recent years, in some instances at least, to assume that if a successful program in medicine was not originated and developed in this country, it is not worth considering. We have turned our scientific backs on some very worthwhile scientific progress made in other countries, to the detriment of our own people and particularly to the detriment of scientific progress in the fields of medicine, because such real progress can only continue in the presence of an open mind.

Japanese B Encephalitis

Japanese B encephalitis is a viral disease that was identified by a Japanese; hence, the name. This disease causes inflammation of the brain and the spinal cord. It is prevalent throughout the Far East. Information received from our Russian medical contacts indicates it is the major problem east of Lake Baikal. It has been identified in Korea, the mainland of China, Formosa, and the islands of the Pacific as far south as Guam. Encephalitis is not limited to the Orient but is prevalent throughout the world. It is particularly interesting from a medical standpoint, because only in very recent years have the efforts of many men in this country and others finally begun to unravel the very complicated way in which epidemics of encephalitis occur.

One of the earliest epidemics in recent years, known as the Saint Louis Encephalitis, occurred in the early 1930s. Gen. James Stevens Simmons was among those sent to find out what the epidemic was and how it spread. Subsequently, an epidemic in New England in 1936 began among horses and was followed a few weeks later by an outbreak among humans. It appeared there might be some method by which this virus was transmitted from horses to humans.

Ray Kelser, a veterinary officer and good friend of mine, who was working in the laboratory in Panama, was able to show that a particular species of mosquito, a *tritaeniorhynchus*, was responsible for transmitting encephalitis to humans. He thought the mosquitoes bit the horses and sucked in the virus; then, as in malaria, the virus passed through the body of the mosquito and was injected into humans when the mosquito bit a human, the injection occurring through the mosquito's salivary glands.

These encephalitis outbreaks in the United States have been designated as eastern equine-encephalitis, indicating an inflammation of the central nervous system of horses; western encephalomyelitis; and Saint Louis encephalitis. It might be stated that these diseases are all related more or less as first cousins to the Japanese B, or Far East encephalitis.

The Japanese had been doing considerable research in past years on the periodic outbreaks of encephalitis among their people. I requested that Dr. John R. Paul, who had worked with me as the head of a neurotrophic virus disease commission in the Middle East, come to Japan with a group to review the work done by the Japanese on the Japanese B encephalitis and see if we could find how it was spread and what could be done to prevent it. Dr. William Hammond of the University of California, later with the University of Pittsburgh, had done outstanding work on the periodic outbreaks of encephalitis which occurred in the central valley of California and the Yakima Valley in the Pacific Northwest. He had found, as so often happens, that the relationship between outbreaks of encephalitis among domestic animals, such as horses, cattle and livestock, and the outbreak of epidemics in humans was not a case of direct transmission from an infected animal to a human host by means of a mosquito. The picture was a little more complicated.

He had found that the reservoir, as it is called, of this virus existed in birds, both wild and domestic. The mosquitoes bit the birds and then bit the horses. Other species bit the birds and bit humans. Mosquitoes have preferences in their biting habits as far as the type of blood they particularly prefer; some, therefore, will bite birds and then bite horses or cattle, while others will bite the birds and then prefer human blood. This accounts for the time interval, since the hatch-out periods frequently differ.

Dr. Paul's group made a very comprehensive study in Japan. It is possible to take blood samples from individuals and determine whether or not they had ever been infected with encephalitis virus. They found that almost all of the adults in the Kanto Plain area, the Okayama area, and the Shikoku area, where the great epidemics of the past had occurred, had been infected. This pattern is typical, particularly with virus diseases such as encephalitis and polio. Of these large numbers of infected people, comparatively few people developed the clinical symptoms of this disease, although infection over the years had been almost universal in the areas where these great epidemics occurred.

The horses, which were raised in Hokkaido and then brought to Honshu, universally acquired encephalitis; a high percentage of them died. Studies were also made by taking blood samples from the work cattle and from dogs; they were also found to be infected with encephalitis. The big problem, of course, was to identify which particular species of mosquitoes were responsible in Japan for transmitting this disease to the various animals and also to humans, since previous research had indicated there were probably two different species. The second problem was to try to identify the bird reservoir.

The species of mosquitoes were identified by catching many, many hundreds of thousands of them and obtaining the virus from their bodies. It was found that one species of mosquito was responsible for infecting domestic animals and that another species, which reached its peak hatch-out some six weeks later, was responsible for the human infections. Because the two species were *Culicines* and *Aedes*, which normally breed in very small collections of water in containers or in gutters around houses, it seemed obvious that the reservoir must be a bird that is found in close proximity to homes. It seemed illogical to believe that the mosquito hatched in a container of water near a building would fly any great distance to bite some bird out in Tokyo Bay and then return to the home and bite a human. Our search, which involved consideration of all migratory birds, in particular, soon narrowed to birds which were found in close proximity to homes. We were interested in migratory birds because this disease is prevalent from Siberia to at least as far south as Guam. If the host were a migratory bird, we could explain the time phasing of the outbreaks.

In cooperation with the people of the Natural Resources Section, we studied the various species of birds. Many were trapped to obtain blood to determine whether they harbored the B encephalitis virus. Dr. Wheeler thought that bird mites, which could be found in the bird nests, might be a means of transmitting the virus from one bird to another, thereby perpetuating the reservoir. This type of research, of course, takes the work of many people and many years to carry out.

A vaccine was developed in the United States by the Army Research Institute, and quantities were shipped to Japan to test its protective capabilities. By agreement with the Japanese after study of the various areas, we believed that the next outbreak would probably occur in Okayama Prefecture or its vicinity. A controlled immunization experiment involving some 250,000 children who had not so far been infected was begun. The children, all of whom were volunteers with the consent of their parents, were immunized. A corresponding control group was kept under observation. They were given booster doses for five years.

Unfortunately, the next epidemic occurred in the Kanto Plain area in the summer of 1948. Some 7,000 cases occurred that year.[12] A second epidemic involving 5,000 cases occurred in 1950. At the time these epidemics occurred, the extensive knowledge that we were trying to obtain about the value of the vaccine was not known. I was concerned during the 1950 epidemic whether we should initiate large-scale production of vaccine for mass inoculation. After seeking the advice of the epidemiological board of consultants to the army medical service, they recommended that it should not be done because we did not have sufficient data at that time to show that it would be protective.

We then attempted to prevent succeeding epidemics by extensive mosquito control. Because *culextritaeniorhynchus* was one of the vectors, the one particularly involved in human cases, this mosquito was attacked by extensive spraying of homes, elimination of breeding places by sanitary teams, and education of the public. Because the livestock industry is of considerable importance to the economic well-being of the nation, extensive spraying programs were carried out in all of the livestock shelters for the *culicines* as well.

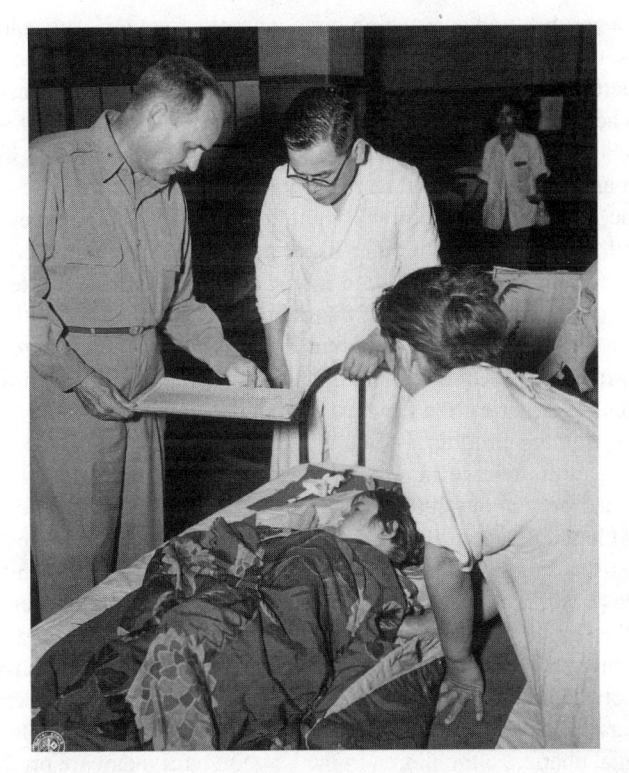

ENVIRONMENTAL SANITATION AND VIRAL DISEASES 99

Figure 16. Brig. Gen. C.F. Sams reviews the Japanese B encephalitis research project at Komagome Hospital, Tokyo, 31 August 1948. Photo credit: U.S. Army Signal Corps, Photographer Leavitt. (Courtesy of the Hoover Institution Archives, Stanford University.)

A review of the data on the vaccine experiment has been made. The number of cases that occurred in the control group as well as in the immunized group was very small, but there was a statistically valid difference. It is believed that the vaccine does offer protection, although, as in the case of most vaccines, far from 100 percent protection.

Polio

Poliomyelitis is also a worldwide disease. It is, you might say, closely related to encephalitis in that it attacks the central nervous system; however, it is spread by a different method. Instead of being spread by blood-sucking insects, such as the mosquito, which directly inoculate the host's blood stream with the virus, polio is spread as an enteric disease by eating or drinking food or water that is contaminated with the virus, which has been excreted in the feces of a carrier or another case. Simultaneously with the study of encephalitis in the Far East, Dr. John R.

Paul and his group found a very high infection rate of polio.[13] The epidemiological patterns and geographic distribution of encephalitis and polio dovetailed: A very high percentage of a cross section of the Japanese population, particularly in the areas where encephalitis was not prevalent, had been infected at some time, probably when they had first been weaned and had begun to take in contaminated water and food.[14] As usual, very few clinical cases occurred.

For some reason as yet unknown, the older an individual is when he is first infected with a polio virus, the more likely he is to become paralyzed. In countries considered underdeveloped with low sanitary standards very few crippled children are seen. If small doses of the polio virus are acquired in infancy, the infant either dies or acquires an immunity; a very low percentage of infants develop paralysis. Consequently, in populations such as those found in the Middle East, Central America, the Far East, and in this case specifically Japan, there are very few crippled children.

In studying this disease in the Far East, we found that among 84 million people, we had only about 400 cases of clinically identified polio; only a small fraction developed paralysis that had been confirmed by laboratory tests.[15] There were almost ten times as many clinical cases occurring in the United States, although the population of the United States was only twice that of Japan.

During the last thirty years in the United States, we have protected our infants and small children through health education of their mothers. We have pasteurized and protected the milk which they have been given in supplementary feeding and afterwards. We have produced sterile, canned baby food. Through such environmental change, our children in the United States today are protected from the small doses of polio virus which children in underdeveloped countries acquire early in life. The age groups in which polio is occurring in the United States are getting older with time. Consequently, we are finding a higher percentage of paralytic cases among those infected in the United States than anywhere else in the world.

This medical problem presents some interesting social and other facets. Americans have become a migratory people on wheels. We have changed from closely knit family groups that seldom ate in public places to loosely knit groups that almost routinely eat in public places, thereby increasing our opportunity for cross infections. Instead of solving the basic problems by extending the improved environmental status to include older groups, we have attempted in this country to use immunization, which is a comparatively cheap and, of course, reasonable approach. It is interesting to note that when a group of Americans who have been protected during infancy are moved into a country like Japan, and there were a good many thousand Americans soldiers and their families there, the attack rate, as shown in identifiable clinical cases among the Americans, was much higher than that among the Japanese.

I think the explanation lies in the basic environmental factor that I have previously mentioned. We have protected our infants and small children better than the corresponding small children are protected in countries such as Japan. Therefore, we have a population which has a lower immunity rate when they are older than the Japanese who acquired their immunity early in life. The question is, of course, Is this good or is it bad? There are arguments on both sides.

In raising the environmental standards to the point we have in protecting our infants, we have reduced the problem of early deaths, that is, deaths in children less than a year old, from all of the diseases, including polio, that are so prevalent among infants in other countries. But we then are faced with the problem, which we have created, of clinical cases, particularly paralytic cases, of a disease in later life among those who did not acquire early immunity during infancy. Is it better to let a fairly high percentage of young infants die in the course of acquiring immunity to many diseases through a low standard of environmental cleanliness? Or is it better to save these infants to have a very high rate of children and young adults live out a lifetime permanently crippled as a result of having acquired a disease later in life because they had not acquired an immunity early in life? This disease presents an interesting philosophical, moral, and medical problem. Perhaps our vaccination program if carried out continuously will give us an answer.

10

The Preventive Medicine Program, Part III: Treatment and Prevention

Of the many diseases prevalent in Japan in which marked reductions in death and disease rates occurred as a result of our programs, I shall mention only a few which might be of general interest. The combined effects of our preventive medicine program resulted in a drop in the crude death rate from a prewar seven-year average of 18.7 deaths per 1,000 population to 10.8 by 1950.[1] Converted into numbers of living people—the difference between those who would have died, had the prewar death rates continued, and the present death rate—millions of people in Japan are alive today who would otherwise have died.

Diphtheria

Diphtheria, according to the available records, had been extremely prevalent in Japan, at least since 1900. Diphtheria was primarily a children's disease: Approximately seventy percent of the cases occurred in children; ninety percent of the deaths occurred in children ten years of age and younger. A total of 94,274 cases occurred in 1944; the rate for 1945 was 122.8 cases per 100,000 population.[2]

The Japanese had produced diphtheria antitoxin, which was used for treatment and occasionally for passive immunization. They were not familiar with the comparatively modern diphtheria toxoid for active prophylactic immunization which had been so successfully used in the United States for this purpose. Pharmaceutical manufacturing companies were taught how to prepare diphtheria toxoid. Requirements were set for the immunization of some 18 million children ten years of age and under.

This particular vaccine is difficult to produce so that it will provide the necessary degree of immunization in the person inoculated without causing a severe reaction. Unfortunately, in the first immunization program, one manufacturer failed to detoxify two flasks of vaccine. Those children who were immunized with this batch of the vaccine became seriously ill; there were a few deaths. This incident led to a complete change in the nationwide control method for standards for assay. Production of vaccine of all types was suspended until satisfactory nationwide controls were established.[3]

After these controls had been established, the immunization program was reinitiated. The Preventive Vaccination Law, which was put into effect in response to directives from SCAP, provides all children between six- and twelve-months old shall be immunized against diphtheria and reimmunized within six months before entering elementary school and six months before completion of elementary school. It takes many years to reap the benefits of this type of mass immunization program; yet by 1951, all children less than ten years of age had been immunized, and the rate of disease had fallen ninety percent to 12.7 cases per 100,000 population.[4]

Pneumonia

Satisfactory preventive vaccines were not available for the pneumonias. The high mortality rate from pneumonias—there were 130.3 deaths per 100,000 population at the beginning of the occupation—was cut in half by the use of sulfonamides and the introduction of antibiotics, such as penicillin, in the treatment of pneumonias.[5]

Venereal Disease

How to handle the venereal disease problem was a controversial issue. From a medical standpoint, venereal disease can be controlled with available modern methods; however, in the minds of many people, there is a moral issue involved as well as a medical issue. Various religious and lay groups, therefore, have taken firm positions as to how venereal disease should be controlled, whether or not the positions are medically sound.

Venereal disease has always been a major problem in military forces. Healthy young men are removed from normal contacts with the female sex, through their dates and social events, when they come into the military service. They are removed from their home environments into a barracks environment. Whether they be in training camps, combat areas, or overseas theaters, they frequently find that it is impossible to establish normal social relations with young women in the neighborhood of their camps or military installations, so many of them are limited to contacts with prostitutes and women who may not be professional prostitutes but who are promiscuous. Many methods have been tried in past years to keep the venereal disease incidence as low as possible. Prior to the introduction of the sulfanilamides in the treatment of venereal disease, soldiers who were infected either with gonorrhea or syphilis were hospitalized. All of our hospitals had one or several wards full of patients under treatment, with the old irrigations and the bismuth and arsenicals, for syphilis. The treatment required hospitalization, during which the soldiers were called "noneffectives" for combat in war or training in peace.

The army had followed a policy that involved not only medical but also disciplinary actions. Under the Rules and Articles of War, if a soldier failed to take a prophylaxis following exposure and contracted a venereal disease, he was subject to two penalties: He lost his pay while he was under treatment, because contraction of venereal disease was considered not in the line of duty under such circumstances. He had also violated an order in failing to take a prophylaxis and was tried by court martial for such violation. The commanding officer of a company or battery that had a venereal disease rate over 60 cases per 1,000 soldiers per year would receive a letter from his military superior requiring that he take disciplinary action and other means to reduce his rate. Sometimes a high venereal disease rate in a command led to relief of the commanding officer.

Prior to World War II, venereal disease rates were always higher in overseas areas than they were in the United States. In foreign countries, the young soldier was usually limited in his associations with women to prostitutes. Because the young women knew that it was most unlikely that a soldier stationed in their country would marry them, they avoided contact with military personnel. If a soldier did contract venereal disease, an effort was made to find out who the girl was. If she could be identified, the girl was examined; if she was found to be infected, she was required to receive treatment.

In the United States at the beginning of the mobilization just before World War II, under our moral standards and mores, the policy was adopted to "suppress" prostitution in the vicinity of military establishments. Cooperation was initiated among the military line authorities, military medical authorities, the police, and civilian health authorities in attempting to establish zones around military installations from which prostitutes would be abolished. Apparently in the eyes of many, this had succeeded because the venereal disease rate among troops in the United States as reported during World War II was reasonably low. When the combat was over, although the same policy was carried out, the venereal disease rate among troops in the United States had a very sharp increase. This fact caused considerable controversy.

One school of thought took the position that the real reason the venereal disease rate had been low during the war was because of several factors. There was great pressure on for troops to be trained as quickly as possible and shipped overseas to combat theaters of operation, so the training schedules were long and arduous. The men had very little free time to leave the military posts and expose themselves to venereal disease. When the war was over, this motivation to carry out intensive training with very little free time no longer existed, so the rate went up; hence, it was concluded that prostitution had really not been suppressed at all. On the other hand, another group maintained that there was a relaxation in the suppression of prostitution following the war.

During the height of this furor, which apparently received considerable publicity in the United States, a Presidential Advisory Commission was established. On the recommendation of this group, the president issued instructions to the secretaries of the army and navy to increase disciplinary efforts to establish venereal disease control councils in all of the military commands at all echelons to attempt to reduce the venereal disease rate. Increased efforts were to be made to suppress prostitution in the overseas areas. Of course, these recommendations were based upon the mores and morals of the United States, not necessarily upon those of the people in the nations throughout the world in which United States troops were stationed at that time.

In the Middle East, for example, we had troops located in friendly nations that, in most cases, were neutrals and were sovereign nations. In the case of Egypt and Palestine, they were nations under the control of the United Kingdom. For commanders of the U.S. forces to attempt to impose on these sovereign governments measures that would require them to suppress prostitution, which, in their eyes, was not only morally but also legally acceptable, simply could not work and did not work. In Moslem countries where polygamy is recognized, if a man wants to divorce one of his wives by the simple expedient of saying, "I divorce thee," three times in the presence of a Sheik, the woman frequently has no means of livelihood except to turn to prostitution in one of the red light areas because females normally do not work outside of their own households. There are no other occupations through which she can earn a living. In all of these countries, legalized prostitution existed. Steps we took to keep our venereal disease rate in those countries at a low level, actually lower than in the United States, were quite different from those which would be acceptable in this country; but they did work.[6]

The situation in the Far East differed from that in the Middle East. We were an occupying power in several areas: the four main islands of Japan; Korea; and the Ryukyu Islands, which had been detached from Japan under the terms of the surrender and were under our direct control. Again, in these three areas, there apparently was not a moral issue involved in the minds of the Japanese, the Koreans, or the Ryukyuans about prostitution. They considered prostitution a necessary part of life to protect the women they intended to marry from exposure to sexual relations prior to marriage. Dating, as we know it, was simply not a part of their way of living. Marriages were arranged; frequently, the couple had not even seen each other prior to the beginning of the arrangements for the marriage. Girls and boys were separated even in classrooms from the fifth grade on, and girls were highly protected from contact with boys outside of their immediate family.

In the rural areas, girls were less an economic asset than boys, who could assist in the farm work. Poor farmers and others frequently sold some of their daughters into prostitution, which was legal. Prostitution was looked upon as a means through which young men might make sexual contacts prior to marriage without exposing the marriageable young women to such dangers and was considered normal and even a desirable part of the social structure.

Colonel Gordon, the first venereal disease control officer on my staff in Japan, made a very thorough study of the situation in Japan and Korea. He found that venereal diseases were considered to be primarily diseases of prostitutes. For this reason, they were not a cause for concern among Japanese physicians, health authorities, or the general public. Japanese physicians, with very few exceptions, were unfamiliar with the epidemiological and clinical manifestations of venereal disease. Control measures were under the jurisdiction of the police and were almost entirely devoted to the periodic examination of the prostitutes. We know this to be practically worthless from a medical standpoint. Clinical measures that were available for the treatment of these infected women were of the pre-sulfonamide days. Contact tracing and case finding were not carried out. Venereal diseases were not even reportable. Prostitution was legal and flourished both in the brothels and, at the time we arrived, also on the streets.

This particular phase of the problem was the result of the war, although we found that prostitution had been carefully controlled and largely limited to the organized brothels. During the war, thousands of young women had been brought into the cities from rural areas to work in the war and other industries. They had been housed in dormitories. At the last stage of the war with the tremendous destruction that had occurred, many of these industries had been destroyed. All war industry production was suspended by direction of the occupation. Many of these girls had lost their families—their families having been killed or dispersed as a result of the bombing attacks on the cities. Because many of them had been school girls before being brought to work in the war industries, they knew no other occupation. There being no longer any war industry, they then turned to prostitution as a means of earning a living. There was, therefore, a major social and economic problem involved in the control of venereal disease in Japan.

There was diverse opinion among the senior military commanders in the occupying forces of Japan. One senior commander felt that the American soldiers who had fought from the Southwest Pacific through the islands to Japan were entitled, as he said, "to enjoy themselves"; in his particular area, the brothel areas were not placed out-of-bounds for some months after the end of the war. Other senior commanders were attempting to carry out the directives received by the Far East commander from Washington, D.C., to suppress prostitution; they had their military police conduct citywide roundups. In the Tokyo-Yokohama area, for example, the military police would round up all women found on the streets after a certain hour in the evening and cart them off to barbed wire enclosures where they were examined. If they were found to be infected, they were then turned over to the Japanese authorities for isolation and treatment. There were some pretty severe repercussions from this attempt to "suppress" prostitution, because even one of the feminine members of the Diet was rounded up in such a sweep while she was on her way home from a late session of a Diet committee. Many Japanese girls who were working in telephone offices and even for the occupation forces were caught in these sweeps. As a result, resentment among the Japanese was very high against the American military authorities.

There was another approach to this problem. As a result of many, many conferences with my counterparts in the medical service and the military forces, we decided to take another approach. General MacArthur felt that we should not try to impose our moral standards and mores upon a nation that held quite different mores and moral standards. On the twenty-first of January 1946, the Japanese were directed to abrogate and annul all laws, ordinances, and other enactments that directly or indirectly authorized or permitted the existence of licensed prostitution in Japan and to nullify all contracts and agreements that had for their object the binding or selling of women into the practice of prostitution. This directive we felt to be quite justified, and the Japanese agreed. Holding human beings in bondage for any purpose could not be reconciled with our attempts to establish the basic premise of democracy, which is worth of the individual in the eyes of the law.

From a health standpoint, these diseases were required to be reported beginning in October 1945. Educational campaigns were begun among the Japanese medical profession as to the diagnosis and modern methods of treatment of these diseases. Within the health center system, venereal disease diagnostic and treatment clinics were established. They were also established in connection with hospitals. At one time, we had some 1,700 modern venereal disease clinics in operation. Adequate quantities of sulfonamides, mepharsin, and bismuth were made available. In addition, a contact-tracing organization was established in connection with each health center. A venereal disease prevention law, originally based on directives and enacted as a law in July 1948, provided for premarital examination for venereal disease as well as prenatal examinations for pregnant women who had come to maternal and child hygiene clinics for examination.

As a result of these steps, 175 cases per 100,000 population had been diagnosed during the first year. As the program improved in scope and the professional capabilities of the Japanese physicians improved, this rate increased to 271 and 273 in 1947 and 1948, respectively.[7]

By 1950, we had sufficient penicillin available so that we could recommend that all cases of early syphilis be treated with penicillin, rather than with the older and longer treatment methods with arsenicals and bismuth. As could be expected, there was a very great drop in the venereal disease rate after 1950, because of the more effective means of treatment available with antibiotics, which reduced the reservoir of infected cases who could spread the disease. As penicillin became available in sufficient quantities to be used in the treatment of many other diseases, including the pneumonias and other infections, the same phenomenon was observed in Japan that Tommy Turner, the venereal disease consultant of the Surgeon General of the Army, told me was occurring in the United States, during one of his visits as a consultant: There was a coincidental prophylactic action taking place in that people were taking penicillin for common colds and all sorts of things and, incidentally, giving themselves a prophylaxis that served to prevent the occurrence of venereal disease when they were exposed.

As time went on, the clinics that we had established for the diagnosis and treatment of venereal disease were not all needed. Certain factors, other than medical, entered into the picture. Particularly in small villages where the people normally do not move a great deal except by foot or by bicycle, the opportunity for exposure to venereal disease is very limited, and the opportunity for spread is limited to a few contacts. In many of these areas the venereal disease rate was so low, nonexistent in many areas, that we could close certain of these clinics in such areas and concentrate our efforts in the large cities, particularly in areas where military forces were located; it was in these areas that the greatest number of infected girls was to be found.

In working on the venereal disease problem in many nations, I found that we sometimes have an erroneous idea of the incidence of venereal disease among foreign people. When we go into these areas, such as Japan or Far Eastern countries, our soldiers usually contract venereal disease for the reasons I have mentioned: Prostitutes are the only female contacts they have. The fact that the prostitutes are highly infected does not necessarily mean that the entire population has a high rate of venereal disease.

In Korea, a unique situation developed, which again involved many social problems. Korean women as a matter of national pride apparently had refrained from social and sexual contacts with their occupiers during the forty years of Japanese occupation. When the American soldiers moved into Korea in the fall of 1945, the Korean girls would have nothing to do with them. In fact, the first girls who were seen in the company of American soldiers were stoned by the Korean people, who had protected their women from sexual contact with the Japanese for so many years. Consequently, the venereal disease rate in the XXIV Corps was much lower than even that in the United States. Tommy Turner came to find out what the commander of the XXIV Corps was doing to have such a low rate when other troops in the Far East and other parts of the world were having skyrocketing venereal disease rates. The simple fact is that, at that time, the American soldiers in Korea were not being exposed to an infected population or to that segment of a population, that is, prostitutes, which is usually highly infected.

Time passed. With the usual gifts of candy and other things, the initial resistance of Korean women to association with foreign soldiers was broken down. A comparatively small segment of the Korean population then became highly infected, as far as venereal disease is concerned, by the American soldiers and, in turn, passed the infection on to other soldiers. It does not take long. The venereal disease rate in the XXIV Corps after a year soon reached that equal to the troops stationed in other areas. I might mention that during the Korean War, the women who had been in association with American soldiers from 1945 to 1948 and who were highly infected soon established contact with American soldiers who, this time, instead of being limited to occupation of a few principal areas, were dispersed all over the nation. Venereal disease, which had been limited to a small segment of the population of Korea, became widespread.

There are two sides to this question of venereal disease control. From the military medical standpoint, we try to protect our soldiers from acquiring infections in foreign lands. On the other hand, people of foreign lands sometimes need to be protected from our soldiers, as far as the venereal diseases are concerned.

The control of venereal disease, particularly in foreign countries, must be adapted to the moral and cultural mores of those countries. Methods that are acceptable in our own country are not necessarily acceptable in other countries, and we can go far astray in our attempts to impose on others our moral concepts. Conversely, we can frequently learn from other people.

I am not sure that our method is necessarily the best; it seems to be the method we prefer. As long as we do not impose it on others, I cannot quarrel with what I consider to be a comparatively ineffective means of controlling venereal disease in a large population. Venereal disease control involves social, economic, and moral factors and is not a simple medical problem.

Tuberculosis

Tuberculosis was the number one killer in Japan in 1945; it had been the leading cause of death in Japan since 1932.[8] While the death rate from tuberculosis had decreased in other countries, particularly western countries, there had been a steady increase in Japan until the beginning of the occupation in 1945, when the death rate reached 282 deaths per 100,000 population. Actually, the number of Japanese who died from tuberculosis among the civilian population that year was greater than the number who died from all of the bombing, the fire raids, and the two atomic bombs.

There are many reasons for the high incidence of tuberculosis and the high death rate. Overcrowding was a factor. In overcrowded areas, in the tenement areas of cities, regardless of where they are, a high rate of tuberculosis is prevalent. In an environment in which only one or two people normally sleep in a room, if one acquires a clinical case of tuberculosis, during his coughing spells, particularly at night, he may spray into the room little droplets which include tubercle bacilli. These may be inhaled by his companion and, in due course, that individual may develop a clinical case of tuberculosis. In a country such as Japan in which many people, from ten to twelve, would lie in rows on *tatami* in a single room that was closed up tight for warmth, one clinical case of tuberculosis could infect all ten or twelve persons instead of only one.

Nutrition is another factor and a very important element in the incidence of tuberculosis. It was been shown—in fact, this knowledge has been used in the treatment of tuberculosis—that a high protein, high calcium diet will assist in helping the body to wall off tubercle bacilli inhaled into the lungs, thereby helping to prevent the development of a clinical case of tuberculosis. In our nutritional studies, we found that the Japanese had a very low protein, low calcium intake. Therefore, they were particularly susceptible to the development of clinical tuberculosis once an individual acquired the tubercle bacilli.

The combination of circumstances, through the disruption of war and the mass movement of people, should have caused a tremendous increase in the mortality of tuberculosis from 1945 until 1951. Such was not the case. This experience was contrary to the experience in wartorn European countries and in past wars.

At the beginning of the occupation, there were only about 25,000 hospital beds available for the treatment of active cases of tuberculosis.[9] The Japanese estimated that there were approximately 1 million to 2 million clinical cases of tuberculosis among the Japanese population who served as a reservoir for infection of others. In this situation, we could not use the methods used in the United States, because it was an epidemic. We initiated a program to identify and isolate all of these cases and place them under treatment; but to build hospital beds, to train doctors, to make the facilities available was a multi-year program. We had to adopt a method in which we could bring this epidemic quickly under control.

In reviewing the available knowledge on the control of tuberculosis, I had come to the conclusion that there was sufficient evidence in the many reported studies which could be compared to justify the use of a vaccine called BCG: Bacillus Calmette-Guerin vaccine. Shortly after the turn of the century, Calmette and Guerin had attenuated the tubercle bacillus, which causes tuberculosis in cattle (bovine tuberculosis). They reasoned that this attenuated cow tubercle bacillus, if inoculated into humans, might produce sufficient resistance in the human to prevent the development of clinical cases of tuberculosis if they were exposed to a human tubercle bacillus. This assumption was not unreasonable. After all, we have successfully used the virus that causes cowpox to inoculate humans and build up their resistance against the virus that causes smallpox in humans.

Unfortunately, in a controlled series of experiments in Europe, some of the children who had been inoculated with BCG had developed active cases of tuberculosis. I can recall the tremendous reaction among the medical profession in the United States during my medical student days against the use of BCG. The Danes and the Japanese obtained cultures from Calmette and Guerin and continued to work on this problem. The Danes carried out very carefully controlled experiments over a period of years; so did the Japanese from 1927 to 1943. A few people in our own country, such as Dr. Saul Rosenthal in Chicago, had also done experimental work with BCG. Many others had worked with this vaccine, and there was disagreement in the reports of the results.

One of the reasons for this disagreement was that during the course of the experimental work various strengths of old tuberculin were used in testing individuals to see whether they had already acquired a human tubercle bacilli. Obviously, if one strength were used which was comparatively weak, a greater proportion of people would be declared to be tuberculin negative than if a stronger solution were used. Those who were tuberculin negative were the only ones to be immunized, because if a person who already had a tubercle bacillus in his body were immunized, a flare-up was caused.

The vaccine was liquid and had a potency of only about six days. From the time of its preparation until its use, it might have lost considerable potency. It was not surprising to me, therefore, that there were conflicting reports about the degree of success in preventing tuberculosis with the use of BCG.

In going through all of the available literature, I found that in those series of experiments in which comparable strengths of old tuberculin were used to determine who should and should not be immunized, and in which comparable strengths of vaccine were used, then comparable results were found. On the whole, about 88 percent reduction in mortality could be expected from the use of BCG and about 70 percent reduction in the occurrence of clinical cases. Like all vaccines, one hundred percent protection does not occur with the use of BCG. I, therefore, made the decision to reinstitute and expand the program for mass use of BCG in Japan as the most effective tool available in stopping this epidemic.

During the war, the Japanese National Research Council had reviewed their experimental work and had declared that in their opinion BCG was a valuable means of reducing the morbidity and mortality from tuberculosis. They had started an immunization program, but it, like everything else, had collapsed. We reinstituted the program.

We began by immunizing the 20-to-24–year age group, which had the highest mortality: a death rate of 617 deaths per 100,000 population. Then, as vaccine became available in greater quantities, we immunized the 15-to-19–year age group, which had the second highest death rate of 403 deaths per 100,000 population, and continued to extend immunization to infants. It must be remembered that everyone in the various age groups could not be immunized.

Tuberculin testing at that time showed that although only two percent of the infants had already acquired human tubercle bacilli, this increased very rapidly. In the 5-to-9–year age group, 26 percent had become infected. In the 25-to-29–year age group, over 76 percent or three-fourths of the people in the age group were already infected and could not be immunized. There were 54,800,000 people in Japan under the age of thirty. A study of this group, by five-year age groups, indicated that 25,500,000, or about 46 percent of those under age thirty, had already acquired a human tubercle infection and, therefore, could not be protected with BCG.

Because of the short life of this vaccine, BCG was produced in some eleven different laboratories. We found difficulty in production and assay control in producing such tremendous quantities of the vaccine. Children were retested with tuberculin at the end of a year, and if they had become negative again they were reimmunized. In studying these reconversions among the children, we found a great variation in the various areas which were supplied with vaccine from different laboratories.

I suspended all immunization programs, including BCG. We established a program of producing a lyophilized or dried vaccine, which had been developed by Dr. Okada and Dr. Hiyashi. This dried vaccine could retain its potency, and

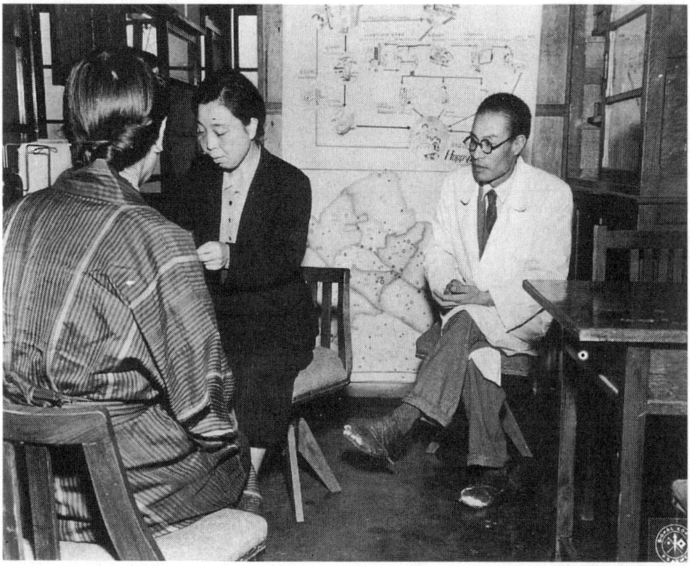

Figure 17. Tuberculosis exemplified the challenges of integrating preventive medicine, medical care, welfare, and social security. Here, a social worker at the Suginami Health Center interviews a woman with tuberculosis as Dr. Tsukahara Kunio, Director of the Health Center, observes. The Division of Medical Social Service acted as a link between the preventive medicine functions of a given health center and the welfare and social security organizations within a given district. The Suginami Health Center was the model for health centers throughout Japan. Tokyo, 4 October 1948. Photo Credit: U.S. Army Signal Corps, Photographer Sarabia. (Courtesy of the Hoover Institution Archives, Stanford University.)

we could distribute it and use it in spite of the limited transportation facilities, which made it most difficult to distribute the liquid vaccine before it became outdated. We were also able to assay this vaccine under very rigid standards to test its potency, sterility, and so forth, before it was distributed, something which could not be done with the short-lived liquid vaccine.

We reinstituted the program in 1949. We immunized 30 million people under the age of thirty with BCG. It takes time, as it did in the smallpox immunization programs and others, to carry out such a tremendous number of immunizations. Among the immunized age groups, we had drastic reductions in mortality and morbidity. As a result of our program of immunization, tuberculosis is no longer the number one killer in Japan.[10]

At the same time, through our health center program, we started the diagnosis of clinical cases with the usual chest X-rays using a small film. Suspicious films were checked with large X-rays. Those who showed evidence of clinical tuberculosis by X-ray among the positive tuberculin reactions were given physical examinations, sedimentation tests, and sputum examinations. Later on when we were able to obtain streptomycin and paraminosalicylic acid, we started a treatment program for those cases uncovered in the case-finding program.

Streptomycin was first imported into Japan in 1949. Then we began a program of production. We needed about 50 million grams of streptomycin per year for the treatment program of those already infected. It was only after this program was inaugurated that the death rate among those who had already been infected but had not been immunized began to drop.

A combination of treatment and prevention is the ideal method of controlling any disease. We can reduce mortality through the use of modern drugs; but, to me, treatment is a poor substitute for prevention.

11

The Veterinarians

Of what interest are veterinary affairs to the health of humans? In many countries, no consideration is given to the relationship of animal diseases to human diseases or to diseases that may be carried from animals to humans or to the health hazard of meat and milk products, which may become contaminated during processing and distribution. There are many individuals who consider the veterinary service as basically of concern only to the Department of Agriculture. Veterinarians are considered essential in controlling diseases of animals, particularly domestic animals, not because of any concern for the health of humans, but because animal diseases represent a hazard to the livestock industry through the loss of animals which might otherwise be sold.

My own experience causes me to disagree with such a philosophy. The diseases of man are the result of his reaction to his environment: whether he breaks his leg in an automobile accident because he had left home in a frustrated rage following a quarrel with his wife; or develops a peptic ulcer because of stress and tension in his work; or develops atherosclerosis with resultant coronary or cerebral thrombosis because of metabolic changes following prolonged stress or faulty nutrition; or develops cancer of the lung from smog and cigarettes; or acquires typhus or encephalitis. These as all other identifiable human ailments are the result of his being part of a given environment. The incidence and distribution of various diseases are modified not only by geographic environmental differences but also by the passage of time and the change in the pattern of living within a given geographic area.

Man is not alone as a living organism in his environment: The plants, viruses, rickettsia, bacteria, parasites, insects, birds, and animals, both domestic and wild, inhabit the same environment. As research expands our knowledge of medicine, we are learning that birds and animals constitute the reservoir from which many human diseases are acquired: yellow fever; malaria; typhus, encephalitis; and others. These human diseases can only be eradicated if man is protected from the bird or animal reservoir from which the diseases are transmitted directly or, more usually, by vectors. Therefore, to me, the activities of veterinarians as members of the health team far outweigh their importance to the economy of agriculture.

Prior to World War I, the U.S. Army veterinary service had been a part of the Quartermaster Corps. It was incorporated into the army medical department because our military medical personnel then felt that veterinarians were not only essential in the care of the many horses and mules, which were the principle means of transport of our military forces prior to World War II, but also had a place in the inspection of food being procured by the army and distributed to our soldiers. Thus, I established a Veterinary Division in my office, initially headed by Col. Oness Dixon, followed by Colonel Scawthorne and then Dr. Beechwood.[1] Their corps of veterinarians, who were subsequently assigned to the various prefectural teams, deserve credit for the inauguration and supervision of the veterinary affairs program in Japan.

The Health Veterinarian

The idea of a health veterinarian was entirely new to the Japanese. The veterinary service in Japan was principally under the control of the Ministry of Forestry and Agriculture, based upon the concept that veterinarians were primarily of concern to the livestock industry, which was very limited in Japan. Their role in connection with human health was not considered: the relationship between diseases of animals and diseases of humans; or the importance of controlling from a health standpoint the processing of meat, milk, and other animal products for human consumption.

During our reorganization and establishment of a nationwide governmental health organization, after many conferences with the Ministry of Forestry and Agriculture and the Ministry of Health and Welfare, the concept was finally agreed upon that the Ministry of Health and Welfare had, or should have, a definite interest in the control of animal diseases as they relate to humans. The Ministry of Health and Welfare was given primary interest in supervising the processing and distribution of products of animal origin, including seafood, for human consumption. A veterinary affairs department was established in the Ministry of Health and Welfare to carry out these functions.

The first task, of course, after the initial surveys of the professional qualifications of the veterinarians and surveys of the domestic livestock industry, which was badly depleted, was to improve the educational qualifications of the veterinarians, following a pattern similar to that which was carried out in the case of medical, dental, nursing, and pharmaceutical personnel. We had to inaugurate training courses at the Institute of Public Health for veterinarians serving not only in the health centers but also in the slaughtering and meat-processing plants and in the inspection of dairy farms and milk-processing plants.[2] In our establishment of health centers, we required the assignment of veterinarians for the control of the animal diseases that might be transmitted to humans, such as rabies from dogs, and for inspection of all processing and retail distribution outlets for milk and for meat and seafood products.[3]

A program paralleling that of the human biologics program, with very rigid standards of assay, was established for the production of biologics for the prevention of animal diseases. Such diseases were not limited to those which might have a direct bearing on humans but included those which would, from an economic standpoint, cause losses among the animal population. Horses that were bred in Hokkaido and shipped to Honshu would acquire B encephalitis. Many of these animals died; however, through the use of encephalitis vaccine, this economic loss was very greatly reduced.

Veterinary health centers for the care of domestic animals were also established throughout Japan. At the end for the occupation, 516 such centers were in operation, in addition to the Veterinary Divisions of the health centers concerned with the food inspection and animal diseases control as it affected people.

The Era of New Sanitation

At the time of World War II, the transportation of the Japanese army was primarily animal-drawn. A large proportion of the veterinarians were, therefore, engaged in military forces and in the government-operated breeding stations for the increased production of horses. So far as we could determine, there was no service in the Japanese army to inspect food products of animal origin during processing or distribution to the Japanese army. The Japanese army had procured and stored very sizable stocks of canned meat for distribution to the army, but, on the whole, meat consumption in Japan was very limited. As for the animals which were slaughtered for human consumption, the draft cattle, small cows which were used for work and gave a very small milk production, served as a source of beef when the animals became injured or too old to work.

Horses were the principal sources of meat products. At the beginning of the occupation, the slaughter of horses far exceeded that of cattle. Very few hogs were slaughtered. It had been the custom to import cattle from Korea and hogs from the Ryukyu Islands, in addition to the domestic cows and horses.

As we improved the sanitary standards, not only in the slaughtering plants but also in the handling of seafood, various plants including retail distribution plants, which adopted satisfactory standards of refrigeration, handling, and storage of these products, were opened to purchase of meat products and seafood for the military forces and for the families of occupation personnel. By 1949, as a result of the incentive of increased earnings given for meeting our high standards, either in the slaughtering and wholesale distribution or in retail distribution, the competition became very keen. Throughout the metropolitan areas, such as Tokyo, Osaka, Nagoya, and other areas where troops and their dependents lived, white tile-fronted meat and fish shops were built with refrigeration and glass cases to protect the meat and seafood from flies, which had formerly covered the unrefrigerated meat and fish in these shops before the era of new sanitation, as it was called, in Japan.

Seafood Inspection

Japan has one of the largest, if not the largest, seafood-handling ports in the world. So far as distribution of seafood products within Japan was concerned, a great deal of dried fish was distributed to the rural areas owing to limited refrigeration; most of the fresh seafood was consumed in the urban areas through local channels and distribution markets because of the spoilage problem. It had also been the custom to export frozen tuna to the United States, where it was processed and canned by American canneries.

Initially, all Japanese sources of food had been off limits to military and occupation personnel because of the low sanitary standards and also because it was the policy of our military forces not to subsist off of the country, which itself, early in the occupation, was very short of food.[4] As the food situation improved in Japan, and through many conferences with our economics people, it was finally agreed that it would be desirable to increase the dollar-earning capacity of the Japanese by procuring fresh seafood and meat from the Japanese, thereby reducing the drain on American taxpayer dollars in GARIOA appropriations for support of the Japanese economy.

Inspection services for the processing of fresh-frozen and canned seafood were subsequently established. As the occupation neared the end and the re-establishment of the export program, particularly of seafood, began to expand, very fine cooperation was received from the seafood processors. Modern methods of handling seafood at the unloading piers and during the entire processing, whether through freezing or canning, made it possible to assure the chief-of-staff that this product met as high a standard as could be procured anywhere in the world.

Human Nutrition and Animal Husbandry

In Hokkaido and in Chiba Prefecture, there were a considerable number of one- or two-cow dairy farms. Some larger farms in Hokkaido were stocked with Holstein cattle, which had been imported years before in an attempt to establish a dairy industry in Japan. Dairy companies processed milk into sweet and condensed milk, which was exported from Japan to the Philippines and other Asiatic countries. Milk consumption by Japanese children was almost nil.

One of our programs in the nutrition field was to increase the protein component of the Japanese diet through the school lunch program. Powdered skim milk was the best source of protein that could be used. We attempted, by working with the Japanese dairy industry and the representatives from the International Dairy Society, whom we invited to the United States, to increase the production of dairy products, specifically powdered skim milk, which could be distributed throughout Japan, in spite of the lack of local refrigeration, without creating a health hazard.

One of the studies in which our veterinary people were directly concerned was the domestic livestock industry in Japan. We attempted to estimate the capacity of the nation to support a domestic livestock industry, which could provide adequate protein for the people without resorting to importation of these products at the expense of foreign exchange in later years. We estimated that some 18 million domestic livestock could be sustained in Japan. The question, of course, was, What type of animal would be most suitable for this mountainous country, the mountains being very heavily vegetated? Sheep and goats were felt to be preferable for increasing the domestic cattle to meet the requirements for increased meat sources. Breeding stock to increase the herds of both dairy cattle and goats were imported from the United States, principally under the Friends Service Program. Artificial insemination was used because of the difficulty of breeding. Animal husbandry in Japan did not embrace the concept of a herd of domestic livestock; rather, it was the case of the individual farmer having perhaps a domestic work cow or a horse or a goat. This animal was highly prized and was stabled adjacent to the house and was tethered for grazing.

I attempted many times to obtain experts in animal husbandry from the United States to introduce to the Japanese the management of herds of domestic animals. It will take many years before Japan can reorient its agricultural economy from one of a grain economy to a combination of grain crops and domestic livestock, which should go a long way forward in making available to the Japanese an adequate balance in diet which will improve the health of their people.

The Canine Population

The canine population had been badly depleted through the war, because there was such limited food: The Japanese policy was to destroy the dogs, because there was insufficient food to share with them. After the war, there was a phenomenal increase in the population of canines. Rabies became a major problem in the Kanto Plain area, so emphasis was placed on the control of homeless dogs. A Society for the Prevention of Cruelty to Animals was established, with the occurrence of one of the interesting incidents in programs of the magnitude of ours.

Two ladies who were wives of occupation personnel, but from different nations, became interested in the dog situation. They repeatedly besieged my office because we had the Japanese rounding up stray dogs, which were impounded and, if unclaimed, later destroyed. These dogs were held under observation for rabies, and many of them were found to be rabid. The transmission of rabies had become a serious problem as a result of deaths of children and adults who were bitten by these rabid dogs; however, the two ladies chose to disregard this aspect. On many occasions, they went to the pound and turned the dogs loose. By virtue of the fact that they were wives of occupation personnel, the Japanese officials felt that they could not resist the demands of these ladies. It took considerable, delicate diplomatic maneuvering to work through the husbands of the ladies involved to attempt to get them to cease and desist from their interference in this particular program.

Another aspect of the problem was in the rapid turnover of the occupation personnel and their families. After 1946, when the families were first admitted to Japan, the inevitable family pet was acquired in Japan. Unfortunately, frequently upon departure of the family, this pet was abandoned to roam not only the occupation housing areas but also the adjacent areas. These dogs were rounded up by the military police in occupation housing areas and turned over to the Japanese dog pounds. The ladies felt this was cruel, so they established a home for homeless dogs. They would obtain many dogs from the pound, which, in turn, were made available as pets to newly arriving occupation families. This home served a useful purpose: It facilitated the procurement of pets by the occupation families. Eventually, through our cooperative efforts, we were able to persuade many people to return these pets to this home upon the departure of the families to the United States on completion of their tour. This program ended what I considered the cruelty of abandoning a pet who had been well cared for in a home but later became a health menace in that he might acquire rabies in his wanderings in search of food.

12

Medicine and Dentistry

The quality of medical care furnished to the Japanese people was an important element of the overall health program. It did little good, so far as the preventive medicine program was concerned, to uncover cases of disease unless there were adequate medical means available to provide care and treatment for people who are already ill.

The Medical Care System

Because the medical care system of Japan was so different from that to which we were accustomed in our country, it was necessary to consider not only the number of doctors and nurses and other paramedical groups available, but also their qualifications.—I have long ago learned that "M.D." after a name does not necessarily mean the holder of that title is trained or has the knowledge that we might consider as the minimum necessary for a Doctor of Medicine.—The same applies to the fields of dentistry, nursing, and pharmacy. In going into any strange country, it is necessary to evaluate the professional education programs in those fields in order to determine the quality of medical care.

Another aspect of medical care in any country is the method by which professional services are made available to the people. It is essential to know the system of practice of medical care—which profession does what—because the division of responsibilities among the various professions engaged in the health care field characteristic of the United States does not necessarily hold in other countries. Also, in many countries, the private practice of medicine, as we know it, does not exist. There are many systems of the practice of medicine.

The Medical Schools

Prior to the war, there were eighteen university-level medical schools with fairly high standards. Seven were associated with the imperial universities at Tokyo, Kyoto, Hokkaido, Sakai, Nagoya, Tohoku, and Kyushu. Six were operated by the national government but were not of the imperial university rank or caliber; although they were first class schools, their faculty and students were looked down upon slightly by faculty and students of the imperial university medical schools. There were four privately operated medical schools: Keio University; Jikkei-Kai Medical College; Nippon Medical College; and Nippon University.

To qualify for admission to one of these university medical schools, a student had to complete six years of primary or grade school and three years in a preparatory school that would be equivalent to our high school. There was a four-year medical course; the first two years in basic science, the latter two in didactic work in clinical medicine. A license to practice medicine was automatic upon completion of the course: No qualifying examination was necessary. Such an educational system was similar to that found in the United States prior to 1910, in which graduates of high schools could enter medical school and upon completion of a more or less didactic course were qualified, following a state examination, to practice medicine.[1]

The Japanese, looking to the German system as the leader in many fields, including medicine, had followed the didactic system of teaching in medical education for many years before the war. Laboratory and clinical methods of teaching, familiar to us in the United States, were neglected. The medical professors often refused to participate in undergraduate teaching, lest they lose face, and preferred to confine their activities to a select group of proteges who were graduate students attempting to qualify for the degree of Doctor of Science in Medicine.

In 1945 and before, Japan had possessed an adequate number of doctors; however, approximately 48,000 of the 77,000 Japanese doctors were graduates of second class medical schools, known as *Semmon Gakko*. These institutions had limited clinical and educational facilities and, in many cases, were not affiliated with a hospital for clinical teaching. The graduates were poorly prepared to practice medicine. The second-rate schools accepted students who were graduates of middle school (high school). After four years of medical school, the graduates were authorized to practice medicine.

There were ten such schools in operation in Japan prior to 1938; by 1945, there were fifty-one. Nineteen were operated by the national government and were attached to national universities; nineteen were operated by prefectural or municipal governments; thirteen were private. At Tokyo Imperial University, for example, we found an interesting phenomenon: There was a first class medical school training one type of doctor and a second class school training second class doctors.

There were many reasons behind this attempt to provide a large number of doctors by lowering the standards for training for most of the doctors. Practically all of the graduates of the university medical schools joined the staff of a hospital; so most first class doctors were to be found in the large hospitals in the cities and metropolitan areas. To meet the need for doctors in the rural areas, it was felt that a cheaper medical education and a shorter one, one with lower standards, could produce doctors in sufficient numbers who could be induced to locate in rural areas. There were, in effect, two types of medical care: first class for the urban people; second class for the rural people.

To me, at least, people being human beings are entitled to the best quality of medical care which can be made available when they become ill or injured. I cannot go along with the philosophy that, because of place of residence or other factors over which people have no control, they are second class citizens and, therefore, should accept a second class quality of medical care in comparison to first-class care acceptable to the people of that country.

Organization of Medical Care

The practice of medicine in Japan is quite different from that in our own country. For instance, the hospital staffs in Japan are full-time staffs. As a group, they practice medicine in the large out-patient clinics which are a structural part of all hospitals. The in-patients for a particular hospital come from the out-patients being served by the staff of the hospital. This particular system has many advantages and some disadvantages. The director of the hospital is a doctor and is responsible for not only the operation of the hospital but also the professional quality of medicine practiced in his hospital, in both the out-patient clinics and in the in-patient departments. Although specialty boards as we have in our country did not exist in Japan, the staff and other specialists form a group clinic—something which we began to use in our country about twenty years ago. The Japanese have used it for some seventy years. The basic difference is that, in the United States, the group clinic is usually quite independent of a hospital staff: Although members of the group clinic may all take their patients to the same hospital, they do not practice medicine as a hospital staff.

The second class doctors felt that they must have some means of earning a living, because they could not admit their patients to the hospitals which were already staffed with full-time salaried members. Under the old Japanese law, they could establish what were called hospitals with fewer than ten beds. These usually consisted simply of one or two rooms with *tatami* on the floor. The doctor made his living partially by keeping his patients who required hospitalization in his rooms; he made some income from the board and room which he charged them. Unfortunately, in many cases, he undertook surgical and other procedures for which he lacked both competence and equipment; many of these patients died.

I visited the clinics and so-called hospitals with fewer than ten beds and observed the quality of the work; it was not a good system. I have resisted attempts to condone such a system of what I consider malpractice.

Economic Incentives

A further method of evaluating the quality of medical care was to analyze the drugs being used by the doctors, particularly the second class doctors. The great majority of the prescriptions which were filled and sold by doctors were made up of baking soda, either in powder, tablet, or liquid form. Under the system of fees which the Japanese doctors was required to accept, it was the custom to receive fifty yen for an office call in 1945. This fee was a very small sum of money, but was, presumably, the fee for the doctor's medical knowledge and his ability to examine and diagnose the patient. The doctor received one hundred fifty yen for a three-day supply of medicine, which it was customary for him to sell to a patient, as the patients felt that they were not properly treated unless they had carried away a supply of medicine. The doctors normally did not write a prescription. The doctor, or his wife, or his children, or some relative compounded the prescription and sold it.

Our analysis indicated that the drugs and containers of this three-day supply of medicine cost about nineteen yen. In effect, the economic incentives to the second class doctor were not to improve his medical knowledge and not to improve the quality of medical care. He was not being paid for that as much as selling as much medicine as possible to the greatest number of patients and to inducing as many patients as possible to board in his hospital. With such economic incentives, the graduate of a second class school made little effort through reading professional journals or by going to any sort of medical scientific meeting to improve his medical knowledge throughout the years.

He was also deprived of the opportunity for professional improvement through the exchange of ideas and association with the better qualified doctors by virtue of the fact that he could not admit private patients to any hospital. As an experiment, I tried to open certain hospitals for the admission of patients by doctors who were not on the full-time staff, but this policy did not work. The custom, which had been in existence too long, could not be changed. Such a change was not acceptable. Consequently, the separation of medicine and pharmacy, in an attempt to improve the quality of medical care by giving an economic incentive to the doctors to improve their medical knowledge, rather than to sell drugs, became a major political battle. It was solved only shortly before the end of the occupation.[2]

Reforming Medical Education

Having studied and evaluated the medical care system in Japan, I was then faced with the problem of what to do about it, if it were to be improved. The first point of attack was obviously the system of professional education. From our experience in the United States, I had a method of approach which might work.[3]

From 1910 to 1920, our medical education system in the United States underwent a major reform. Our schools, like the Japanese schools, were of several categories, so far as the quality of the graduates was concerned. A Council on Medical Education was established by the American Medical Association. Our schools were surveyed and classified into three types. Through improving licensing requirements by statutes and other means, our medical schools had been brought up to what might be called the first-class standard of teaching.

I did not have ten years to accomplish such a gradual evolution in Japan; but knowing the pattern, which I thought would work, I established a Council on Medical Education. There was a group of about sixty doctors in Japan who had been trained in European and American medical schools and who were the more highly trained professional men. After many consultations, I selected a group for the Council on Medical Education, which was established under the auspices of the PHW Section, and later was legalized as an Advisory Council to the Minister of Education.[4] This council was headed by a very courageous Japanese doctor, Dr. Kusama Yoshio, who I hope will become known as the father of the new era of medical education in Japan.

I indoctrinated this group in the principles of first-class medical education for all medical students. A curriculum was devised giving emphasis to proper allocation of the hours between what we call basic science and clinical subjects. A set of standards was formulated to be used for classifying the existing medical schools. The Minister of Education, the Minister of Health and Welfare, SCAP's Civil Information and Education Section, as well the PHW Section participated in many discussions and finally agreed on a method to revise the system of medical education.

All of the schools were inspected. Those schools that had adequate equipment, laboratory facilities, and hospital affiliations, so that clinical teaching could be carried out properly, as well as a faculty of high standards who, with proper guidance, could carry out the new curriculum, were rated as class A schools. Schools that through the acquisition of additional faculty or through construction could, within a period of several years, provide sufficient laboratory space adequately to teach, through laboratory methods and demonstrations, those subjects that require such procedures were placed on probation; they were designated as class B schools. Certain schools which, either because of location, physical plant limitations, or limitations on faculty, could not hope even in the future to meet the new requirements were closed.

Because it took some time to actually implement such a program, this transition, which began in 1947, had to be a gradual process, otherwise the medical education system would have become completely chaotic. It was agreed, for instance, that as a transitional step freshmen should have two years of university training instead of three before they were eligible for medical school. Those schools on probation were permitted to continue the classes which they already had in the sophomore, junior, and senior years, but were not permitted to accept new freshmen classes until they had succeeded in reaching class A status. Thus, by 1951, the number of medical schools was reduced to forty-five class A schools, which were producing only first class doctors. They were producing a sufficient number of graduates to achieve a ratio of one doctor for every one thousand population.

Medical Licensure

A national licensing law was placed in effect, which is a tool used for regulating professional educational standards. This law required medical graduates to be graduates of class A schools before they could take the national examination, which would be required for a license to practice medicine. The license would permit a qualified doctor to practice medicine in any of the forty-six prefectures. When this examination was first held, only about forty percent qualified; by 1952, the percentage had risen to over ninety-two percent.

The benefits of this long-range program should become apparent in improved quality of medical care over a period of fifteen or twenty years. The 48,000 second class doctors were permitted to continue their practice under a grandfather clause. In the next fifteen or twenty years, most of them will have retired from practice. Eventually, there will be only first class doctors and first class medical service for the people.

Two of my staff deserve great credit for this major reform in medical education: Maj. Sylvan E. Moolten, who was first a laboratory officer and who became interested in this problem, helped in the initiation and establishment of the Council on Medical Education. Col. Harry Johnson, chief of the Medical Affairs Division, carried the work to its completion. I consider this program one of the major long-range accomplishments of the occupation.

Internships

Because the study of medicine had, in previous years, been so didactic, I thought it might be desirable to institute an internship system in Japanese hospitals. In 1948, we established an internship system for the first time in Japan. A one-year internship was required after graduation before a medical student could become eligible to take the national licensing examination. I am not sure this was a wise decision, even at this late date, as many Japanese doctors pointed out they, in fact, had an internship system in that practically all of the graduates of class A schools joined a hospital staff as junior members and, therefore, were under the supervision of older doctors on the staff.[5] On the other hand, there were still many thousands of doctors who, even under the revised system, had to be encouraged to enter the private practice of medicine, particularly in rural areas. Unless they had some period of training under supervision in which they applied the knowledge that they had received during their medical education, I felt that we would not accomplish the aim of having a high standard of medical care throughout the country.

Because this idea was new to the Japanese, it is not too surprising that, for the first several years, the staff of a hospital devoted very little time to teaching the young interns and supervising their practice. I was most disappointed that there was a lack of such training afforded these young men. Most of them took the year to study very hard for their national licensing examination. As time passed, the idea began to be accepted by the senior members of the hospital staffs that these interns would not all remain on their staffs but some would go into private practice. They, therefore, had an obligation to supervise and give additional on-the-job training to the entire group. I believe that the situation has improved. Only because I felt that the man who would not remain on a hospital staff needed this additional training did I feel justified that the establishment of intern training was beneficial.

The PHW Section attempted to interest the U.S. military medical service in accepting a limited number of selected Japanese graduates to serve their internship under American supervision in our military hospitals. This program was agreed to, and twenty-four young Japanese doctors were admitted as interns in eleven American military hospitals. There they could see firsthand what we had been trying to teach about modern hospital care and medical service. This program was subsequently expanded; fifty-four Japanese doctors assisted as interns in the American military hospitals to the mutual advantage of the U.S. military medical service and the Japanese medical care program.

The Medical Examiner System

At the beginning of the occupation, there was no law in Japan that required an autopsy to determine the cause of death in the case of death from violence or among individuals who were unattended by a physician or who had a questionable diagnosis. Likewise, it was illegal to use cadavers for teaching anatomy. This situation was equivalent to that in the United States not too many years ago.

I do not know how anyone can teach anatomy or learn anatomy without actually having the opportunity to conduct dissection and study a body and its organs. Likewise, when causes of death are not known, it is certainly desirable to attempt to find out the cause by autopsy, if for no other reason than to improve medical knowledge for the future.

Consequently, we established a nationwide medical examiner system to conduct autopsies in November 1945; in December 1946, a directive was issued requiring the establishment of a nationwide system, which was later incorporated in law. This system also applied to the use of cadavers for teaching anatomy, in the case of unidentified, unclaimed bodies.

The Teaching Missions

Early in 1950, after revisiting many of the medical schools and observing the progress being made in the revision of the curriculum, I was somewhat concerned about the quality and methods of instruction, despite the proper allocation of hours between basic and clinical work and between didactic and laboratory work. Teaching methods such as clinical pathological conferences were unknown to the Japanese. Through the Unitarian Service Committee, a group representing faculties from various medical schools in the United States came to Japan and held two institutes in 1950: one in Tokyo for the faculties of the medical schools of northern Honshu and Hokkaido; one in Osaka for the faculties of schools in southern Honshu, Kyushu, and Shikoku. For example, an American professor of pediatrics would not only go over with the Japanese professors of pediatrics the subject matter which was being taught in modern pediatric medicine, but also demonstrate to the Japanese faculty how the many subjects were taught. When I first proposed these institutes, many of the Japanese professors were doubtful about whether they would be of value. After the institutes were completed, they became quite enthusiastic.

In 1951, a second group of professors from the leading medical schools in America was brought to Japan for a two-month period. This time they did not conduct institutes but visited the Japanese medical schools to evaluate the teaching problems of the particular schools and to assist and advise the professors concerning their particular problems. The work of these two missions, obtained through the Unitarian Service Committee, was most valuable in completing the reformation of medical education in Japan.

The Question of Training Specialists

Throughout the occupation, many visiting groups suggested that we institute a postgraduate training system and specialty board certification system, such as we had evolved in the United States. For two reasons, I did not institute a graduate training system for the development of specialists and board certification in Japan.

First, I was unsure that we were entirely sound in our own country. At the time, we had reached a peak in which every young medical student was sure that he had to take three-to-five years of additional residency training leading to specialty qualification and board certification. In other words, practically all medical students were aiming to become specialists. I was quite sure that this would not lead to a good system of practice of medicine in the United States. It must be clearly understood that we do need to develop qualified specialists in many fields of medical knowledge in any country which is to attain a high quality of medical care; however, there must be balance between the number of specialists and the number of first-rate doctors who are looking after the whole patient and not just a part of the patient.

From about 1946 to 1953, there was considerable controversy and ill feeling within the medical profession in the United States and between the medical profession and patients, because the pendulum had swung too far. Many patients complained that no doctor was looking after them as a patient and that they frequently had to make the rounds of half a dozen specialists before they could find out what was wrong with them.

We had the same problem in the military medical service. We had difficulty attaining a balance among the specialists which we required in the numerous fields. Sometimes we had too many surgeons and not enough pediatricians; sometimes not enough anesthesiologists and too many obstetricians. It was very difficult to administer a medical service under such a situation and provide a high quality medical service. With every doctor trying to be a specialist, the nursing profession took over, by necessity, much of the total patient care, which properly belongs within the practice of medicine.

Recognizing how the trend was building up in the United States, and feeling the impact in our military medical service, I was not sure in 1945 and 1946 that we were on the right track; therefore, I did not feel that we should adopt the extreme position of trying to train every Japanese doctor as a specialist until we could foresee a method by which some balance could be attained through economic or other incentives between the specialists and the well-qualified general practitioner, who should and does handle about eighty-five percent of the medical care in any civilian community, if it is of high quality.[6]

The second reason I did not adopt such a system was because I felt that the medical reforms, which we had compressed into a very few years, and which corresponded to those that had evolved over a period of at least ten years in our country, were a severe enough shock. If I had achieved the goal of producing first class doctors in the short time available, that in itself, if I could be sure of the result, was a sufficient accomplishment in that field at the time. If it became desirable to institute graduate training leading to specialty qualification and specialty boards, this could be done later; but it should not be done until first class doctors were the foundation for such a system. I was not too popular with some of my American medical colleagues for a number of years because of my views.

The Japan Medical Association

So far as we could determine in 1945, the Japan Medical Association, like the dental and nursing associations, was a national organization for the control of the profession. It established fees in connection with the insurance system. Its officers were appointed by the government.

According to my philosophy, a professional organization has one basic reason to exist: to promote the exchange of professional knowledge, which the individuals making up that profession hold and which identifies them as a profession; and to attempt to continually raise the professional qualifications of its members. Such a philosophy does not mean that the society will not be concerned with economic and other programs which may arise between that body and some other group or between the profession and the government or lay public; but its basic purpose is one of promoting medical ethics and improving the quality of professional knowledge and standards. It took quite a while to sell such philosophy to the Japanese professional groups. In the case of the Japan Medical Association, with the assistance of a group of consultants from the American Medical Association, this task was finally accomplished.

By March 1948, the first national election of officers was held for the newly reorganized Japan Medical Association (JMA). For the first time, a scientific assembly was incorporated into its activities, which finally took over with legitimate interest the medical education council which I had established.[7] In January 1947, the JMA began publishing a monthly journal for the first time in its history. We also received permission from the American Medical Association for the monthly publication of a Japanese translation of the *Journal of the American Medical Association*, the first issue appearing in August 1948.[8]

Professional Publications

The initiation of a profession-wide journal containing scientific articles was important because there was a rare rigid compartmentalization within the educational system of Japan.—A young man could go through the university and complete his medical education there. Then, for the rest of his life, his professional knowledge was limited to what we might call alumni publications. Any advances in the profession of medicine, so far as he was concerned, were carried out by his medical school; he received his information through only their publications. There were no professional publications which spread throughout the medical profession in Japan advances made in all of the medical schools.— Breaking down this compartmentalization, I believe, was an important and fundamental step forward in improving the quality of professional knowledge of the Japanese medical profession. Similar steps were taken in the professions of dentistry, nursing, pharmacy, and veterinary medicine.

Another step taken in this direction was to attempt to bring professional journals into Japan from the United States and other countries. On my first trip through Japanese medical schools, I found on the library shelves their school publications and certain German publications. German was the second language as far as the scientific medical group was concerned. Germany had lost its leadership in medicine with the advent of Hitler; medical progress subsequent to that time had been carried out in other western European countries and the United States. I believed it was important to bring modern knowledge to Japan.

We began by obtaining donations of publications since 1941, as well as texts that were surplus to the various medical schools and libraries. The American Medical Association put on a drive for us. The library of the Surgeon General of the U.S. Army sent us extra copies of various journals and textbooks. The Rockefeller Foundation sponsored subscriptions and also donated books to the library of the Institute of Public Health and Tokyo Imperial University Medical School. Through many, many sources and many contacts, we were able to gradually bring into Japan modern medical knowledge which could be disseminated through their journals and through their scientific meetings to the professions.

We ran into some interesting difficulties in the translating business. Initially, we intended to obtain permission from various publishers to have their books translated into Japanese and published in Japan; but I ran into difficulty with another SCAP section that was concerned with patents, copyrights, and royalty rights.[9] After much communication between SCAP and Washington, D.C., we were up against a stone wall; under a very, very old treaty, the United States and Japan had agreed that either nation could take the books of the other, translate them, and publish them without regard to copyright or payment of royalties to the originating company. The publishers and authors in America wanted to change this treaty during the occupation. Because this was a matter for diplomatic negotiation after the occupation and after a peace treaty, we were in a difficult position.

It was finally agreed, after several years of negotiations, that we could translate publications into Japanese and publish them in Japan, because we had no dollar exchange to pay out for royalties. Accounting would be kept of all of the documents or books sold. When the occupation ended and there was free exchange of currency among yen, dollars, and other currency, then the author, if the State Department decided to abrogate the old treaty, could put in a claim and recover from the Japanese publishers. This situation was one of the many difficulties that one encounters when trying to initiate programs of the magnitude we were undertaking.

During this interim period, we were obliged to literally beg from every available source in the United States, the United Kingdom, and elsewhere, for textbooks and professional journals. The Japanese attempted to read these in English; until English became more widespread, the degree of dissemination was not as good as we would have liked it to have been.

Acupuncture and Moxacautery

Every country has its problems of quasi-medical practices, including our own.[10] There were some 250 quasi-medical practices in Japan, ranging from acupuncture to bone setting to moxacautery. Acupuncture is a very old Chinese system in which needles are inserted into the parts in which pain is present.—Of course, we fire and needle horses today when they have bowed tendons and similar ailments. The local irritation counteracts the pain and perhaps does ultimately help in some cases through stimulation of circulation, in the opinion of many.— Moxacautery is also a very ancient practice. It involves placing a piece of fluff over an area of pain and setting the fluff on fire.

This procedure was done to some of the Americans who were held prisoner when they developed pain. Consequently, when they were released from prison, they immediately charged that they had been tortured. When the prosecutors came to interview me about pressing war crime charges against Japanese doctors who had used moxacautery or acupuncture on American prisoners, I was forced to point out that this was an acceptable practice in Japan; under the provisions of the various Geneva Conventions and other rules of war, such practices could not be considered a war crime. If the holding nation treats its prisoners as it treats its own individuals, then there can be no legal perpetration of an atrocity.

This provision also held true in the use of anesthetics. The Japanese performed many operations without the use of anesthetics, which are routine in our country. When they carried out such operations on American prisoners, they were again charged with torture. None of these charges could stand up legally on the grounds that they were torture in the eyes of the holding power, in this case the Japanese.

In an attempt to eliminate these various quasi-medical practices, we investigated their status. We found that acupuncture in Japan was a prerogative of the blind. Certain very interesting political battles developed. If we attempted to do away with it through a licensing law that would prohibit the practice of acupuncture by its converts, we would deprive the blind people of their livelihoods. As a result, the inevitable compromise had to be made. Through legislation, the standards of training of these various cults were raised and limitations were placed on the scope of their practice. We have followed this pattern in some of our own quasi-medical professions at home.

Dentistry

The Japan Dental Association had been a governmental organization for controlling the dental profession. Apparently, its principle function was the allocation of gold to dental practitioners. The use of gold, which is seldom seen nowadays in American dental practice, was widespread in Japan, much of it being put on teeth for decorative purposes. Because dentistry is an important element in improving health, it was necessary to define and separate the functions that properly belonged in the field of dentistry from those in medicine and pharmacy.

Gen. Dale Ridgely, chief of the Dental Division, undertook a reorganization of the dental profession as a scientific profession along lines similar to those for the medical profession. He was assisted by a mission from the American Dental Association, which we invited to Japan to act as an advisory body in reviewing the program and recommending improvements through education, licensing standards, and reorganization of the dental association into a truly professional group.

A council on dental education was established. The eight dental schools in Japan were classified. Two of the eight were unable to meet the standards for improved professional education and were closed. Courses in preventive dentistry were established at the Institute of Public Health for training dentists to staff the Dental Divisions of the health centers, which were primarily engaged in preventive activities. Mobile dental clinics were built, and schools were established to train dental hygienists. In November 1948, the Japan Dental Association began publication of a journal.

13

Pharmacy and the Pharmaceutical Industry

Separation of the professions of medicine, dentistry, and pharmacy in Japan was a real problem. The Japanese had made attempts to take steps in this direction but without success. They had been unable to formulate a code of ethics for their respective professions or to arrive at an agreement of what functions each profession should undertake. Until the Diet passed the Pharmaceutical Affairs Law in July 1948, pharmacists in Japan were permitted to prescribe and to sell potent drugs without prescriptions; second class doctors were making a considerable portion of their living through the compounding and dispensing of drugs; and dentists were making a considerable portion of their livelihood through the installation of gold for decorative or other reasons.

The Pharmaceutical Affairs Law established standards for licensure, which elevated the standards of training for pharmacists.[1] The pharmacy schools were inspected and classified, and a four-year course in pharmacy was established as a requisite for eligibility to take the licensing examination. The Japan Pharmaceutical Association was also organized as a professional organization.

A mission from the American Pharmaceutical Association visited Japan at our invitation in July 1949. The mission included representatives of various areas of professional concern: education in pharmacy; the manufacture, control, and distribution of pharmaceuticals; and the practice of pharmacy in general. Their recommendations were of great assistance in carrying out the pharmaceutical program.

Separation of the Professions:
Medicine, Dentistry, and Pharmacy

In the United States, the evolution of the definition and separation of functions among the three professions has taken place over a period of almost one hundred years. Occasionally, we still find, in isolated areas of the country, doctors who are doing their own compounding, dispensing, and selling of drugs. That is quite different from a doctor on a call who may dispense drugs as an emergency measure. The public as a whole has not been quite aware of the gradual step-by-step evolution and separation of the three professions into their respective but closely allied activities with the result that medical care has improved.

In an effort to accomplish this definition of functions in Japan, by agreeing on what should constitute the field of pharmacy and what should be the field of dentistry and the field of medicine, I established a council comprised of representatives from the three professional associations after their reorganization had been completed. This group recognized the need for such a step, if the quality of medical care provided to the Japanese people was to be improved. Known as the Medical and Pharmaceutical Systems Deliberation Council, it was established to study the problem. In addition to representatives of the three professions, this council included so-called learned men and certain governmental officials, as the government itself was very much concerned with this problem.

I emphasized to this council that the economic incentives in Japan had led to the continuation of the existing conflict: A doctor could make more selling drugs to his patients than he could from his medical knowledge; a dentist could make more by installing gold than he could by practicing good dentistry. Therefore, economic incentives should be re-evaluated, and a man paid properly for his professional knowledge. Whether drugs or gold, the material was an adjunct to the application of this professional knowledge and should become the secondary consideration.

A second council was established to study and review the fee scales in all three professions, because they were tied in with the overall health insurance system in Japan, which had been developed over the years. This review was an effort to provide economic incentives to improve the quality of medical care by the doctors and the quality of dental care by the dentists and to provide incentives for the pharmacists to improve their own qualifications so they could make a living through the dispensing of drugs on the prescriptions of the doctors, rather than by the over-the-counter practice of medicine through nostrums and patent medicines, as they had been doing in the past.

This separation of the three professions could have been done, of course, by edict; however, if change were to endure, our policy was to study the situation in a given field to attempt to determine the reasons which had led to the situation that existed at the time we entered Japan. If principles such as I have mentioned here, which are found to be essential in improving the quality of medical care provided to a people, were to be put into effect, then the change would have to be made in a manner which would be acceptable to the Japanese people and to the professions involved, if they were going to stick and be durable. Otherwise, such change would be a transient phase of an activity imposed by the occupation on the people to be repudiated immediately upon the end of the occupation.

This problem took a great deal of my time in discussions with the various groups concerned. It became a matter of discussion in the Diet and the press. The various proponents and opponents freely discussed their positions, as we attempted to encourage them to do as an illustration of a democratic process.

On 24 June 1951, the Diet passed the law amending the Medical Practitioners Law, the Dental Practitioners Law, and the Pharmaceutical Affairs Law. The amendments provided economic incentives through changes in fee scales for a gradual transition. For instance, if a doctor decided that his patient required medicine after his professional examination and diagnosis, then he would prepare a prescription. The patient then was free to take this prescription to any qualified pharmacist for compounding. On the other hand, pharmacists were prohibited from dispensing so-called powerful drugs over-the-counter without a prescription. The dentist, in turn, was also required to write a prescription for any medication that he felt was required pertaining to the field of dentistry.

Recognizing that this would take some time—because we could not suddenly deprive the second class group of doctors of their livelihood without creating chaos, and we could not suddenly redistribute all of the first class doctors and all of the qualified pharmacists so there would be a qualified pharmacist to fill prescriptions in rural areas as well as urban areas—the law allowed a transition period: It would take effect the first of January 1955. Incentives for each of the three professions have been developed as a result of this law. Each group now knows its clearly defined responsibilities to improve the quality of medical care through professional reading and continued study by the practitioners in postgraduate seminars. The importance of this agreement and this law, in spite of opposition by certain groups, will be felt for many years in the future. The Japanese people should benefit from this reform for many years, as other nations have benefitted when they have developed such a separation through a process of evolution over many, many years.

Redirecting Production and Distribution of Medical Supplies

The pharmaceutical and medical supply industries of Japan had been developed to a degree that permitted an extensive export trade throughout the Orient, principally to China and Southeast Asia; however, the emphasis was on quantity rather than quality: We found large stocks of patent medicines of doubtful value in the country at the beginning of the occupation. These stocks were for export to other countries. In addition, the patent medicine salesman was an institution; he regularly visited the rural homes and areas, replacing the stocks of herbs, tigers' teeth, bears' gall, and other medicaments to which people were accustomed as home remedies.

Surgical instruments, X-ray equipment, and other hospital supplies were ordinarily produced in small factories. Approximately fifty percent of the factories that had been engaged in the manufacture of medical supplies and pharmaceuticals before the war had either been destroyed or converted to the production of other war materials. We estimated the remaining factories could produce only twenty percent of the prewar requirements.

During the war, Japan, like many other countries in wartime, had established rigid controls over production, including the production of pharmaceutical supplies and equipment. Various control corporations were established. The limited available stocks of raw materials were allocated through one control corporation, and production quotas were established. The government purchased the bulk of the products for the armed forces: The Japanese army and navy took approximately sixty-five percent of the medical supplies; the civilian population received a very small share.[2]

Distribution was also accomplished through a series of control associations and companies. Each controlled a specific commodity group. Such distribution might result in a doctor receiving drugs of a type and quantity which he did not use or being unable to acquire drugs which he did use and need.

We received numerous requests for importation of pharmaceutical and medical supplies. These requests were frequently forwarded by American military commanders who were moving into various areas of Japan and who were responding to appeals from Japanese doctors, particularly directors of hospitals who were, at that time, almost destitute of supplies; however, we found very large stocks of medical supplies and pharmaceuticals in the depots of the Japanese army and navy. After discussing the problem with the chief of the Economics Section and the chief-of-staff, I recommended that we limit the importation of finished products to a minimum. We believed that we had sufficient stocks, if the Japanese military medical supplies were distributed to civilian doctors and hospitals, to tide us over until we could place the pharmaceutical industry on its feet.[3]

Because of the dispersed and isolated locations of the medical depots, it took some time to inventory and locate drugs and to move them into distribution channels. We initially had to utilize existing control associations, because there was no other means available for distributing the existing supplies to civilian hospitals and doctors. Subsequently, these control associations were dissolved. Upon the establishment of the Economic Stabilization Board by the Economics Section of SCAP, the Pharmaceutical and Supply Bureau of the Ministry of Welfare was designated as the agency under SCAP supervision, that is, under supervision of the Pharmaceutical Division of my office, for allocating raw materials to medical supply industries. Prior to the end of the occupation, all controlled items were eventually eliminated, and normal commercial distribution through wholesalers to retailers and users was in effect.

Introducing New Drugs

Simply importing a new drug, or an old drug in a new form, into a country is not a solution to the problem of improving medical care. This new product must also be accepted through training and education of the profession and as well as the public. Otherwise, as I have often seen, American drugs and other modern drugs and supplies will rot on the shelf for lack of use by those who need them.

We initially imported some forty drugs in finished form in fiscal year 1946; within the next four years, this number was reduced to three. To understand the introduction of new drugs in Japan, it must be emphasized that the problem had to be approached from many angles, if it were to succeed. Hexylresorcinol is an example.

Medical surveys showed there was almost one hundred percent infection with intestinal parasites. In previous years, the Japanese had routinely given santonin to their children in the spring, as a sort of spring tonic. Santonin was no longer available because Russia had control of most of the sources; hence, we decided to introduce a modern and more effective anthelmintic called hexylresorcinol. This drug is far more effective in the treatment of intestinal parasites than the old santonin.

We first imported hexylresorcinol in comparatively small quantities in finished form. It was tested on a group of volunteers, under the supervision of the Ministry of Health and Welfare and the Japan Medical Association, to demonstrate its effectiveness. Regardless of the fact that the scientific literature from other countries, including our own, was full of reports on the efficacy of hexylresorcinol, it had to be demonstrated to the Japanese doctors and Japanese children that it was effective. We must always remember that in dealing with people, there is a certain national pride, and an attitude can be adopted that if it is not done in our country, it is not so. The demonstrations created a demand for its use. The Japanese manufacturers were then instructed how to produce it and, in due course, were licensed by the Ministry. It was then distributed. When production met demand, we stopped importing the finished item.

In the case of penicillin, the Japanese had been experimenting with litter lots of penicillin that they had put into five hundred unit ampules, which, of course, are totally ineffective. We were eager to begin the production of penicillin, and I was fortunate in obtaining the services of a consultant, Dr. Jackson. Because penicillin was produced under a government license, we received authority from the U.S. Government to begin production in Japan. Because of the tremendous popular demand for penicillin which was sweeping the world at that time, its production required strict control. The inevitable black market developed, which can only be liquidated by providing sufficient supply to meet demand. We accelerated supply, maintaining adequate standards, until we were able to remove controls of penicillin in 1948. Fortunately, Japanese production under Dr. Jackson's guidance was of high quality, and we were able to meet production requirements for use in Korea when the Korean War started in 1950.

Streptomycin in combination with paraminosalicylic acid had been under testing for the treatment of tuberculosis by various agencies in America. We had followed the results of their controlled studies for a number of years; through close liaison, we received reports as soon as they were available. We decided to use this combination of antibiotic and drug in the therapy of active clinical cases of tuberculosis in Japan. As is usually the case, various American manufacturers had developed their own particular production methods. I wanted to accelerate the production of streptomycin, so I attempted to interest

American antibiotic manufacturers in coming to Japan in 1949 and 1950, to enter into licensing agreements with Japanese manufacturers under which the Japanese would receive the benefit of the technical advice of the American manufacturers in return for a royalty payment. If we could make such royalty agreements, it would save us several years of work.

I was unable to obtain such an agreement, although I made a special trip back to the United States for conferences with various manufacturers. They did not have sufficient foresight to realize that, after the occupation, Japanese production could be used for export to other areas in the Far East, to their mutual advantage with increased financial benefit. I was forced to obtain a basic culture and a licensing agreement from Dr. Waksman at Rutgers University. We then developed production methods in Japan and were able to meet our requirements of approximately fifty million grams per year. At the same time, we began production of paraminosalicylic acid. Streptomycin and other antibiotics of high quality are now being produced in Japan and exported to other countries.

In the treatment of leprosy, we were able to introduce the sulfone drugs, which had brought such promising results in the treatment of leprosy in America. We began a controlled study on the use of these drugs. I am very happy to report that prior to the end of the occupation, a joint project for controlled studies was undertaken, which has produced some valuable scientific information on the efficacy of the sulfone drugs in the treatment of leprosy.

Assay of Vaccines and Drugs

The Pharmaceutical Affairs Law, which is similar to the Food and Drug Law of the United States but far more rigid and comprehensive, established a legal basis for quality standards for all pharmaceuticals and medical supplies. As a result, the extravagant claims of various nostrums and patent medicines to cure anything from flat feet to pregnancy are no longer permitted on Japanese labels. This improvement in quality standards has been a great step forward and has subsequently made Japan a formidable competitor with other modern nations in the export of pharmaceuticals and medical supplies.

The National Hygienic Laboratory was established as an agency of the Ministry of Health and Welfare to assay drugs, to establish assay requirements, and to make periodic checks on quality standards on all pharmaceuticals and medical supplies produced by the pharmaceutical industry, with the exception of antibiotics and biologics, which were assayed by the National Institute of Health. During 1948 and 1949, very rigid assay standards were established for all biologics.[4] During the period of re-assay of all vaccines, we used all of the laboratory animals in Japan and had to make an emergency request for some 20,000 guinea pigs from the United States in order to complete the program.

Supplies and Demand

The policy we carried out throughout the occupation was to keep to a minimum the importation of finished supplies and to import the raw materials, which could be processed in Japan, particularly in the case of new drugs and antibiotics with which they were unfamiliar, until we could develop sufficient production in Japan.[5] Besides the raw materials for production, there were other facets to the rehabilitation of the pharmaceutical and medical supply industries. Owing to the shortages of fuel, power, and building materials, we had to be claimants for a fair allocation of these materials for the pharmaceutical industries and for the rehabilitation of hospitals; otherwise, we would have been unable to carry out our programs. We received the finest cooperation from General Marquat's Economics Section, which controlled such allocations.

In the early days of the occupation, we had a very large requirement for the insecticide DDT, which had been made available to the United States under a Swiss patent. Initially, we had to import DDT in finished form to Japan; however, it was not long until we were able to import only the concentrate and use talc produced in Japan as a mixer, thereby saving both dollars and shipping space.[6] Eventually, we were able to produce DDT concentrate in Japan to meet all requirements, not only for control of flies and mosquitoes as disease vectors but also for insect control on crops for agricultural purposes. Fortunately, the production capacity was so sufficient that we could obtain from Japan all of the DDT we required for the Korean War. Records were kept on production so that royalties could be paid under a licensing agreement at the end of the occupation.

For reasons unknown to me, there was apparently some difficulty in the United States immediately after the war in meeting requirements for X-ray film for the military services. As we were re-establishing the X-ray film industry in Japan to meet civilian requirements, we also produced, at the request of General Martin, who replaced General Denit as theater surgeon, sufficient film to meet requirements of the military medical service in the Far East, until adequate supplies could be obtained from the United States.[7]

The Pharmaceutical Industry

No matter how well trained a professional group may be, without adequate tools it is handicapped in the application of its knowledge. In the case of the medical and allied professions engaged in health work, unless they have the tools—the modern tools produced by the pharmaceutical and medical supply industries—to apply their knowledge, little progress will be made in improving health and preventing disease among the people in an underdeveloped country, such as Japan was at the beginning of the occupation. Our Pharmaceutical Division, headed by Col. Bernard Riordan, and subsequently by Dr. Band, made a tremendous contribution to the pharmaceutical industry of Japan. Today, the Japanese doctor has the armamentarium of any modern medical practitioner.

Our basic policy was to place the Japanese industry on its feet, to establish high quality standards, and to import only finished products in sufficient quantity, in the case of new drugs, until we could meet our requirements through Japanese production. I believe the American pharmaceutical industry missed the boat in adopting what I consider to be a shortsighted view. I am quite sure that some of my friends in the industry resent the activities we undertook because they themselves were unwilling to take certain risks with regard to the Far East. They were only interested, as far as I could determine, in the export market for their finished or semi-finished items and a quick profit. Immediately after the war, it may be recalled, the eyes of the United States were principally on Europe. Most of the manufacturers were apparently interested in establishing branch plants in Europe. Dr. Draper, who had been in charge of the economic rehabilitation in Germany, subsequently visited Japan and was quite astonished to find that we were producing by that time our total requirements for penicillin, when he had been unable to get production underway in Germany.

I believe that if our industry had been foresighted enough and had been willing to wait for the establishment of free currency conversion, in which yen profits could be converted into dollar exchange, they would have entered into licensing agreements with Japanese manufacturers, in many cases to the mutual advantage of the American pharmaceutical and Japanese pharmaceutical industries. The American manufacturer could have developed and expanded a Far East and Southeast Asia export market by using as a base of his production the Japanese production capacity. They would now be in a mutually advantageous position instead of a competitive position. Today, Japan is highly competitive in the pharmaceutical and medical supply industries with the British industries and our own, because the quality of their products is as high as ours and their production costs are comparatively low. They are able to produce on a competitive basis as far as price and quality are concerned.

These facts are pertinent to our present economic war with Russia. I have found too often in foreign countries that some of our American producers may have a surplus of certain commodities, which they want to dump at a quick profit, and they are not too concerned with establishing a firm re-order base. This practice does not give us too good a reputation in certain foreign countries. If we mutually developed a given production in a foreign country, then we have not only followed sound, long-term business methods, but also made a mutual friend and a staunch one. I am also well aware of the fact, unfortunately by personal experience, that some manufacturers are not adverse to dumping on foreign markets products that have been rejected under quality standards of the U.S. Food and Drug Law as unsalable in the American market. Such practice does not help the prestige of our business. I hope, in due course of time, such practices will no longer continue if we are to win the economic war in underdeveloped countries.

14

Nursing

Prior to the occupation, nursing, as we knew it, had not really been recognized as a profession in Japan. There were some 166,000 nurses who had graduated from all kinds and types of training courses in Japan.[1] In many of the nursing schools, the girls were used as attendants for the doctors or as cleaning women. The Japanese Red Cross, which, like most national Red Cross societies, continued its basic concept of being a medical organization, provided training for nurses who had been used by the Japanese military medical services. Most of the graduate nurses worked for various insurance associations and private corporations. It was difficult for girls of good families to be induced to enter the nursing profession because it was not recognized as a professional group.

One of our problems was to get the families out of the hospitals, where they frequently became infected from the patients through cross infection. To do so, we needed to teach the hospital directors and the medical profession that one of the responsibilities of the hospital was to provide bedside nursing and nursing care.[2] Few hospitals utilized nursing services as such.

There was one exception: St. Luke's Hospital in Tokyo, which was built by funds donated by the Episcopalian Mission of the United States.[3] It maintained a nursing program that was comparable to an average modern hospital in the United States; but, the number of St. Luke's graduates was a drop in the bucket compared with the total number of nurses in Japan.

Reorganizing Nursing Education

I was most fortunate in having Maj. Grace Alt, who later became a civilian, as head of the Nursing Affairs Division.[4] In training professional nurses, we again followed the pattern that we had used in the other professions. A Nursing Education Council was established.[5] By agreement with the staff of St. Luke's Hospital in Tokyo, which was taken over by the military medical services as a U.S. military hospital, we consolidated the faculty and nursing classes of the Central Red Cross Hospital and St. Luke's Hospital. American nurses were put in key positions as instructors, and a model nursing school designed to raise nursing standards and to train leaders for other schools in modern nursing requirements was established at the Central Red Cross Hospital in Tokyo on 1 June 1946. It became known as the Tokyo Model Demonstration School of Nursing.

There were initially some 420 trainees. A three-year course in clinical nursing was established, and the first class graduated in June 1949. The empress of Japan interested herself in this program, and the graduation exercise was attended by the empress and by Prince and Princess Takamatsu and other members of the imperial family. The Ministry of Education granted recognition to the school as a college of nursing.

As the Japanese instructors developed capability in carrying on the instruction, the American staff was then used to start other model nursing schools. In 1948, a second school was opened in Okayama Hospital. As graduates of the new courses became available, additional model schools, similar to the model health center program and the model hospital program, were established with the object, eventually, of having model nursing schools in each prefecture.

By agreement with the military surgeon's office of the Far East Command, two hundred selected Japanese nurses were employed as nurses aides in the twelve U.S. Army hospitals in Japan. They were instructed by American nurses. This approach was similar to that used to show the young Japanese doctors how American medicine was practiced and what we were trying to teach them. It served the mutual benefit of the military medical service, which was then short of American nurses, and assisted in expanding the program of elevating nursing education standards for the Japanese.

Prior to this reorganization, training in public health nursing was considered more or less as an undergraduate course, instead of special training to be given after completion of basic training as a nurse. The concept of public health nursing was given new emphasis in 1947, when courses for public health nurses were established at the Institute of Public Health.[6] American public health nurses were also assigned to the forty-six prefectural civil affairs teams to assist in the expansion of the nationwide nursing program.

As in the medical and dental professions, modern texts and journals and literature in the nursing profession were very limited. Initially, American nurses working with Japanese nurses translated texts, which were published for the use of the Japanese nurses. Procedure manuals for clinical nurses, public health nurses, and midwives were also published. Subsequently, it was possible to obtain texts and professional journals from the United States and other countries for the use of Japanese nurses in bringing them up-to-date in modern professional training.

Standards for Licensure and Education

In November 1946, the three government-controlled nursing associations, which had been in existence for controlling midwives, nurses, and public health nurses, were dissolved. A new professional association was established with officers who were elected by the membership. A professional journal was also established by the association.

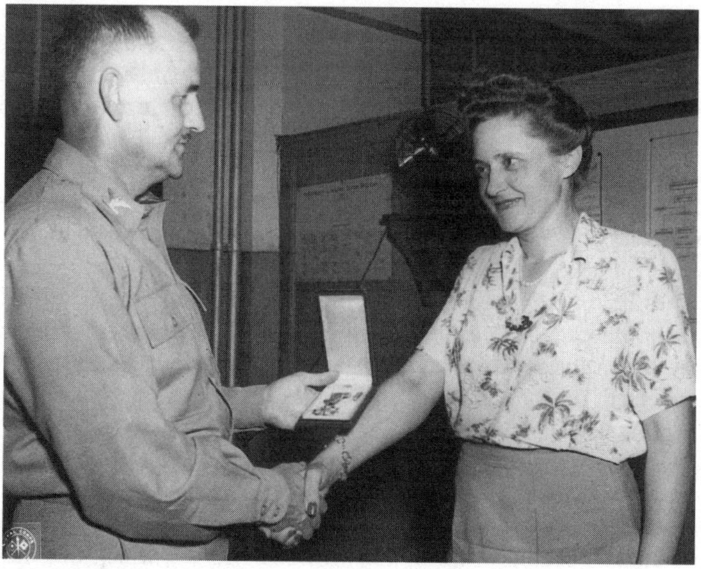

Figure 18. Brig. Gen. C.F. Sams presented the Legion of Merit Medal to Grace E. Alt for her work in establishing the first demonstration school of nursing in Tokyo. Grace Alt, formerly a Major in the U.S. Army Nurses Corps, was the first Chief of the Nursing Affairs Division, PHW Section, SCAP. Tokyo, 21 August 1947. Photo Credit: U.S. Army Signal Corps, Photographer Lemire. (Courtesy of the Hoover Institution Archives, Stanford University.)

In July 1947, a Japanese Cabinet Ordinance, in compliance with SCAP advice, established standards for licensure and registration of clinical nurses, public health nurses, and midwives. On 3 July 1948, the Diet incorporated this ordinance into new law, which provided the necessary permanent legislation to maintain and control nursing standards and education. The law required twelve years of schooling before licensure, which consisted of six years of primary school, three years of lower middle school, and three years of upper middle school. In addition, it provided that clinical nursing courses would be of three years' duration and that public health nursing and midwifery programs would be on a post-graduate level after graduation from the three-year clinical course, to ensure that such nurses had a sound background in nursing.

Under the new law, the nursing schools were classified. By 1951, three were 116 Class A training schools and 132 Class B schools. In revising the law on nursing education standards, the inevitable grandfather clause had to be incorporated so as not to work undue hardship on those who had been trained under older standards. Those who had practiced under the old standards for thirteen years were not required to take an examination but were automatically licensed.

By 1954, only graduates of Class A nursing schools were designated as nurses in Japan. Consequently, nursing as a profession, rendering bedside care to patients, has become a reality in the majority of hospitals. Hospital directors and doctors have been trained to accept the new nursing program and have come to recognize the nurse as an integral part of the hospital staff, rather than as a personal servant to the doctor or as a cleaning woman. The public health nurse has also become recognized as an integral part of the public health team in the community and is turned to for advice and guidance by patients and their families.

15

Hospitals

Although we undertook reforms of the systems of education and practice for the professions of medicine, dentistry, pharmacy, and nursing, these programs alone are not sufficient to improve the quality of care to people. The facilities, drugs, and equipment available to the professions must also be studied and improved. Otherwise, we would be guilty of having overtrained the individual for the tools available to him. It was, therefore, necessary to become involved in the hospital system of Japan.

The State of Hospitals

During the war, a total of 1,027 hospitals in Japan, with a total capacity of 53,000 beds, had been destroyed. Approximately one out of four hospitals was destroyed through fire and high explosive and atomic bomb raids in the last year of the war. At the start of the occupation, only 2,852 hospitals of more than twenty-bed capacity were left in Japan. The remaining hospitals had a capacity of 244,709 beds. There were also 320 army and navy hospitals with approximately 78,000 battle casualties in operation at the time of surrender.

The hospital situation was not unlike that of our own country and of Europe many years ago in that a hospital was a place to which one went as a last resort: It was a place where one went to die. So even the limited number of hospital beds in the civilian hospitals were occupied.[1]

Yet, "hospital beds" in Japan did not mean the nice white metal hospital beds of our country. In most cases, a bed in Japan was a *tatami* on the floor. The hospitals had been without soap; they were filthy dirty, because they could not be cleaned. There was a lack of fuel, even for heating water. They were short of medical equipment and drugs; they had not had X-ray film for at least three years. They had to wash and reuse such cotton dressings as they had, and they usually resorted to paper dressings.[2]

The hospital buildings ranged from very large modern buildings to some very ancient rickety structures. In those hospitals which had high-priced private rooms, there were separate little alcoves for the body servant of the patient to sleep. Again, we must turn the pages back to visualize that this also existed in America in past years, although they had some interesting differences from many of our hospitals. In our country, the university teaching hospitals had large out-patient clinics, but the average local hospital did not have an out-patient clinic as such, unless it was a city or county hospital. In Japan, all hospitals had a large out-patient service; the staff usually treated three out-patients for each in-patient.

Japanese hospitals were quite shocking to many American visitors. They found the rooms and wards cluttered with families and relatives gathered around the bed, frequently living and sleeping there and cooking at the patient's bedside. It was the custom for the patient's family to provide the nursing care and to prepare the patient's meals. Very few hospitals had what we call central cooking facilities, so the patient's family brought the food and a little hibachi on which to cook. The place of diet and nutrition in the therapeutic armamentarium of the Japanese doctor simply did not exist. Apparently, the doctor had no interest in what the patient ate or how he obtained his food.

The Demilitarization of Hospitals

Prior to the war, the Japanese had established the Medical Treatment Corporation as an emergency mobilization measure. This corporation took over all hospitals. During the occupation, steps were undertaken to gradually eliminate the Medical Treatment Corporation and to turn hospitals to previous or new ownership. We established a pattern of hospital ownership and operation that included nationally operated hospitals, prefecturally operated hospitals, and privately owned hospitals. The tuberculosis sanitaria were usually operated as national hospitals. This reorganization took considerable time, but the Medical Treatment Corporation was liquidated before the end of the occupation.

In accordance with overall policy directives received by SCAP, no preferential treatment could be given to Japanese veterans. Those hospitals which would correspond to our Veterans Administration Hospitals in America, under their civilian status, could not be so classified. Therefore, they became national hospitals and were required to accept patients from all categories of personnel and were not permitted to give any preferential treatment to military veterans of the war. I also received approval to turn over to the Ministry of Health and Welfare the 320 army and navy hospitals, which for the time being were to be operated as national hospitals for Japanese civilians.[3]

Another overall policy directive we received required a complete demilitarization of Japan; it directed that all career military personnel should be purged. Sometimes these overall broad directives that are issued for political reasons have repercussions which are a little difficult to solve. This directive gave me considerable trouble in the case of the former army and navy hospitals with 78,000 battle casualties to treat. If I complied with this directive, I would immediately have had to throw all of the doctors who staffed these hospitals out of jobs, because they had been in the army or navy during the war. On appeal to General MacArthur through the Government Section and by agreement of General Whitney, we obtained permission to retain on the staffs of these former military hospitals the doctors who had been in the army and navy but were now civilians, if they were below the grade of lieutenant colonel. This waiver on the purge was given for about a year and a half. We were then directed to complete the purge down to the lowest former lieutenant. The waiver did give a breathing space in which we could gradually replace these former military medical officers with civilians without completely throwing all of the patients out in the street.

The Model Hospital Administration Program

We had some major problems. To rebuild the hospitals that had been destroyed was very costly and could not be done all at one time; but plans were made and the program was inaugurated. We expanded the tuberculosis hospitals from 25,000 beds to 101,000. Part of this expansion was done by new construction; part of it was done by changing the requirements for the types of hospitals.

Every community of any size in Japan had an infectious disease hospital. We emptied them. In our preventive medicine programs, we had practically emptied the hospitals of cases of infectious and communicable diseases; the comparatively few cases still occurring could be handled in isolation wards in general hospitals. Many of the largest hospitals in Japan, which had been infectious or communicable disease hospitals, could then be converted into either tuberculosis sanitaria or general hospitals. We were able, thereby, to reuse buildings which had formerly been required for a type of patient who no longer existed in the numbers existing prior to the occupation.

Another problem was to attempt to orient the Japanese people to the concept that the responsibility of the patient's family was to impress on the hospital director that the feeding and nursing care of the patient was really a responsibility of the hospital staff. Obviously, such a program required long-term effort. Like the model health center program, we introduced a school of hospital administration. Some of my own staff, including myself, taught the first courses. We undertook to train hospital administrators in modern concepts of hospital administration and care, professional and otherwise.[4]

We used a former army hospital, known as the First National Hospital, as a model. It was re-equipped, repainted, and refurbished as a modern hospital.[5] Following what I call "the pebble in the pool" pattern, we established forty-six model hospitals, one in each prefecture. As in the case of the health centers, the competition among hospitals to improve their standards became keen: to establish central cooking; to have some responsibility for patient feeding; to establish proper nursing care standards as well as standards for cleanliness and other measures which are necessary for provision of the first-class care in a first-class hospital.

Establishing Standards for Hospitals

Hand-in-hand with this school of hospital administration, it became necessary to develop a law which would provide a legal basis for hospital standards and also an educational program according to the new concept. This law, like the others, was initially a SCAP directive executed by Japanese Cabinet Ordinance. It was later passed as a law by the Diet, known as the Medical Service Law, in July 1948. Medical service districts for the administration of this law were established. Because the population unit and distribution of medical resources were similar to that desirable for the health center districts, these medical service districts coincided with the health center districts.

The criteria for classifying a building as a hospital were also established under the law. All of the hospitals were reinspected and classified. Those which could meet the standards under the program were classified as Class A; others were placed on probation. Hospitals with fewer than ten beds were abolished, because they could not provide normal minimum standards, such as laboratory service, operating room service, and so forth.

As in other major programs, a period of transition was required. A five-year period was established for the elimination of the hospitals with fewer than ten beds. They could no longer be hospitals, but they could be designated as clinics. Patients could not be kept in such clinics longer than forty-eight hours, unless an emergency existed which had to receive the approval of the local health officer.

The reporting of available and occupied hospital beds was changed from a weekly to a monthly report. I had required the reporting of such information when it was necessary that I know how many beds were immediately available to meet the epidemics during the early part of the occupation. By 1951, the change in attitude of the Japanese people through increased confidence in the quality of medical care being furnished, and through the improvement in hospital standards, caused an increase in the occupancy of hospital beds to an average of 334,000 beds. In 1945, there was an occupancy rate of less than 25 percent; this rate increased to 78.4 percent in 1951. In the eyes of the Japanese people, the hospital is no longer a place of last resort where one goes to die, but is a place where one goes with the expectation of receiving proper and adequate treatment leading to the probability of an early recovery. This change in attitude was the goal we hoped to attain when we began the program.

An Integrated Approach

I have frequently been asked, Why did you engage in all of these activities? Couldn't you carry out your basic mission of preventing disease and unrest simply by going around and sticking needles into people and inoculating them with vaccines? My answer is that disease and unrest cannot be prevented by applying only what in the past have been considered preventive measures, such as improved environmental sanitation, immunization, and so forth. There are many, many diseases—in fact, more diseases—that cannot be prevented through immunization than there are those that can. Unless one can also prevent the frequently fatal, but more often disabling, effects of these diseases by providing high-quality medical care through the early recognition and treatment of such diseases, then the overall mission of preventing disease and unrest fails.

In the case of hospitals, if an attempt is made to improve the standards of hospital administration through teaching the director not only to more closely supervise the quality of his professional staff, but also to improve the quality of nursing care, so that people will enter hospitals for treatment leading to recovery, rather than to die or to linger out a terminal illness, then you must provide that director with nurses who can produce proper nursing service. It is ineffective to attempt to train nurses in high standards of nursing and then send them into hospitals to carry out those standards, if the hospital director tells them that these are not in accordance with the way he wants his hospital run, because he does not know what high nursing standards are. He has not been trained. An endless set of situations must be met, almost simultaneously, if overall progress is to be made in such a nationwide program. They range all the way from revision of professional education to medical economics. There is no single line of approach in any one of these major reforms which will be successful unless additional approaches are undertaken simultaneously.

Too many times, a beautiful hospital building is built and completely equipped by American or other foreign funds in what I call a single approach to improve medical care.—I have seen this in Japan, Korea, the Ryukyu Islands, and the Middle East.—The hospital is turned over to people who know not what to do with it. It is a waste of time to attempt to improve standards in underdeveloped countries by building a building and furnishing it with fine equipment and considering the job completed. The problem must be attacked from many angles, which I have outlined in our attempt, through reorganization of professional education, improvement of hospital standards, and other means, including education of the public as to their attitude toward the services offered, before a lasting change occurs. For this reason, we engaged in many ramifications in each of these major programs. It was an effort to develop programs that would be lasting and acceptable and adaptable to the Japanese people. So far, they are still sound and still in effect. Of that I am proud. I believe it justifies the concept of a many-faceted approach, such as our approach to the broad field of health and welfare in Japan.

In addition to the training and educational program in which we were engaged in Japan, we also sent Japanese to the United States and other countries to see firsthand the things we were talking about. This procedure has been used over many years by various governments and private foundations, such as the Rockefeller Foundation, by granting fellowships to foreign nationals to go to America, receive training, and then return to their home countries. Used alone, this method is not too successful: In the case of many doctors I have seen who have come to the United States or who have gone to Europe and returned to their own countries, they found they could not carry out what they had learned because the tools were not available or the new procedures were not acceptable. But if used in combination with a program carried on in the homeland, this tool of sending foreign nationals to America is most useful in furthering progress in raising standards, at least in the fields of health and welfare.

Such progress as we have made in Japan, and I believe it is substantial, was possible because we used this multiple line of approach in every major problem. We have integrated the efforts; so instead of pushing on one wheel of the wagon, we started it moving by pushing on all four wheels at the same time.

16

The Atomic Bomb Casualty Commission

The situation at Hiroshima and Nagasaki was of great interest to the United States at the beginning of the occupation. Between the fall of 1945 and the spring of 1946, numerous groups came to Japan to study the effects of the atomic bombs. There were some six groups or organizations, as I recall: the Atomic Energy Commission; the Joint Commission on Atomic Effects; the U.S. Public Health Service; the Strategic Bomb Survey; the Army Medical Corps Intelligence; and the Navy Medical Corps Intelligence. After a time, it was decided that, because these studies were concerned with the health of the Japanese people, which was my responsibility, these activities should be placed under the control of the chief of Public Health and Welfare.[1]

Dr. Stafford Warren and Dr. Shields Warren, in particular, and I had numerous discussions.[2] As a result of thinking back in America and our thinking in Japan, the Atomic Energy Commission of the U.S. Government made a contract with the National Research Council to study the effects of atomic weapons on humans. The National Research Council set up a corporation, the Atomic Bomb Casualty Commission, which was to carry out the studies on behalf of all interested U.S. agencies.[3] This group then was sent to Japan and attached to my office. We established temporary laboratories initially in Hiroshima and a control area in Kure. I had hoped to establish a similar group in Nagasaki, but this was not considered desirable at the time by the people with whom we were consulting in Washington, D.C.

Eventually, a very fine and beautifully equipped laboratory was established at Hiroshima. Lt. Col. Carl Tessmer was its first Director. The Scientific Director was Dr. Grant Taylor. A staff was built up in my office for logistical and other support.[4]

I felt very strongly that if such an organization were to continue studies under the program which was mutually agreed to, the delayed effects of radiation, such as the development of cataracts, malignancies, shortened life span, and genetic effects, could only be observed if the studies were carried out over many, many years. If we imposed this organization in Japan, disregarding entirely the Japanese professional interest in this subject, it was quite likely that on the termination of the occupation it would be claimed that this group had been brought into

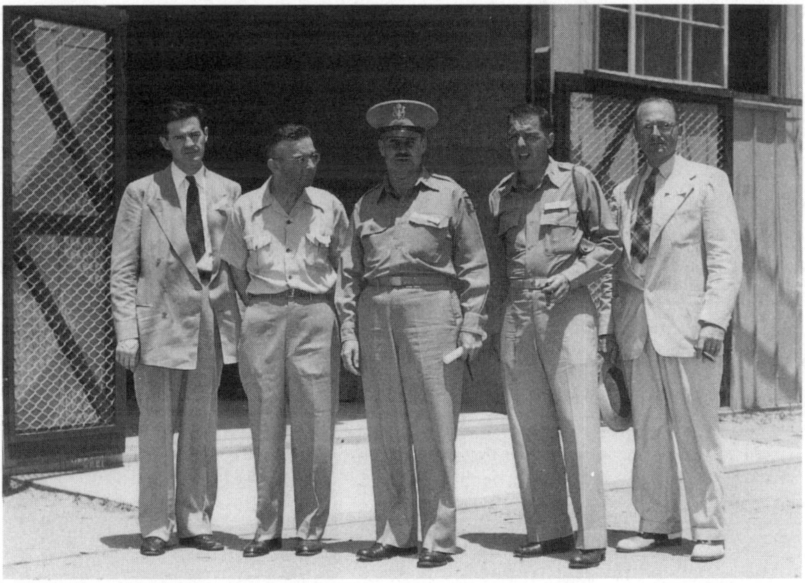

Figure 19. The PHW Section, SCAP, provided logistical support to the Atomic Bomb Casualty Commission, which studied the long-term effects of radiation on survivors of the atomic bombs and their offspring. Officers of SCAP and ABCC paused for this photograph at the entrance of the ABCC motor pool at Ujina machi during a visit to the ABCC's initial facilities in Hiroshima, 14 July 1949. Left to right: Harry Kelly (Science Advisor, SCAP), Walter Cheslak (Motor Pool Supervisor, ABCC), Brig. Gen. C.F. Sams, Lt. Col. Carl F. Tessmer (Director, ABCC, 1947–51), Dr. Henrik Luykx (Principal Statistician, ABCC). Photo credit: ABCC Photo Lab. (Courtesy of the Hoover Institution Archives, Stanford University, and the Radiation Effects Research Foundation, Hiroshima.)

Japan in the interest of the United States alone and they would be promptly thrown out.[5] After consultation with the State Department representatives and others, it was agreed to set up a Japanese counterpart under the auspices of the National Institute of Health, which I had established for research under the Ministry of Health and Welfare.[6] This group was to work with the Americans in the study of the Japanese people in the Hiroshima-Kure areas. Apparently this decision was sound, because when the preliminary negotiations for the peace treaty were begun, a special agreement was made for continuation of this activity after the termination of the occupation.[7] It is still in existence, supported by the U.S. Government, as far as the American participation is concerned; the National Institute of Health of Japan supports the Japanese counterparts who are working with the American professional people in the Atomic Bomb Casualty Commission's long-range program.[8]

There were many consultants who came and went in connection with this program. During the period of the occupation, many of these consultants recommended various changes in the program, which went so far as to consider using clinical facilities of the Atomic Bomb Casualty Commission for providing free medical care for the Japanese who were being examined there periodically.[9] Other recommendations included using this as a teaching institution for Japanese professional personnel.

In 1951, representatives of the National Research Council visited my office for a frank discussion of whether, in view of the fact that the occupation was nearing termination, the program should be discontinued entirely.[10] I felt very strongly that if the basic mission of the Atomic Bomb Casualty Commission was adhered to, and many of the side programs were eliminated or curtailed, the financial expenditure, which was considerable—a number of millions of dollars per year—would be justified. I also felt that a favorable atmosphere had been created among the Japanese agreeing to work with the Americans in this activity and that it should be continued. Today the Atomic Bomb Casualty Commission is a very important element in the total atomic energy biomedical programs.[11]

17

Narcotics Control

One of the missions assigned to me as chief of Public Health and Welfare of General Headquarters, SCAP, was the control of narcotics. The question that immediately arises is, Why should this law enforcement activity be placed with health and welfare activities? In our own country, the control of narcotics at the federal level is carried out under the Treasury Department under the guise of collecting internal revenue. Because the legitimate use of narcotics is basically a function of the medical profession, the U.S. Commissioner of Narcotics, Mr. Anslinger, had suggested the enforcement of narcotics control in Japan should be undertaken in the health and welfare field. Therefore, it became my responsibility.[1] Fortunately, Mr. Anslinger supplied for my staff, on a loan basis, some of his top agents; Mr. W.L. Spears headed the Narcotics Control Division.[2]

Disregard of International Obligations

There was no control over narcotics in Japan prior to the end of World War II. An estimated two hundred farmers grew opium poppies as a side crop. Their opium was purchased by the Government Monopoly Corporation. It was processed and distributed not only to the Japanese population but also to the occupied areas which Japan had seized in Manchuria in 1931. Later on, the Chinese mainland and on down through Malaya and Singapore were areas in which they distributed narcotics. Coca leaves were imported from the Ryukyus. We found a large coca plantation there, which was subsequently destroyed.

Opium smoking in Manchuria and the Chinese mainland and among Asiatic people was a common practice and had existed over many, many years. People who are on a semi-starvation level frequently turn to smoking or eating opium to dull the pangs of hunger. It is possible to control large segments of a population through encouraging addiction to opium or opium products, because once an addiction is established, the individual will resort to any activity to ensure continuation of his supply. It was charged that the Japanese had used narcotics and encouraged their use in areas which they had occupied. The Japanese were also charged with establishing distribution centers throughout these areas under the guise of treatment centers for narcotics, which actually encouraged the spread of drug addiction. I raise this point because in our own country I have recently read proposals of some poorly informed individuals in and out of my own profession advocating that such treatment centers be established in our country where addicts can obtain their supplies at a nominal cost. I wish that these individuals could see as I have the result of such a practice in other areas where such a procedure actually encourages the widespread use of narcotics.

The Japanese Government, while a member of the League of Nations, had subscribed to the provisions of the supervisory body for the control of narcotics production. The Japanese Government files showed that they had submitted to this international body figures representing only one-sixth of the production of heroin that their manufacturers' files showed was actually produced in Japan. Heroin was shipped from Japan and Korea to Manchuria in quantities that would more than suffice the total world requirements.

The Japanese reported that, in spite of the fact that narcotics were uncontrolled in Japan and one could perfectly legally pick up a pound of opium most any place, addiction was not a problem among the Japanese. This was contrary to our assumption, because any doctor or pharmacist in Japan could purchase and dispose of any amount of narcotics without being required to maintain records. It seemed illogical to assume that, under such conditions, they would not develop a considerable number of addicts.

Controlling Production, Processing, and Use

We immediately directed the Japanese Government to prohibit the planting, growth, and cultivation of narcotic seeds and plants and to prohibit the manufacture and export of narcotics. We also directed the establishment of strict centralized controls over the processing and distribution of narcotics. Heroin, which existed in large quantities throughout Japan—in caves, medical depots, army and navy hospitals, and other military, civilian, and industrial establishments—was seized and destroyed. Some of this heroin formerly reached the illegal markets in the United States and other countries.

Following this instruction, all crude and semi-processed narcotics were taken into custody by the occupation forces in the fall of 1945, whether they were formerly in the hands of the Japanese army or navy or in the hands of civilian processors. A centralized control system, similar to that used in the United States under our Harrison Narcotic Law, was established. Strict reporting and recording systems were developed for distribution and dispensing of narcotics used legitimately by the medical profession. The control regulations were enacted into Japanese law by June 1946; they were incorporated in a new law passed by the Diet on 28 June 1948. Responsibility was placed within the Ministry of Health and Welfare, where a Narcotics Section was established. Subsequently, regional offices were established in eight major regions of Japan.[3]

After the United Nations was organized and took over the responsibilities of the old League of Nations narcotics control body, reports on the production, processing, and use of narcotics were submitted to this organization by SCAP on behalf of the Japanese. Prior to the end of the occupation, the Japanese Government, after having adhered to the new agreement of the United Nations, was given the responsibility for such reports.

As the sources of narcotics began to dry up, the presumption that addiction was not prevalent among the Japanese people was soon shown to be false. It was not long until some five thousand addicts were identified.

Once the enforcement and control program for distribution had been well established, which took several years, it was decided that under this program it would be possible, under our supervision, to process some of the stocks of crude or semi-crude products into finished products for legitimate medical use in future years by the Japanese. This carefully controlled program was begun.

Illicit Trade

As control within Japan was established, our next problem became that of limiting the importation of illicit narcotics from Iran, the Chinese mainland, and other sources. As Japan's trade expanded, smuggling, which is carried on worldwide principally through shipping, became one of our major headaches.

It soon became apparent through information obtained by our agents and the Japanese agents, whom we had trained and supervised, that the Japanese Communist party was smuggling narcotics into Japan by way of North Korea.[4] The yen currency realized through this illicit sale was helping to finance the Communist party activities in Japan.

As frequently happens in the enforcement of narcotics control, information of illicit activities is received through informers. A special entrance had been made in my office for such informers to have access to our narcotics agents. Tips were received that narcotics were being run into the Communist party headquarters at Yoyogi, but raids invariably would prove fruitless. This situation provided an interesting sidelight on some of the methods of operation of the communists.

The chief of my Translators and Interpreters Division had brought to my attention a post card that was addressed to one of our Japanese employees, a clerk-stenographer in the Narcotics Control Division, notifying her of a communist cell meeting. This information was immediately turned over to our counter-intelligence people. After thorough investigation, they determined that this girl was not involved in communist activities and gave her a new clearance.

Later, an anonymous letter addressed to me pointed out that this girl was acting as a spy in my Narcotics Control Division and that she was tipping off the Communist party when raids were about to be made on any of the establishments that we had been informed might be holding smuggled narcotics. Again, an investigation was carried out, and the girl was cleared. Subsequently, I received a second letter.—This time it was signed.—It pointed out that this girl was pulling the wool, as it was stated, over our eyes.

A further investigation showed that she was one of the cleverest espionage agents with whom I have ever had contact. She spoke English fluently and had made many contacts among the American girls who were secretaries and clerks in SCAP headquarters. She also carefully avoided any direct contact with any known communist cell or agents. She would sit in our office and listen to the tipsters or informants and then, through a very roundabout transmission chain, would transmit information to the Communist party that such information had been received and a raid was projected. When this case was finally brought to a close and this girl was discharged, many of her American friends came to me demanding to know why I was persecuting this young girl by discharging her, because she was such a lovely young lady. After she was eliminated from our personnel as one of a number of communists who had been planted there, we no longer had difficulty making successful raids on Communist party headquarters and other locations which were distributing illicit narcotics smuggled from North Korea. We, thereby, were able to seriously depress the yen funds available to the Communist party to carry on their activities.

I was notified that some five hundred tons of opium were being offered by the Chinese Communists after they had swept over China and forced the nationalists to withdraw to Formosa. I contacted our narcotics people in the United States, recommending that this opium be purchased by the U.S. Government and held in storage in the United States or destroyed. I felt that if this opium were not purchased through legitimate channels—and the cost of opium through legitimate channels was really very low—then it would be distributed through illicit channels and eventually would reach the United States as well as Japan and, thereby, complicate the enforcement of our narcotics laws at great expense to both nations. For reasons unknown to me, my recommendation was not favorably considered. Shortly thereafter, our problem of trying to prevent the smuggling to narcotics from the mainland of Asia was tremendously increased.

18

Welfare

There are four basic elements to a nationwide program that has as its objective the health of the people: public health or preventive medicine; medical care; welfare; and social security. No one of these elements should dominate the others, as occurs in many governmental organizations. The need for integrating co-equally these four foundation stones of a sound health and welfare program is illustrated by the example of tuberculosis. Preventive medicine programs uncover or discover active clinical cases of tuberculosis. Removing a person from circulation during the infectious state can prevent additional people from becoming infected. Therefore, we desire to treat this person in a medical care program. We must provide the necessary integrated medical care program to arrest his case, so that he can return as a useful citizen to his community and, in the meantime, will not serve as a source for infecting new cases. Though a high quality medical care program has been provided, if the individual is unable to take advantage of this treatment because he will be without income and will be unable to look after his family, we immediately enter into the realm of welfare in its broader sense. Social security is one aspect of using an insurance principle to provide financial support under such circumstances for the industrial portion of a population. It is an important element in providing a balance among the activities necessary if we are to prevent disease and unrest and improve the health of the people of a nation.

Welfare was one of our major activities.[1] Some 2.5 million homes in Japan were destroyed and some 8 million individuals dispersed into the countryside during the war. The food-rationing system had broken down. There was a constant movement of people into and out of the burned-out areas. Those remaining in the areas or those who had returned were without homes and without food. There were thousands of orphans living in the rubble of the cities, without parents, without homes, or without means of sustenance. In addition, 6.5 million individuals were due to be repatriated to Japan. Many of these individuals had been born in Manchuria or the Philippines or other parts of the Far East, and they had never lived in Japan. They could bring only that which they could carry and the equivalent of one thousand yen. This situation resulted in a gigantic welfare problem, which, in magnitude, equalled or exceeded that in any other part of the world that we know of, with the exception perhaps of Russia.

Nationwide Relief and Population Movement

There were several possible solutions to this problem. We could have gathered together the refugees and the war-sufferers, as they were known, in huge concentration camps. This solution would have involved an accepted principle of handling refugees in which the people are maintained in idleness in these encampments. Food is brought in and soup kitchens are established. Unfortunately, it is bad for the people concerned; the years pass and there is little incentive for them to seek to be self-sufficient. Frequently, a residual portion of the refugees become permanent residents of a refugee camp.

After considerable study, I decided to try a different approach, which had its advantages and its disadvantages. If we kept the refugees dispersed in small communities, they could, at least, assist in growing food, which was an advantage.[2] Then, as the cities were rebuilt and industry re-established, they could become self-sufficient in their old environment. The disadvantage to this plan was that instead of having a limited number of tremendous refugee camps to which food could be distributed and clothing and medical care provided, it involved setting up a nationwide relief organization for the distribution of essentials of food, clothing, medical care, and preventive medicine throughout the nation.

Therefore, with the approval of the Supreme Commander, I directed a population movement order prohibiting the return of refugees to the destroyed cities unless the individual had a job and a place to live.[3] This order could be enforced not only because such individuals were unable to buy rail transportation tickets but also because they had no ration cards to use in obtaining food if they walked into the cities. It was so effective that, although I felt the need for this order was probably over by 1947, the Japanese Government requested that it be extended. It was extended until 1949, when the major portions of the cities had been rebuilt and jobs had been re-established, and population movement restrictions were no longer required.

The second action which had to go hand-in-glove with the restriction of population movement was a revolutionary step for Japan—in fact, for any nation —to take. To briefly indicate why this was revolutionary, it is necessary to understand the Japanese attitude toward public assistance. The very closely knit and strong family system required, under a system of obligations, that the individual take care of his own. The family took care of its relatives who became destitute and needy; but there was no obligation to take care of a stranger who might be starving and literally dying in the street in front of your door.

There had been some private welfare work in various welfare institutions established in Japan before the war. They were literally charity institutions and had been subsidized by grants from the emperor or empress or from wealthy Japanese industrialists. They apparently sufficed to meet the needs to a degree under the prewar conditions; but the magnitude of the public assistance problem at the end of the war was far beyond the capabilities of any such concept of charity based on categories such as the aged or homeless children.

In the fall of 1945, we directed the Japanese Government to establish a program in which the government accepted responsibility—in this case, the national government—for the provision of the essential food, clothing, shelter, medical care, and subsistence needs of the indigent, who were indigent through no fault of their own. The indigent population was approximately 14.5 million people. This program later became established under a law known as the Daily Life Security Law, which was passed by the Diet in response to a SCAP directive of February 1946.[4] The administration of this law operated in conjunction with other steps we took.

In the many conferences held with the Japanese concerning this problem, we could not for some time understand each other. We found later that, literally, there was no Japanese word equivalent to the English or American concept of public assistance. Under our concept, "public assistance" differs from "charity," which was the Japanese word. Charity, under their interpretation and under our interpretation, was based on the old concept of crumbs from the table of the wealthy being given to the destitute. In our country prior to the great depression, the Thanksgiving basket of groceries or the Christmas basket which was taken around by the well-intentioned individual to the destitute represented such a concept. A modern concept of public assistance under a democratic interpretation considers that the government as the tool of the people, rather than the master, acts on behalf of the people, if they so desire, in assuming responsibility in carrying out a program of public assistance to those who are indigent through no fault of their own.

Eventually, the modern concept of public assistance was understood by the Japanese, and the law was passed.[5] Approximately 150,000 *minsei-iin*, who were volunteers in the local communities, administered this public assistance law. The initial sources of supplies were the confiscated stocks of the Japanese army and navy clothing and food supplies, which were distributed to the prefectures and local communities for distribution to the destitute.[6]

Because of the continued inflation in Japan, it was necessary to increase the grants of money in lieu of assistance in kind to keep in step with the inflation. Dealing closely with people in the Economics Section, we were able to keep these grants just a little behind the inflation, thereby encouraging people to leave the public assistance rolls as quickly as possible, rather than to live in comfort in idleness.

After this law had been in operation for a number of years, the residual group of people on public assistance represented about 1.5 million people, including those in institutions as well as those receiving assistance in their own homes or the homes of neighbors or relatives. This final hard core of public assistance recipients was largely made up of widows and orphan children and aged people. Then came the difficult decision about what to do about able-bodied, young war widows with children. One of my welfare staff members felt that such widows should be required to accept a job, if one were made available, and that the children should be placed in nurseries or institutions. Eventually, I decided it was more desirable for the mother to raise her own children; it was certainly most desirable for the benefit of the children that they should have a home rather than become wards of the state and become institutionalized. I decided that a young mother who had children would remain entitled to public assistance until the children were able to assist in the support of the family. It was one of the difficult decisions about a controversial subject which must be made and which can have very far-reaching effects on many people over the years.

Rehabilitation of Repatriates

In conjunction with this public assistance law, which also provided for the medical care of the indigent, a program was developed particularly for the rehabilitation of repatriates from other countries who had returned to Japan, so they could become self-sufficient as quickly as possible. A system of loans was begun so that a man who had a trade before he came back to Japan could acquire tools and re-establish himself in his trade. If he had been a farmer, he could obtain a loan for the simple hand tools used by Japanese farmers and for seeds and the acquisition or rental of land. If he had been in business, as many as thirty such individuals could get together and pool their loans and re-establish themselves in business. This program worked. The loans were initially for five years, but the repayment was very rapid. At the end of some four years, eighty percent of the initial loans made during the first year had been paid.

Rehabilitation of Handicapped People

We also undertook a rehabilitation program for some 600,000 physically handicapped people in Japan. Miss Helen Keller, the world famous physically handicapped lady, was invited to Japan to stimulate interest and public awareness of the need for such a program. A model center for physical rehabilitation and vocational training was established. Under the rehabilitation law which was passed and placed in effect, this center was expanded to eighteen such centers at the end of the occupation.

Child Welfare

One of our most significant accomplishments was the establishment of a child welfare program. This phase of the welfare program was to provide for the thousands of so-called war orphans who were living in the cities in squalor. Our first progressive measures were to round up these children, examine them for illness, clean them up, and place them in institutions. As a matter of philosophy,

I have felt that it is not good for a child to live out his entire youth in an institution without the benefit of a family life. Although we initially gathered these children into institutions, our subsequent program was to attempt to find foster homes for these children into which they could be placed.

This program involved then, for the first time in the history of Japan, the passage of a Child Welfare Law. Following the passage of this law, child welfare centers were established, people were especially trained in handling children, foster homes were carefully inspected, and supervision was maintained over the welfare of children who were placed in these foster homes. I might add that a Child Welfare Bureau was established in the Ministry of Health and Welfare. The first chief of this bureau was a Japanese woman, the first female bureau chief in the history of Japan. This lady was a graduate of the New York School of Social Work and was one of the few qualified social workers who had been trained outside of Japan.

The sale of children into indenture was one of the problems which we encountered in Japan. It is not necessarily peculiar to Japan and is found in many other underdeveloped countries. This problem, of course, existed in our own country years ago when children were placed to work in a trade, as an apprentice, or on a farm, as a farm hand, under agreements for a given sum of money. With the progress of civilization, such procedures have been considered practically immoral. The abolition of the sale of children, like the sale of girls into prostitution, was carried out.

One of our techniques in inaugurating a new program such as the child welfare program was to bring to Japan as a consultant an outstanding representative in the field. In this case, Father Flanagan of Boys Town was the consultant. He was taken on a tour of Japan, in which he gave many talks to various groups pointing out the importance of the welfare of the children. He aroused public interest and support for the program. It is a valuable technique when such a program is to be inaugurated in a country in which the concept is entirely new.

Welfare Districts

As time passed, and as progress was made in rebuilding the cities and rehabilitating the industries, it became apparent, as it has become apparent in the United States, that the local political jurisdiction is not necessarily the ideal unit for the administration of such a program. In 1951, the Daily Life Security Law was amended to establish welfare districts. Because we were dealing with population units, as in the health field, these districts coincided with the health center districts. Also, it was found that for greater efficiency in the administration of such a program, a much smaller organization could be utilized if the members of the organization were well trained in the various aspects of social work. Full-time staffs were eventually trained not only for the administration of the public assistance law but also for the child welfare law and other welfare laws that we

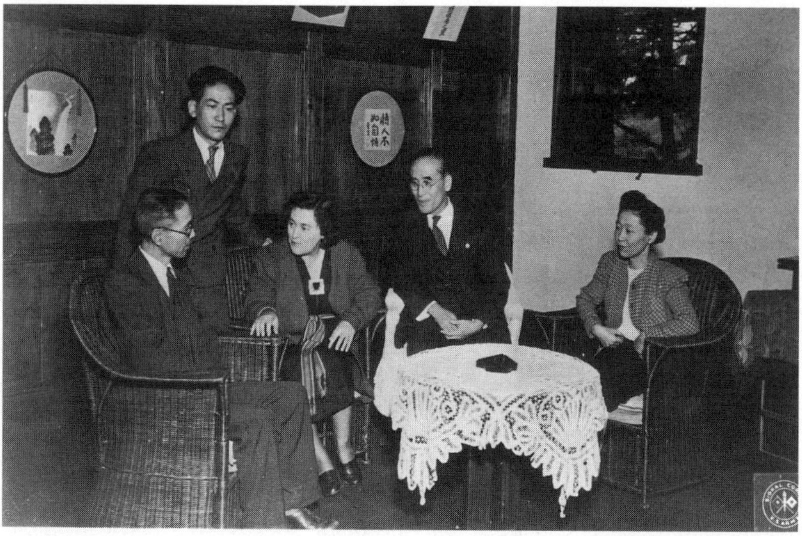

Figure 20. Although social work was not recognized as a profession in Japan at the beginning of the occupation, SCAP's social work consultants worked with social work and welfare organizations to develop schools of social work, establish public assistance and child welfare laws, and develop welfare and rehabilitation programs for war widows, orphans, and repatriates. Tokyo, 7 October 1948. Left to right: Aoki Hideo (Head, Japan Social Work Association), Imaoka Keniichiro (Head, Japan School of Social Work), Florence Brugger (Social Work Training Supervisor, PHW, SCAP), Hara Taiichi (President, All-Japan Welfare Association), Ohata Tane (Technical Advisor on Social Work in Japan to PHW, SCAP). Photo Credit: U.S. Army Signal Corps, Photographer Sarabia. (Courtesy of the Hoover Institution Archives, Stanford University.)

inaugurated. As in the field of preventive medicine and medical care, it took time to establish training centers, because social work training as such and social work as a profession were not recognized in Japan prior to the occupation.

The Profession of Social Work

The usual steps were taken in attempting to gain recognition for social work as a profession. A national professional association was organized. Licensing requirements were set up for social workers. We followed the pattern that was used in other fields, which has now become familiar.

We established a school of social work in Tokyo, and then expanded this program to a second school in Osaka. Subsequently, we were able to introduce an emphasis on training social workers into the universities to meet the requirements of a continuing program in the field of public assistance, child welfare, maternal and child health, and other aspects of welfare.

Private Welfare Organizations

In addition to the nationwide governmental programs in welfare initiated by SCAP, I would like to indicate my philosophy on the place of private welfare organizations and programs in relation to governmental activities. Japan had a few charity organizations. I felt, however, that the establishment of well-run privately sponsored institutions and programs should be encouraged in Japan, because, to me, the basic purpose of a private welfare program is to pioneer a new program to meet a need which has been identified. If the approach to the problem is sound and the need is met, then extension of the program may well be carried out by turning that program over to government organizations which can finance such expanded programs. The private welfare organization should then go on into new fields. I recognized, in studying social work, that such a procedure is seldom carried out. Frequently, we find in some of our communities at home a multitude of private welfare organizations which have been in existence for years and have outlived their usefulness; yet, I still feel that private welfare organizations should be encouraged to pioneer in new fields and programs.

A law was finally passed in Japan for the encouragement of private welfare activities, which involved the inspection and licensing and establishment of standards for homes for the aged, children's institutions, and other organizations to ensure adequate services. One of the basic differences between Japan and our country is that in Japan it is not permitted under the current Constitution to utilize government funds to be expended by private welfare or other private organizations. This, I think, is a good law. It does minimize what might be called racketeering through the utilization of government funds and diversion of those funds for the benefit of certain individuals or groups.

To meet the need for funds for private welfare, we inaugurated for the first time in Japan the concept of a public fund drive for private welfare. The first such drive was carried out in 1947. It became known as the Community Chest Organization, in which a fund drive is established on a nationwide basis for all private charity organizations. The allocation of these funds among the various private organizations is carried out by community committees.

International Relief Organizations

After the end of the war, many American relief organizations, religious groups, and other agencies, desired to send relief supplies to Japan, as they had sent to Europe. After considerable negotiation through Washington, D.C., Licensed Agencies for Relief in Asia (LARA) was established, which represented all of the various relief organizations, particularly private organizations, which desired to donate supplies of food, clothing, and medical supplies to the Japanese people. By agreement, such supplies were shipped to Japan on government transportation, regardless of their source; the PHW Section of SCAP was then responsible for their distribution.

It was the natural desire for a given religious organization in the United States to ship food and clothing directly to its religious affiliates in Japan. We in SCAP, however, were in a difficult position. Japan was not a Christian organization; there were only about 100,000 Christians in the population. If we diverted our relief activities to that small segment of the population, the implication would immediately arise that we were giving preferential treatment to Christians. Therefore, we as a governmental agency would be charged with favoritism. It was agreed that, although many of the supplies came from religious organizations, they would be distributed without regard to religious or other affiliation among the destitute in Japan on a priority basis of need, rather than religious or other beliefs. Three representatives of LARA—one representing the Catholic Church; one the Friends Service Committee; and one the World Church Alliance, a Protestant group—were attached to my staff to provide liaison to their parent organizations as to how we were utilizing the donated gifts.

I felt this was a very important part of our welfare program. Although the quantity of supplies, measured in tonnage, which was received in Japan through private charity organizations was a drop in the bucket as far as meeting the needs, it still represented, so far as I was concerned, something far more important than the actual physical items supplied: It represented to the Japanese people that the American people as such had an individual and personal interest in their welfare. By 1950, when recovery of the Japanese nation was well under way, we felt it advisable, because all of the basic needs of the people had been met, to do away with this restriction on the distribution of supplies from various private groups in America to their counterparts in Japan; yet, LARA had worked so well to the satisfaction of both the Japanese and the Americans involved that they decided to continue the organization. We, therefore, stated that they would then be free, as the occupation was nearing its end, to negotiate an agreement directly with the Japanese Government, which was about to become a sovereign government, for continuation of the program. An agreement was made in which pooled supplies would be shipped to Japan and distributed by the Japanese governmental welfare organizations without regard to the religious or other beliefs of the recipients after the end of the occupation.

CARE, the Cooperative Agencies for Remittances to Europe, Inc., also desired to extend its operations to Japan. In August 1947, an agreement was reached whereby CARE was authorized to ship its packages to Japan for distribution. The first shipments were received in July 1948.

In my constant efforts to seek sources to meet the requirements for powdered skim milk to extend the school lunch program, I had noted in a press release that the United Nations Children's Emergency Relief Fund (UNICEF) was shipping powdered skim milk to Germany. Their previous activities had been limited to relief for children in so-called liberated countries. No supplies had been shipped to former enemy countries, such as Germany or Japan. I immediately sent a message back through Washington, D.C., requesting that UNICEF be invited to come to Japan and to contribute powdered skim milk to the school lunch program.[7] Miss Marguerita Strahler, who was an old Japanese hand whom I had first met when she was with the International Committee of the Red Cross in 1945, came to Japan again, this time as the Japanese representative of UNICEF.

The Red Cross

In accordance with the original concept of the national Red Cross societies, the Japanese Red Cross had been a medical organization concerned with the care of wounded soldiers in time of war and, as such, operated hospitals and clinics throughout Japan. Because the Japanese army and navy were abolished, a reorganization and reorientation of the Japanese Red Cross was undertaken. By agreement with representatives of the American Red Cross, my staff was loaned a group of highly qualified people who then carried out the reorganization of the Japanese Red Cross. The Japanese Society, which was then the second largest national Red Cross Society in the world, retained its basic function in the operation of hospitals and clinics and training schools for nurses as part of the overall privately operated medical care program in Japan; but, in addition, emphasis was given to other functions of the Red Cross, such as life saving, Junior Red Cross, and disaster relief. The Japanese Red Cross became the organization to coordinate the relief activities of nongovernmental agencies in time of disaster.

Disaster Relief

Japan is a nation of disasters: typhoons; fires, which destroy entire cities; and earthquakes, which are constantly occurring. On Christmas 1945, an earthquake shook some fourteen prefectures of Japan, including the major island of Shikoku and the neighboring prefectures along the Inland Sea. Prior to the end of the war, the Japanese army and navy had carried out disaster relief activities; however, under policy directives issued to SCAP, both of these organizations as well as the Japanese navy were to be abolished.

As there was no Japanese organization then in existence to handle this widespread disaster, disaster relief was another program in which I became involved. It became necessary then for my own staff to undertake the emergency relief activities. We utilized relief supplies of food, clothing, and medical supplies, which we had imported and held as a reserve for emergency distribution. As a result of this experience, in which a considerable number of lives were lost and much widespread property damage resulted, particularly from a tidal wave, we realized that we must establish a nationwide civilian disaster relief organization.

I believed certain basic concepts were necessary if such an organization were to function. First, there must be a governmental organization established to cope with national disaster; it must be in existence at all times. Second, there must be available in regional or other warehouses existing stocks of food, clothing, and medical supplies which could be utilized in any part of the country when required by disaster. Third, there must be an appropriation of funds by government to finance national disaster relief, rather than to depend upon a fund drive after a disaster.

Ralph Riordan of my welfare staff deserves great credit for outlining a National Disaster Relief Organization, which was an entirely civilian organization. It required a law that made it possible to have funds and personnel and supplies available in order to function. Such a law was passed in 1947. An important safeguard was incorporated into this law. The safeguard states that as far as the national treasury is concerned, financial contributions will be made only if the total relief costs exceed five percent of the total property value and business tax income of the communities. This safeguard encourages the handling of local disasters by local agencies and the funding of local disasters by local and prefectural agencies rather than running with a hand out to the national government when a house burns down.

The National Disaster Relief Organization included the establishment of organizations at the national, prefectural, and operating levels: a National Disaster Board, which was headed by the prime minister and included all cabinet ministers; Prefecture Disaster Boards; and operating teams comprised of police, health officials, welfare officials, economics officials, transportation officials, firemen, and engineers. We felt this National Disaster Relief Organization established a pattern which was new among nations.

The first test of this organization occurred with the great flood of the Kanto Plain area in September 1947, when some 1.7 million families were flooded out. The second test occurred in the Fukui earthquake in June 1948. The organization was successful. It is now a permanent part of the civil government and social structure of Japan.

By the end of the occupation, Japan had undergone a revolution from a very backward concept of welfare to one of the most modern concepts. Commander Bouters, followed by Mr. Nelson Neff and Mr. Markuson, were, in turn, chief of the Welfare Division. To them and the members of their division staff goes great credit for the success of the welfare program in this wartorn country. During the rebuilding of a partially destroyed nation in which one out of five persons was destitute, they were able to provide the emergency relief required and, at the same time, inaugurate permanent welfare programs which will benefit the Japanese people throughout future years.

19

Social Security

Social security can ruin a nation or be of great benefit, depending on how it is handled. The modern concept of social security was developed in Germany in the days of Bismarck, to meet certain hazards inherent in the evolution from an agricultural into an industrial society. When an individual enters the work force of an industrial society, he is subjected to certain hazards which do not exist, at least to the same degree, in an agricultural society or which he can protect himself against through his own efforts. The basic hazards inherent in an industrial society are four in number: unemployment; sickness; temporary or permanent disability that prevents the individual from earning an income; and old age and the provision of some financial security for survivors in the event of death of the wage earner. When a man is no longer acceptable in an industrial work force because of old age, he has a hazard not inherent in an agricultural society.

Japan had copied in form the western ideas of social security using the insurance principle, thereby spreading the risk against these hazards through the institution of insurance systems, to which both worker and employer contributed, to provide against the four major hazards characteristic of the industrial age. The legal basis for this system extended back many years before the occupation and was a hodgepodge of legislation.

By the end of the occupation, after considerable study and reorganization and the passing of additional laws, some 68 million individuals in Japan had some form of coverage under one or another of the various social security programs.[1] During the occupation, a Workmen's Compensation Law was placed in effect, providing for benefits to be paid to injured or disabled workers. Another law providing for unemployment insurance was placed into effect by the Economics Section of SCAP.

Health Insurance Programs

In the field of health insurance, there were several programs. First, there is a health insurance program for industrial workers in which the employer and the employee make their joint contributions through payroll deductions. This program provides medical care for the employee and his family. The way in which this medical care is provided is through one of several systems. The individual may go to any doctor or hospital of his choice, and the expenses within the fee scales are paid out of the insurance fund. The employees of the particular plant, through their own council, may establish a clinic and hospital of their own and employ doctors to provide this medical care, or they may contract with existing hospitals or doctors.

For the nonindustrial worker, there is a system in which any community that desires to establish a local health insurance society may hold an election and, if the majority so desires, establish such a society. The contributions in the form of premiums are paid by the members and, under the principle that the majority shall prevail, this contribution is obligatory on all of the members of this local community once the people have voted. The benefits are provided either by the members going to any doctor or hospital of their choice, or the society itself (if it is large enough) may, if it so desires, establish and operate its own hospital and employ its own medical personnel.

One of the important elements of this particular coverage is that it applies nationwide, so that an individual may belong to a society in one town and then move to another and his benefits are transferred to the new society. There is a federation of local health insurance societies which makes it possible for all nonindustrial workers to provide themselves with insurance against medical care expenses. In the case of the medically indigent who cannot afford to pay premiums to such a society, their medical care expenses are provided for, again, through any doctor or hospital of their choice through the Daily Life Security Law.

I had an important decision to make after the Daily Life Security Law had been in effect for a number of years and the immediate postwar relief problem had been met. A considerable proportion of the total funds of the Daily Life Security Law was expended in paying the medical bills of the medically indigent.[2] One solution, of course, to this problem would be to pay premiums to one of the local health insurance societies, thereby spreading the risk, using the Daily Life Security Law funds for such premium payments. It is believed that, ultimately, the cost would be less so far as that particular program is concerned.

It is interesting to note that, under such a combination of systems, every Japanese has medical care provided under a system of health insurance, either through industrial health insurance, the voluntary local societies, or the Daily Life Security Law. The principle that doctors should carry the burden of charity work in the medical field out of all proportion to their numbers no longer exists in Japan. The financial burden is spread where it belongs, among all of the people who benefit from such medical service.

I want to emphasize that this reorganization, which took some six years, adhered to the principle of avoiding a national system of compulsory health insurance in which freedom of choice of doctors and hospitals is denied to the recipients of such a service. We did not like the idea of state medicine, which is so common in many countries. It tends to stifle the initiative of the medical and allied professions in improving the quality of medical care, because there is no economic incentive for such improvement. It overburdens the professional groups with endless routine and excessive numbers of patients who are not really ill. It leads to many abuses. We have also maintained the principles of the freedom of choice of doctors and of nurses and the principle of the private practice of medicine. We have reconciled such a principle with avoidance of the financial catastrophe that may occur to anyone or any family through illness or injury.

Inflation and Taxes

One of the problems I had, of course, was the effect of inflation upon the reserves which had already been accumulated, because with the depreciation in the value of the currency, we could not hope to provide the benefits which they had been established to provide. There had been some ten thousand local health insurance societies, about two-thirds of which went broke during the period of rapid inflation immediately after the end of the war. They ceased to function for the simple reason that the contributors had paid in premiums insuring against sickness when the yen was worth 4.5 to the dollar, but the total funds available to the societies were not enough when it came to paying out benefits under an inflation of 390 yen to the dollar. Likewise, for old age benefits, the money that had been contributed over the years, which was to provide an income for the laborer who had passed the working age, was sharply losing its value by simply being held in trust during inflation.

After consultation with many of our financial experts and others, I adopted a principle that had been tried and that had worked successfully in other countries which had sound social security programs, without being socialistic, and which had gone through a period of inflation. The principle was to use general tax money to make up the deficit between the value of the currency at the time it was paid in, as premiums or payroll deductions, and its lowered value at the time it was paid out in benefits. This principle was carried out during the period of rapid inflation. It was no longer needed when Joseph Dodge so successfully stabilized the value of the currency in Japan from 1948 through 1950. It was a temporary expedient which saved the financial stability of the entire social security program.

Unemployment, Inflation, and the Family System

The *zaibatsu*, the great industrial family combines, which actually controlled most of the wealth of Japan and most of the commerce and industry, were very paternalistic. During the period of comparatively little industrial activity at the beginning of the occupation, when war plants were closed by edict, these companies kept an excessive number of employees on their payrolls. It was a case of stretching out the work, a device which was used in our own country during the days of depression.

In discussing the effect of some of the fiscal policies to be undertaken by SCAP on our health and welfare programs, we had to resolve an interesting controversy. One group of the economics and labor people in SCAP thought that it would be wise if the big industrial corporations would reduce their payrolls. They felt that these payrolls were excessive in relation to production demand, which was undoubtedly true under the circumstances. This employment was quite obviously a major element contributing to inflation. On the other hand, if these people became unemployed (and I had my social security people make studies in connection with the labor people of the Economics Section), it was felt that there would be a tremendous impact on the welfare program; that is, the public assistance program as well as the social security program. If the estimated number of unemployed developed, subsequent to ringing the water out of the payrolls in industry, our costs for public assistance then would increase tremendously. This sort of thing raised an issue that required a very fundamental decision. Was it better to keep a man actually working at fifty percent capacity on a payroll?—He at least produced something for the money received, which in turn enabled industry to contribute taxes to the government.—Or was it better, as an anti-inflationary measure, to discharge this man and place him on unemployment benefits for the limited time provided by the social security law and, subsequently, on public assistance rolls, whereby he would receive certain benefits and produce nothing?—If he were placed on public assistance, then the tax cost for the whole country would increase. This increase would occur at a time when we were putting pressures on industry that would reduce their capacity to contribute to the tax revenue.

This very fundamental issue is a question which any country going through a period of either inflation or deflation frequently has to ask itself, although I am afraid many measures are taken without such soul-searching decisions actually being made and without knowing the full impact of the decisions. It was felt, after many discussions, that the continued padding of the payroll and its major contribution to inflation was a greater detriment in the long run to the economy of the country and the welfare of the people than any temporary increase in public assistance costs which might result from such increased unemployment. Steps were undertaken to implement this decision. We very carefully watched increases month-by-month in our public assistance load. There was a temporary increase, which fortunately did not last more than a year.

This increase was an interesting phenomena. There were many reasons, we believed, behind the fact that there was not a larger increase, such as had been anticipated. My personal belief, after going over many studies, is that the close family system which has been a part of Japanese society made it possible for men temporarily out of work to be helped by other members of the family. The family in Japan is not simply a father and mother and four children; in Japan, brothers help brothers and sisters, young people look after the old, and they all look after the cousins and aunts. It is a very closely knit group, this family unit, which then is amalgamated into what we might call a clan. I believe that the public assistance load would have shown a very large and sharp increase in a country such as the United States, or in Western Europe, where the family system largely has broken down and dependence on government has replaced such family self-sufficiency.

In Japan, it was the strong family system that prevented such a peak. People were unwilling to go on public assistance after unemployment benefits ended until the entire family resources had been exhausted. I think it is a great tribute to the willingness of the Japanese to attempt to retain self-sufficiency and stand on their own feet under very arduous and adverse conditions.

Controversies of State Medicine

I have noted our policies and philosophy in the social security field, which were approved by General MacArthur, because in 1946, a labor advisory group visited Japan at the invitation of the Labor Division of the Economics Section of SCAP. This group recommended that SCAP undertake a study of the social security system to protect it against collapse as a result of the inflation which was well underway at the time. Subsequently, in 1947, a second mission, from the old Federal Security Agency in the United States, was invited to visit Japan to make a study and give us their advice and recommendations.

While this mission was in Japan, a certain American congressman thought that he had discovered a deep dark plot on the part of certain individuals in the Federal Security Agency of the United States to work through my section of SCAP and impose state medicine and compulsory national health insurance in Japan. This issue became a matter of public controversy back home. We were immediately besieged by the proponents and opponents in the United States. As a result, we invited a mission of the American Medical Association to come to Japan and review the situation and to make their recommendations. It must be recalled that during the years from 1946 through 1949, a great controversy in our country was underway between the medical profession and those who would impose socialized state medicine on the American people. It was this controversy that apparently led to suspicion of a plot to impose such a system on Japan.

We were able to show to the various groups concerned what we were doing and why we were doing these things. We received not only the endorsement but the support of the American medical profession in carrying out our program. I have been particularly interested in the gradual evolution of a pattern in our own country which is paralleling that which we developed in Japan. I believe it is sound. I believe it is economically sound. I believe that it is socially wise without being socialistic and that it is free of elements of compulsion that are characteristic of the dictatorship known as a welfare state.

Another one of the issues at the time of the controversy in America, which unfortunately through the press and other means was extended to our activities in Japan, was an attempt on the part of the Social Security Commission, which was part of the Federal Security Agency, to dominate the preventive medicine (known in the United States as public health), the medical care, and the welfare fields through financial control. I cannot emphasize too often or too strongly my feeling that no single element, either the medical or the welfare or the social security element, should dominate any of the others. They should all be coordinated by a chief and should be considered as co-equal and integrated programs. That principle has been constantly emphasized in my conversations and talks with various groups. I believe it to be sound to this day. It was a principle that we carried out in our programs in Japan.

Lessons for the United States

I would suggest, however, these cautions in our country as a result of lessons I have learned in my own experience in having such a program in another nation. First, we found that if complete nationwide coverage were carried out against the four hazards which are characteristic in industrial societies, some 27 percent of the total national productive income would be required to finance such a program. Such financing of total nationwide coverage can only be accomplished under a managed currency system with a gradual creeping inflation that ultimately has only one end, whether measured in years or decades. That end is financial collapse.

The basic weakness in such a philosophy, which is being carried out step by step in our own country following the pattern of certain socialistic European countries, is to gradually extend coverage against a hazard to the total population when the hazard actually exists for only a small segment of the population, the industrial workers and their families. The risk of unemployment, disability, and old age and survivors benefits under social security should be limited basically to that segment of the population in the industrial work force which even in our own country represents less than 30 percent of our population. To attempt to extend protection against a hazard that does not exist in the same magnitude to the total population can lead to utter financial collapse.

An explanation of this assertion is perhaps desirable. Under any system so far devised to provide financial security to the people of an industrial society, there are usually governmental programs and nongovernmental social security programs. The nongovernmental programs are usually health and welfare and pension plans developed through labor union and employer negotiations. They may be operated and controlled by labor unions or employers. They supplement the governmental programs in the provision of benefits. Whether they are governmental or nongovernmental, they can be financed only by contributions from industry or payroll deductions of labor or both.

As time passes, there are constant pressures both on government and private industry for greater benefits. Greater contributions are required to provide these benefits. These lead to pressures for wage increases by labor to offset the loss in take home pay. These demands in turn lead to price increases by industry in order to pass on to the consumer the increased contributions and increased wages. If increased productivity accompanies such increases in wages, the inflationary pressures generated can be kept under control; but when such increased productivity has reached its limit, then a vicious inflationary cycle is established, which can only accelerate. The decreased purchasing power of the currency accelerates the pressures for increases in benefits, and the Frankenstein created to provide benefits is out of control and, ultimately, financially destroys itself and those whom it was designed to benefit. There are, of course, other factors. When coverage is extensive, there is little incentive to save for a rainy day or old age. Money is, therefore, spent more freely, increasing the demand for goods, again generating additional inflationary pressures.

The sums of money involved in nationwide governmental and nongovernmental social security programs are so vast that they can be one of the major elements in the economy contributing to inflation. In Japan, as I have emphasized, the equivalent of one out of four dollars of the total national production would have been required to give complete financial security to the whole population from before birth to the grave, as advocated by some of the extremist proponents of the welfare state.

There are some excellent examples in Western Europe of the final stages of such social security programs, which lead to economic collapse. On the other hand, there are examples to be studied in other nations, including Japan, where the social security programs have been kept in balance, and pressures for unreasonable expansion beyond needs have been checked. I suggest that those in our government, industry, and labor who are interested in social security study these examples before the Frankenstein gets out of control or, to mix metaphors, before the goose that lays the golden eggs is killed by demanding too many golden eggs. Human greed is a terrible thing.

20

The Communist Activities

Our nationwide programs in the health and welfare fields were carried out with some difficulties. One of the difficulties was the attempt of the communists to discredit, undermine, and eventually overthrow the occupation. We in the health and welfare field were constantly on guard, because we knew very well that the programs which the communists desired to infiltrate, and to eventually control, were those that affect the fundamentals of the daily life of the greatest number of people. Such programs, of course, include those in health and welfare. They also include programs involving educational and information fields and, of course, labor activities. I shall try to illustrate a few of the instances which were of direct concern to me.[1]

The Sources

The principal sources of communist activities were three in number. First were the Russian Communists who were members of the Russian Mission, headed by General Dryvenko. Second were the Japanese Communists. Third were the American Communists who served in the occupation. Actually, all three groups worked together.

The Russian Communists

When we first moved into Japan from the Philippines, there was a Russian military liaison group, headed by General Dryvenko, attached to General Headquarters, because the Russians had entered the war on the eighth of August, a few days before the surrender. When the occupation began, the Russians attempted, on the diplomatic level, to take over Hokkaido and to have the Japanese islands divided into zones similar to the pattern adopted in the occupation of Germany. Dryvenko attempted to bring in some five hundred people from Russia as part of his staff. As they began to come in, it was apparent that they were very highly skilled technical people in all fields from communications to medicine and engineering. There could be little doubt that they were there for technical intelligence purposes. They were a nucleus, actually, of anti-occupation and anti-American propaganda and intrigue. As soon as this became apparent, General MacArthur limited their request from five hundred to some three hundred people.

The Japanese Communists

The Japanese had thrown their communists into jail as political prisoners. Some of the leaders had been in jail for several years before the occupation. Under the directives which SCAP received from Washington, D.C., all political prisoners were to be released. One of the first things that was done under these directives was to take the communists out of jail and dust them off and set them up in business. The Japanese Communist party became very active.

The American Communists

During the process of recruiting civilian employees to staff the many activities of SCAP, and later the military government teams, when civilians replaced military personnel, a considerable number of people, let us say, were recruited in Washington, D.C., many from government agencies which had been in existence for some time or which were going through a period of readjustment following the war and were cutting down on personnel and making other readjustments. Many of these people then came to the Far East as civil service employees. Along with their records came information on their status in the Communist party or in communist activities. Of course, this information came through channels.

We could not discharge these people: No U.S. Government employee could be discharged for race, creed, or political beliefs. Until President Truman issued an executive order in 1947 making it possible to get rid of known communists in our own ranks, our hands were pretty well tied. All we could do was to try and protect ourselves by circumscribing their activities, one might say. It was not too successful.

Several had come to my section. One was found to be an active espionage agent after we became suspicious of his activities. Prior to his discharge, he was properly observed over a period of time by the counterintelligence people. He led them, of course, to his contacts with the Russian Mission, the Japanese Communist party, and to certain Americans who they had not suspected of being communists.

It does not take large numbers of communists in key positions to do a great deal of harm. SCAP had been directed to establish and promote a democratic labor organization to begin a nationwide labor organization activity. There was the need and desire for a good strong labor organization in industry to protect the Japanese workers from exploitation, which industry had admittedly done, particularly shortly before the war and during the war. Among the people sent to staff the Labor Division of the Economics Section were some communists.

This particular group of Americans, interestingly enough, began some new activities—going far beyond the directives. They began to organize all government employees into labor unions, as had been done in certain European countries, which was a very dangerous thing to permit. If government employees are permitted to organize into unions and a few unscrupulous leaders get control of that union, the government of a nation can be paralyzed; and the nation can, thereby, be seized. This technique has been one of the means of communist subversion in taking over, apparently without violence, the governments of presumably sovereign nations.

If one placed himself in the position of the Japanese, he would begin to wonder about the attitude of the Americans toward communism. We had released the Japanese Communists from jails where the Japanese had placed them for safekeeping during the war; we had set them up in business. The Japanese through their own system of open ears knew pretty well every move we made. They knew, of course, of the activities of American Communists. Many Japanese apparently believed that Americans were pro-communist. They were somewhat puzzled as to what we were trying to do. This situation reached a climax in the spring of 1946.

A Test of Strength

Health and welfare fields are usually considered somewhat innocuous, but they are the fields most often used to establish precedents, legal or otherwise. The first test of the communist-inspired and communist-organized labor activity was in the health and welfare field. It was a test that involved several principles.

Under the new Labor Standards Law, which had been put into effect and which was the desirable law, the communists organized unions of doctors, nurses, and patients in hospitals. We knew pretty well what was going on: The communist leader of the Doctors, Nurses and Patients Union in the Central Red Cross Hospital had used intimidation procedures and so forth to force nurses to join the union. I raised the question whether a patient in a hospital was an employee or an employer. You could look at him both ways; but I could not for the life of me see where patients could be members of a Doctors, Nurses, and Patients Union.

The Doctors, Nurses, and Patients Union demanded that they should take over the management and control of the Japanese Red Cross hospitals. This demand tested two things: Were the unions strong enough to demand to take over the entire management? Could they get away with it in a non-governmental group of hospitals, such as the Japanese Red Cross hospitals?

The doctor's union demanded simultaneously that they should take over the operation of the Tokyo Health Department. This demand also tested a principle: Could organized labor take control of an activity of a local government? The third prong of this attack was to test the policy of SCAP.

Prince Shimadzu, as president of the Japanese Red Cross, came to me with his problem when these demands were made. The questions in the minds of the management element of the Japanese Red Cross were twofold: Was SCAP promoting an economic and social order which involved labor unions taking over control of management functions? Was SCAP supporting the communist element in such labor unions? The Minister of Health and Welfare and the chief of the Tokyo Health Department came to me with the same problem: What was SCAP's policy?

In America about this time, our labor unions were beginning their drives in the health and welfare fields to establish labor union-operated medical programs and health and pension programs, which subsequently reached the point of becoming the subject of congressional action, because of the inevitable corruption which such programs develop when they are uncontrolled by law. The Japanese, frankly, were very much puzzled.

I immediately went to General Whitney of the Government Section, to the Supreme Commander, General MacArthur, and to General Marquat, chief of the Economics Section. I outlined the situation and what I believed these tests signified: Who were we supporting? Which way were we going? I was asked for my recommendations.

I was wholeheartedly in support of a democratic labor movement in industry. I specifically recommended that I be authorized to inform the Japanese who had come to me from government and the private medical fields that SCAP's policy in this situation was to limit the activities of labor unions to negotiations with management in the fields of wages, hours, and working conditions; and that it was not SCAP's policy to support two aspects of labor activity which were now at issue: namely, labor's demands to take over management and policy in private industry and to take over a part of government.

There were extended discussions. I was authorized by General MacArthur to call in the Japanese and to state that the recommendation I had made was SCAP's policy. A written memorandum outlining this policy was handed to the Japanese on behalf of the Supreme Commander, as I had been authorized to do. Within less than twenty-four hours, this policy had swept through Japan like a whirlwind. My office was immediately besieged by a delegation from the Japanese Communist party who wanted to know how it came about that the chief of the Public Health and Welfare Section of SCAP was announcing a labor policy, instead of this coming from the Labor Division of the Economics Section. I immediately reported this to the Supreme Commander, because we had to be on guard in such a large organization, as one does in any large governmental organization, against having one element played against the other. We all had to pull in the same direction and have a united front in dealing with the Japanese. General MacArthur recognized this and directed that the head of the Labor Division should come to my office and, in the presence of the Japanese Communist party delegation, add his signature to the memorandum. That was done.

This particular episode was not widely publicized. It was simply a test of strength; however, it set back the communist activity for some time. Unwilling to admit defeat, they began their activities again. Eventually, they felt that they had sufficient strength to call a general strike the following year. It is well known that General MacArthur forcefully stopped the strike to prevent the overthrow of the Japanese Government. At that time, he reaffirmed the policy that government employees in a democratic country should not be organized into labor unions, because to do so creates a great hazard in which a small group can very quickly paralyze the government and seize control of a nation. For the protection of the people in a democratic country, such a practice should not be permitted.

Propaganda and Public Health Statistics

There were three highly trained Russian medical officers in the Russian Mission who were authorized by the chief-of-staff to be in contact with my section at the beginning of the occupation. In due course, because we were repatriating many Japanese from Russian-held areas, I desired information on the health conditions in the country from which they were coming, with regard to the presence of epidemics of smallpox, typhus, typhoid, and, possibly, plague. We also desired as much information as we could obtain about the Russian medical service. With proper authorization, an agreement was reached whereby we would obtain certain information from the Russian Mission; in turn, we would give them what was actually public information on the disease conditions in Japan, because there was nothing classified about that particular information. Unfortunately, the Russians misinterpreted some of the data.

General MacArthur had informed the Allied Council in Japan that it was an advisory group and not a control body, and that it was not in a position to review his policies unless he requested such advice. It became then a sounding board for Russian propaganda; General Dryvenko, in due course, attacked the programs of each SCAP staff section. When our health and welfare programs began to show a rather dramatic effect after a couple of years and they became the subject of favorable support by the Japanese people as a whole, the Russians began their direct attack on the health and welfare programs in the Allied Council. One of the charges concerned the high tuberculosis rate in Japan, which was admittedly high at that time, but which was dropping very rapidly under the BCG program and other programs we had placed in effect. The Russian propaganda line had been that Russian tuberculosis rates were so low that this situation in Japan was the result of American bungling.

I was called on, of course, to prepare a counterstatement and present it before the Allied Council. This statement was very carefully reviewed by all concerned within SCAP. We were able, in our presentation, to refute all of the statements of the Russians; we believe we made a very effective counterattack. Without disclosing any secrets, I can state that I had received through some roundabout channels the official morbidity and mortality figures of the Russian commissar of health, from the beginning of the Soviet regime after World War I until 1947. I presented a chart showing the Russian rates, the Japanese rates, and the American rates. Of course, the contrasts were striking: The Russian rates had been going up steadily since 1918; the Japanese rates, which had been very high, were rapidly dropping; and, of course, since World War I, the American rates had been steadily dropping.[2]

I thought that General Dryvenko would have apoplexy when he asked where I obtained such information and what was the basis for such statistics. I stated it was the commissar of health of the USSR who had unwittingly furnished the Russian statistics. That promptly terminated any further attempts of the Russian Mission to publicly attack health and welfare programs.

Sabotaging BCG Vaccine

Communists had also infiltrated the Oisa BCG laboratory, which was just outside of Tokyo, where I had concentrated all BCG production of lyophilized vaccine in one laboratory. We had found a very high percentage of this vaccine was being discarded upon our assay tests because of bacterial contamination and other reasons. A very frightened director came to my office and admitted that communists in his organization had threatened his life if he disclosed the fact that they were trying to sabotage this program. Such things are hard for Americans to understand. Human life is so worthless in the eyes of a communist that for simple propaganda purposes they will not hesitate to jeopardize masses of human lives.

This was a very critical program in our health and welfare field. After receiving approval from SCAP, I personally went to the Oisa laboratory and took control of it. We discharged all communist members of that laboratory. Had it been necessary, I would not have hesitated to request that American troops be placed around that laboratory, because of its key position, to ensure that the communists did not again enter its doors. Any individual who will deliberately contaminate vaccine with pathogenic bacteria, hoping to kill people and thereby discredit a program for propaganda purposes, is beneath contempt, as far as I am concerned. We had no further difficulty after this one-man "show of force." Our rejects on assay then dropped very remarkably.

The communists tried one other attack on the BCG program, after issuing public statements that the Russians had a new way of curing tuberculosis by transplanting chicken livers into humans, which was better than the tuberculosis control programs of the Americans. This statement was issued by the Communist party cell in Sendai. The first I knew about this incident was a report that a number of children who had been immunized at one health center in Sendai with BCG had come down with active clinical tuberculosis. I immediately went up there and found that this was true. We immediately put the children under streptomycin therapy and began a very detailed investigation as to what had happened, which took a long time.

We found that these children had been inoculated from one vial of vaccine. The organisms were human tubercle bacilli and not the bovine strain of BCG vaccine. We were eventually able to find a communist who had deliberately inoculated this vial with virulent human tubercle bacilli. To my mind, hanging and drawing and quartering is too lenient a punishment for such individuals.

The Fukai Earthquake Relief

The Fukai earthquake disaster illustrates another aspect of communist activity. Some six hundred or seven hundred people were killed when they were trapped in buildings. Then when the town caught on fire, the death toll ran to about seven thousand. Our disaster relief organization was immediately moved in.[3] Gen. Joe Swing, commander of the I Corps in Kyoto, moved in American military assistance as well. The communists moved in, not with medical assistance or with food and clothing for relief, but with signs. They proceeded to place signs adjacent to all of our aid stations and food distribution stations saying, "This is a gift of the Communist Party." That made me slightly irritated, to say the least. We put on an immediate drive to remove the signs. They kept popping up though, almost as rapidly as we could remove them.

The Case of the Foreign Doctor

There are frequently many individuals in foreign countries who pretend to be doctors of medicine and get away with it for a long time. In one particular case, there was a "foreign doctor" who presented his curriculum vitae to the Japanese at the beginning of the war in 1941, knowing the Japanese could not check its validity in the United States. He claimed to be a graduate of one of our outstanding medical schools. He claimed that he had been employed by one of our outstanding research foundations and had built up a beautiful personal history. Under the old Japanese law, he could not be licensed to practice medicine in Japan without evidence of his graduation from medical school. He became a close friend of the prime minister at the time, who directed that he be permitted to practice in spite of the law. He practiced medicine in Tokyo, and later in Karuizawa, where the European foreign nationals were held during the war.

Immediately after the war, on our arrival in Japan, he came to my office with a curriculum vitae in which he claimed to be a graduate of a well-known Russian medical school. He also claimed that he was a Russian citizen and demanded that I direct the Ministry of Welfare to authorize him to practice medicine and to grant him a license under the new licensing law which we established. As soon as I did a little checking and found that the curriculum vitae which he had given to me was quite different from the one which he had given to the Japanese Ministry of Welfare some five years before, I told him that under the new laws we could not even authorize his appearance before a licensing examining board until he presented photostats of his graduation certificates from medical school. As a Russian citizen, he should present this information through the chief of the Russian Mission, General Dryvenko.

A formal demand was made to SCAP in due course of time that this doctor be licensed to practice as a Russian citizen and a graduate of a medical school under the Russian control. Our reply was that we would be very happy to have him appear before the licensing board just as soon as the Russian Mission forwarded photostats of his graduation from medical school. Nothing was heard officially for several months.

Then we had a report from one of our agents that a member of the Russian Mission had visited this doctor one night. When the Russian Mission member left, this doctor committed suicide. I found out later what I had originally suspected and had been able to verify through channels that I will not disclose, which was that the Russians had found this man was a fraud. He had not graduated from any medical school in Russia or Russian-controlled East Germany. I had checked, at my own expense, the American medical schools and the foundations and the licensing boards mentioned in his previous curriculum vitae and found his claims to be entirely fraudulent. In typical Russian fashion, because he had caused a senior member of the Russian Mission to be publicly embarrassed, he had been visited by a Russian Mission member and told in effect that he was welcome to blow his brains out or to be removed to a slave labor camp in Siberia. This case illustrates a typical Russian Communist technique that just happened to be one of the little things in which I had a direct concern.

The Individual and the State

The communists always took advantage of any error we made, such as in the food shipments of sugar and soybean flour, in which they took a situation and perverted it into a propaganda to their advantage.[4] They were always on their toes looking for any means by which they could discredit or undermine the objectives of the occupation. I do not want to give the impression that they limited their activities to health and welfare programs. They did not. They infiltrated the information and educational fields as well as labor and other activities. They were willing to import and smuggle narcotics into Japan for sale through illicit channels and to use the funds for their Communist party.[5] The mere fact that their funds for propaganda activity came in part from human misery, which accompanies narcotic addiction, was of little or no concern to them.

I mention these things because of my great contempt for the communists. I have dealt with them at firsthand. I have seen their ruthlessness and brutality. I will describe more of it in discussing Korea.

And when our so-called intellectuals in the United States discuss with me, as they have from time to time, the inevitability of communism sweeping the world and its desirability in uplifting the masses, to me they fail to see the bitter pill beneath the sugar coating or they are unwilling to accept reality. So far as the brutality of any dictatorship is concerned, in which the state is the master of the individual, under whatever name it may be—communism, naziism, fascism, romanism, any name—it is bad for the people concerned. Our constant effort in Japan was to attempt to sell the idea that the individual was worth something and that government should be the servant, not the master, of the individual.

21

The Big Question

Our health and welfare programs were having an impact on the daily life of every individual in Japan, and the Japanese were well aware of it. Their children were no longer dying before their eyes. Their communicable disease hospitals were being emptied. There were many other manifestations, including the fact that no one had died of starvation. By so doing, we were literally demonstrating to the Japanese that we considered individual human life worth something as a principle of democracy. This principle was new to their concept, because under their form of dictatorship the state was the master, and human life was to be sacrificed for the emperor or the government without question. We were teaching the principle of democracy by demonstration, which is the only way that I know to make any teaching last or be really understood or be accepted.[1]

During the occupation, the crude death rate dropped: It dropped from an average annual rate of 18.7 deaths (per 1,000 population) for the seven years prior to the occupation, and from a peak rate of 29.4 deaths in 1945, to a rate of 10.8 deaths in 1950. In the six years from 1947 to 1952, life expectancy at birth increased from 54.0 to 63.0 years for women, and from 50.1 to 59.6 years for men. These changes are attributed to the elimination of early deaths from communicable diseases.[2] Such an accomplishment took about sixty years in our country. It was done in Japan in a very few years.

There had been a great propaganda barrage about population pressure in Japan. It was felt that the population increase in Japan before World War II had caused her to desire to expand; so, many people asked "the big question": "What is this man Sams doing by cutting the death rate so drastically in Japan and saving literally so many millions of lives? Is he creating a new problem? What are you going to do with all the extra people?"

The Far East Commission, the thirteen-nation body which was organized to establish policy for the occupation of Japan, visited Japan just after its organization. In briefing this commission, I discussed our programs and was asked specifically this "big question." Their next question was, "What are you going to do about the birth rate?"

There were two directives that had been adopted by the Far East Commission as their policy directive, which had been initially written in the United States by the State, War, and Navy Coordinating Committee (SWNCC). One directive stated that we should produce a peaceful, stable, democratic Japan, capable of taking its position among the family of nations. The second directive stated that we should keep the level of industrialization in Japan below that of Korea, China, and the Philippines, as I recall, which were all agricultural nations. SCAP could not, as I outlined to the Far East Commission, hope to establish a peaceful, stable, democratic Japan, unless we could stabilize the population. The two directives, therefore, were inconsistent.

Demographic Trends

We had invited some very good demographers to come over as consultants, including Dr. Warren S. Thompson, Dr. Frank W. Notestein, and Dr. Whelpton. In our studies of the birth rates, death rates, marriage rates, and family patterns and their distribution, we had evidence that the birth rate in Japan had dropped by approximately one-third in the nineteen years from 1920 to 1939. This observation was important. In demography, and I shall oversimplify it, if one studies the family pattern—the birth and the death rates—of a nation which is primarily agricultural and is gradually going into the phase of urbanization, one finds that the birth rate eventually drops. Likewise, if one compares the family pattern for urban areas and rural areas of a nation, there is a higher birth rate in the rural areas and a lower birth rate in the urban areas. We might say, therefore, that one of the principles of demography is that children are an economic asset in rural or agricultural communities: There is work for one more pair of hands. There are many variables involved, but the economic risks which led to the development of social security when a man becomes a part of an urbanized industrialized area also tend to cause him to limit his family size, because children are then an economic liability, not an economic asset.

We had found that the rapidly dropping birth rate in Japan between 1920 and 1939 coincided with the shift in population from rural to urban areas. In this period, Japan was going through her industrial expansion. All of these facts, plus the fact that the urban family pattern in Japan consisted of a mother and father and two-and-a-fraction children, while the rural family pattern consisted of a mother and father and four-and-a-fraction children, confirmed my interpretation of the data, which differed from our consultants' interpretations. I believed that if the industrialization of Japan were to be re-established, instead of prohibited, then the population would shift again toward urbanization. Incentives would again be provided for the individual family to limit the number of children and the population could be stabilized.[3]

Some of our highly competent consultants maintained that this would not occur in Japan, although it had admittedly occurred in Europe and was occurring in the United States, until certain other factors developed, such as mechanization of farms, which might change the pattern. Increasing the general standards of living, which we were doing, was a factor which would also tend to minimize a reduction in the birth rate as a result of urbanization. When talking about demographic trends, we were dealing in decades.

The Morgenthau Doctrine

The directive limiting reindustrialization was based on the ill-famed "Morgenthau Doctrine," which Henry Morgenthau had tried to apply in vengeance to the Germans. The same directive had been issued to SCAP, simply changing the word *Germany* to *Japan*. If this directive remained in effect, we could not re-establish those demographic factors which would cause the families voluntarily to limit their size.

General MacArthur asked that I go into considerable detail with Gen. Frank McCoy, the American representative on the Far East Commission, as to these ideas, which I did. Eventually, instructions were received from the Far East Commission to authorize reindustrialization in Japan. This policy was opposed, of course, by Japan's industrial competitors; but in the long run, it was a sound procedure.

Birth Control

One group in America put pressure on us, both in America and through their representatives in Japan, to take no steps to cause a reduction in birth rates. This group was the Catholic Church. Another group representing the Margaret Sanger school of thought, Planned Parenthood, demanded that they be invited to Japan to campaign throughout the country with propaganda demanding the Japanese to limit their families.[4]

In my opinion, both groups were wrong. My contention, after studying the demographic factors which cause nations to grow and change and die, was that it would do no good whatsoever to propagandize and preach birth control, as it was called, if the economic and social structure discouraged birth control. That would be true if we kept Japan an agricultural country. On the other hand, if we set up the necessary demographic factors, then family size would be limited by one means or another by the families themselves, in spite of the religious beliefs of any group of Americans.

During this two-sided propaganda barrage in which I found myself involved and frequently the target, the Japanese were quite amused. To them there was no moral religious issue involved at all. The Japanese, as many other nations, and this goes back throughout history, will limit their families one way or another when the factors are established to provide such an incentive. Abortion, infanticide, and other methods have been commonly practiced to limit family size throughout the world for many, many centuries. The Japanese had used abortion and infanticide to limit families during the period from 1920 to 1939; in fact, they had done so long before the Meiji era. It was not a matter of how to limit the family size in their minds; it was a question of should we or not.

My position was that we must stabilize the population. Our projections showed that it could be done, if we simply did two things.—I should not say "simply," because they were tremendous jobs.—One was to reauthorize and encourage the establishment of industry and urbanization. The other was to make available to the Japanese modern medical means and knowledge for limiting their families when they decided to do it. I maintained that no man and his wife will be dictated to by anyone as to how many children they shall have, whether he is a Hindu, a Japanese, an American, or anyone else. If children are an asset to him, he will have lots of them. If they are not, he will limit the number.

In the meantime, I was attacked in the American press. I received extracts from Catholic journals from little children saying I was going against the way of God, and that I was advocating birth control. I was not propagandizing one way or another about the modern concept of birth control. Through the Institute of Public Health and through the maternal and child hygiene centers, we made available to Japanese professional people modern knowledge on how families can be limited through medical means without harm to the health of mothers or children, if the parents desired to do it. The necessary materials were produced in Japan to meet all demands.

Abortion

I had been taught in accordance with our moral concepts in America that abortion is a terrible thing. I had been taught medically that abortion leads to infections and deaths in the mothers and that it is morally wrong; and, of course, infanticide is legally murder. In some states in the United States, to limit families through the use of modern contraceptives is against the law. I say this only to emphasize that this is our view. The Japanese and other nations do not think that way at all. The most unwise thing we could do in this problem, as in the venereal disease problem, would be to attempt to impose our moral concept in this matter by edict.

In recent years there has been a great hullabaloo in our press about the high abortion rate in Japan. By choice the Japanese preferred abortion to contraception. In Japan, a child is not alive until he or she is born. There is no moral concept as to when life begins, which is still, incidentally, from a legal standpoint, a matter of controversy within various jurisdictions in our own country.

Japanese homes are crowded and frequently ten or twelve people sleep on *tatami* in one room. Under such circumstances, it is quite difficult for a Japanese wife to go through the maneuvers and have the facilities for the use of a cervical cap and jelly contraceptives and the necessary activities later. Many Japanese women prefer to become pregnant and have a legal abortion rather than to use modern contraceptives to prevent the pregnancy in the first place. We must understand that is her choice. Modern contraceptive knowledge is available to Japanese women; all they have to do is to go to a maternal and child hygiene clinic and receive it. Within the last few years there has been a gradual increase in the use of the contraception rather than abortion.

I had been taught, as had all American doctors, that abortions were a very dangerous thing to the health of the mother. Maternal death rates would rise. They did not. The textbooks, again, are wrong. A Catholic priest-correspondent came to me to obtain evidence to show that with the increased abortions in Japan the maternal death rate was rising. It was not. He was disappointed. Abortion is done under aseptic conditions in Japan, where it is legal, and does not increase maternal death rates. When it is done in some dirty back room, as it is done by the hundreds of thousands every year in our own country because it is illegal, maternal death rates and morbidity rates from infection do increase.

I do not advocate legalization of promiscuous abortions in our own country. Our moral and ethical standards do not condone such a practice. I use this as one more illustration of the fact that from a medical standpoint our teachings on the hazard are not borne out under the conditions I have described in another country.

A Demographic Bet

As the reindustrialization of Japan was accomplished, I won a small bet with one of my consultants. The birth rate in Japan had reached a postwar high, as it did in every country when men and women came together again after a period of separation during the war, and the marriage rate had increased. I knew that the marriage pattern had leveled off, that the postwar peak had been completed, and that the first half of the two-child family had already been born.[5] So, I was fairly close when I bet that within three years, once we started the population shift from rural to urban, the birth rate would drop by one-third: The birth rate dropped from a postwar peak of 34.3 births (per 1,000 population) in 1947 to 28.1 in 1950.[6]

22

Summation of the Occupation

Let me sum up the activities of a "medic" in the health and welfare field in Japan during the occupation. The record is documented in voluminous reports with many volumes of statistics. This record, which I have barely touched on here, indicates that in terms of measurable criteria that are usually accepted in evaluating the progress of health and welfare programs, a major revolution was accomplished in Japan from a medical and welfare standpoint. This revolution was conducted in a manner that was acceptable to the Japanese. If it were not, sufficient time has elapsed since the end of the occupation for them to have terminated or drastically modified these programs. To this date, the programs have stood the test of time. The benefits, as I have tried to point out, in the lowered death rates and lowered disease incidence and improved standards of living have continued and will go on for many, many years so long as these programs are continued.

Had we attempted to impose on the Japanese our way of doing things just because we do things a special way in our own country, I am quite sure we would have failed. I emphasize this because I think it is important in our future relations with other countries with whom we desire friendship. As I have tried to show, most underdeveloped nations are underdeveloped for many reasons, but one of the reasons is that the bulk of the population is sick, chronically infected with diseases that may cause mental retardation, loss of physical stamina, and many other things. If we desire to improve the standard of living of some undeveloped nations as a policy in our foreign relations, hoping thereby that they will understand our version of democracy and the worth of the individual, then the place to start is in the health and welfare field, which is fundamental to the success of any such improvement.

Health and welfare programs themselves should be carried out; but without them, no other program in the economic, financial, commercial or other fields will have any lasting effect. And if we attempt to build monuments to ourselves in our health and welfare fields in the form of elaborate buildings that are beyond the standards of those the country can even hope to attain for a hundred years and that are not adaptable to their standards, then we are again wasting our money.[1] We have to start with the multi-angle approach to each one of the major fields that I have mentioned in my very, very brief discussion of our activities in Japan. If we do, it will pay dividends.

We think we sold democracy—not our form of democracy, but the principle of democracy—that is, the worth of the individual, to the Japanese people. It was worth doing. Only the test of time will show how well worth doing it was.

23

Life in Japan

Much has been written during and immediately after the occupation about the living conditions of military personnel and their dependents in the occupied countries of Germany and Japan. It is not my intention to repeat the information and material in these books and articles. I intend only to briefly outline the life in Japan of one medic and his family.

The Early Days

From September 1945 until the summer of 1946, life for the military personnel in Japan was much as it had been during the war. I lived in the billets for senior officers of General Headquarters at the Imperial Hotel, which had been partially destroyed by fire. In Tokyo, as in all of the large cities, light, potable water, heat, and the usual comforts or even essentials of peacetime living were not available in quality or quantity comparable to peacetime standards. In any partially destroyed or burned-out city, utilities are always damaged, and it takes time to rehabilitate the power plants, to restore water purification systems, and to repair sewage disposal systems. It was also some time until we were supplied with rations other than the wartime C rations. In the late fall of 1945, reefer ships were made available to bring frozen food and fresh vegetables to the troops in Japan. Continued efforts improved living conditions: Buildings were rehabilitated, and furnishings for both offices and billets gradually improved. The primitive beat-up furniture which was salvaged from burned-out buildings was gradually replaced with new furniture or furniture which had been newly manufactured.

By the spring of 1946, the time was rapidly approaching when wives could join their husbands in the occupied area and bring their dependents. The plans had reached the stage of surveying existing and surviving apartment buildings and individual homes which might be requisitioned, rehabilitated, and made fit for occupancy by these families. In addition, temporary buildings were constructed, usually of quonset hut type, in housing areas such as Palace Heights. Later, buildings were constructed by Japanese contractors to meet the standards of the army engineers, at Washington Heights, Grant Heights, and other housing areas where occupation families were moved. This construction required several years, and the first quarters available were the quonset huts at Palace Heights, requisitioned private dwellings, and a few apartments. Because there were many oriental-type houses with limited lighting and plumbing facilities, extensive modification and rebuilding were required. European-type homes usually required only repainting and a few repairs. Boards of officers were established to survey these buildings and to classify them for occupancy by officers and their dependents according to rank, which is the usual custom on military posts in peacetime. Those officers who desired to bring their families to Japan were then permitted to select from the available quarters one which they desired, according to seniority within their grade.

Making Plans

In the summer of 1946, I had returned to the United States to represent Japan and Korea at the organizational conference of the World Health Organization in New York. I obtained a leave to be with my family in Washington, D.C., where they had been living since 1944. During this period, our older daughter, who had transferred from the University of California to Sweetbriar College in Virginia, in order to be closer to her mother and younger sister, who were living in Virginia, married a young medical student whom she had known since her high school days in San Leandro, California.

Like many officers who had served during the war and who were senior in grade, I had to decide whether I should stay on in the service; and if I decided to stay on, whether I should return to Japan or accept one of several assignments in the United States, which were offered to me by the Surgeon General of the Army. Because of my length of service overseas in several theaters during the war, I had been informed by the office of the Surgeon General of the Army that under the "point system," I was eligible to remain in the United States for some time on a new assignment, if I so desired.

After a few shifts in the staff sections of General Headquarters, SCAP, General MacArthur had interviewed each of us. I had been flattered by his expressed desire that I should serve on his staff during the period of the occupation. Under the circumstances, these selected senior staff officers were to serve during the entire occupation, which was of unknown duration at that time, in order to complete the job and, thus, were to be exempt from the usual rotation criteria for return to the United States. Because I felt the work in Japan of helping to rebuild this devastated nation, at least in the health and welfare fields, was the greatest challenge professionally which any man could hope to find, I felt I should return to Japan.

We decided to sell our home in Virginia, and plans were made for my wife and younger daughter to join me as soon as priorities on shipping space could be made available. The availability of quarters in Japan for dependents and the amount of shipping space on transports were the limiting factors, so far as the time of arrival of dependents was concerned. Accordingly, I returned to Japan and began going through the routine of attempting to secure a set of quarters for my family. The first dependents had already arrived during my absence; however, I was fortunate in obtaining a western-type house which had formerly been occupied by a member of the Italian Embassy. It was a two-story frame and stucco building, which rocked and groaned and creaked during the frequent earthquakes but did not fall down.

A Great Day

My wife and younger daughter arrived on the hospital ship *Hope*, after a very rough trip, in early January 1947. They had left Seattle before Christmas. It was a great day for me when they arrived at the port in Yokohama.

An American school had been established for the children of occupation families. Because our younger daughter was a junior in high school, she immediately entered the American school. As time passed, there were many activities established which could be enjoyed by the families of the American military personnel.

Taisa

Because I was doing a great deal of travelling throughout Japan, and as the Japanese army and police had been abolished and there were not sufficient American troops available to guard each individual isolated set of quarters, I was concerned about my family being alone so much when burglary and robbery of occupation homes were then at their peak. I obtained an Akita dog to be trained as a watchdog. They are a fine breed of dog: first cousins, I have been told, to the Alaskan Husky. They were brought to Japan from Siberia, where the parent strain developed and which subsequently produced the Husky, the Akita, and Chow dog in China. They grow to tremendous size—about 120 to 130 pounds—and are most powerful. The Japanese used them for watchdogs and for bear hunting; in Hokkaido and northern Honshu, they pull carts as well.

This dog was to earn his food many times over in driving away robbers and helping me on three occasions to round up burglars who were trying to break into our home. At least, I felt more secure as far as my family was concerned during my absences when "Taisa" was looking after them. Taisa was the name selected for this dog by my Japanese driver: In Japanese it is translated to "Colonel."

A Japanese Garden

We had moved from our first home to another building, which was a ferro-concrete building, as the Japanese called it, located in a very beautiful garden. This home was one of a number of homes owned by a wealthy paper pulp manufacturer and had been requisitioned for senior officers in the occupation. To me, it was a never-ending pleasure to go into and through this lovely Japanese garden. The Japanese gardens are designed for a series of "views," and within the garden was one view of a small mountain and running stream in which we raised goldfish. Another view of the lawn and small pool could be obtained from the glassed-in sun porch.

The house was large, and we had the usual complement of a household staff, including a cook and a number of maids. Originally, the household staff was furnished as part of the service requisitioned from the Japanese Government by the occupation forces; but shortly afterward, we took over the payment of these people. As in any country where a number of people work together in a household staff, personal jealousies and difficulties occasionally arise. We were most fortunate in obtaining the services of Iwashita-san. She was a very lovely Japanese lady, the widow of a wealthy Japanese industrialist whose estate had been frozen, as one of the zaibatsu, under policy directives sent to General MacArthur. She was an elderly lady whose family had grown up, and she came to us to help run the house as a housekeeper and supervise the maids and household help. We were very grateful to her for her kindness in joining us. We learned from her many interesting things about the culture of Japanese society. It was with real regret after my wife returned home that we learned that Iwashita-san had become ill.

Peacetime Social Life

Officers clubs were established for General Headquarters personnel where dinner parties were frequently held. The Imperial Hotel ballroom was rehabilitated and became the place of many beautiful evening parties. A number of very fine golf courses were rehabilitated. They, of course, had been sadly neglected during the war. My wife and I began to play golf again after a lapse of many years. Until the arrival of the families, the seven-day week wartime duty hours had been in effect, but after the families began to arrive this was relaxed to a certain extent and it was possible for even staff section chiefs of General Headquarters to have an occasional Sunday free.

Horses

Our family pleasure had, throughout our military service, been concerned with horses.[1] I was able to lease from the Japan Racing Association horses for my wife, my daughter, and myself. These horses were kept at the Racing Association stables in Setagaya, a beautiful location where the training stables were located. There was beautiful countryside where we could ride during our free time, which we enjoyed doing, of course, very much.

I had become acquainted through mutual friends with Colonel Kido, who was in charge of the imperial household stables, and was frequently invited to the imperial stables to watch the top Japanese riders perform and to watch the Japanese version of polo. Colonel Kido, himself an outstanding horseman, had been a member of the 1932 Olympic team, and I had first met him during his visit to the United States. We enjoyed many pleasant times at the imperial household grounds at parties given by our Japanese friends. There is a cup, which is still in existence so far as I know, known as the General Sams Cup, for which the student riding teams of the various medical schools compete.

Duck Netting

One of the interesting activities in which we participated each year was the duck netting at the imperial duck preserves. The imperial household maintained these preserves and invited various senior officers to participate in this unique ceremony, for that is what it really was. An elaborate feeding area had been developed to attract wild ducks on a rather large body of water where live decoys, of course, lived. Around this pond, concealed by live bamboo screens, small ditches, six-feet wide and perhaps thirty-feet long, radiated out. The guests who were to net at a particular canal lined up behind a bunker at the end of the canal where they were not seen by the ducks. Decoys followed by wild ducks would then swim into this canal from the main feeding area. They were assisted in their desire to enter the canal by a various ingenious feeding system in which grains of rice were dropped down a chute and distributed on the water ahead of the ducks; then an attendant, pumping a billows with his foot, gently blew air under the water, which rose as bubbles behind the ducks. When the master of this particular group of guest netters was convinced that all of the ducks that were going to had entered this little canal, he silently dropped the gate behind them and signaled the number of wild ducks in the canal. Each guest had a large net on a pole and a number; and on a signal from the master, ran around to the sides of the canals and took his proper position. The wild ducks in the canal, of course, became alarmed and flew up out of the water. The job of the guests was to try and net the ducks before they escaped. A falcon was always present on the wrist of another attendant, and it was amazing to see the speed with which this falcon could strike down a duck that had eluded the netters and which might alarm his companions in the main feeding pond if he returned.

Part of this interesting ceremony, of course, was a lunch of sukiyaki duck. I had never before eaten duck prepared in this manner, and I have never eaten duck, before or since, which equals in flavor sukiyaki duck. The meat is removed in small bits from the carcass of the wild duck. The small bits can be handled with *hashi*, which we know as chopsticks. The pieces of duck are soaked in *shoyu*, which we call soy sauce, and *sake*, and then are broiled individually on a flat ungreased plate over a small charcoal hibachi.

Hunting

Because my second pleasure after working with horses has always been hunting, the Japanese imperial household was most kind in inviting me to hunt ducks and geese. I was invited by other friends to hunt the wild boar in Ito peninsula. Pheasant and quail are largely found in the foothills of the mountains of Japan. The flat lands, although offering ideal cover for these birds, had been pretty well hunted out for food during the war. I have enjoyed many a pleasant hunt with my Japanese friends and my shooting companions, Col. Tommy Taylor and, later, Col. Pete Connor.

I have hunted duck in a number of parts of the world, but the method of hunting ducks in Japan, besides the unique imperial pastime of duck netting, was also unique, so far as I was concerned. A long narrow boat with an inboard gasoline motor, known as a duck boat, was suitable for two hunters sitting abreast in the forward part of the boat. Tommy and I would go out with the boatman on Tokyo Bay well before daylight. There were literally millions of ducks resting on the open waters of the bay. The tactics, which, of course, are contrary to both custom and law in this country, were to approach one of the large flocks of ducks resting on the water as closely as possible before they were alarmed and took to the air. Because there were always a few laggards who were a little slow in getting off the water, the boatman then turned the boat quickly into the area formerly occupied by the mass of ducks; it was possible to get a shot at the laggards who took off while still within range of our guns. Unfortunately, Tokyo Bay can kick up a storm in a very few minutes, and a certain hazard existed in that these boats, which were perhaps twenty feet long and only about four feet at the beam, could be easily swamped when a squall came up, as it frequently did, and the water became very rough. After some friends of ours unfortunately were drowned during one of the unexpected squalls while hunting, my wife put a ban on my going into the bay again; so, Tommy and I and, after Colonel Taylor returned to the United States, Pete Connor and I went up to a small lake in Chiba Prefecture, where we would go in a small boat, which was poled by the boatman, and either hide in a blind or attempt to stalk flocks of ducks which were not so plentiful on this comparatively small body of water. The hazard of rough water was non-existent there.

In the pheasant shoots, the innate courtesy of the Japanese in their desire to entertain their guests can sometimes be almost embarrassing. Of course, because of my position and the work I was doing as a senior member of General MacArthur's staff, as was true of other senior officers, whether it was on business or for simple pleasure such as hunting, if I went into a prefecture, the Japanese governor and the local officials always met me; and there were the usual ceremonies and entertainment and usually a dinner. On pheasant shooting, the Japanese friends were so anxious that I would be sure to get pheasants, which were admittedly scarce, they had hunters not only abreast of me but also in front of me; I actually had no opportunity to get a shot when the dogs would flush a pheasant. Nevertheless, the Japanese courtesy was such that, as their guest, I must have a full bag of game and my hosts would insist on pressing on me the birds which they had shot. After a few trips of this type, I asked my friends if they would permit me to take a dog and go alone for a little time so that I might get a few shots myself, which had to be done very diplomatically so they would not be offended. I have never known people quite so courteous and solicitous of their guests as are the Japanese.

Karuizawa

On my staff visits and business trips, I did not make it a practice, as did some officers, of having my wife accompany me. I have always felt that business and pleasure should be two separate things. Nevertheless, we were able to enjoy a few trips together which were only for pleasure. When my older daughter and her baby came to visit us in the summer of 1949, my wife's mother also came. Because they were not my dependents, it was necessary for me to arrange, of course, commercial transportation on the American President Lines. I arranged for a weekend up in the mountains in Karuizawa. This area was high in the Japanese mountains in which a small European colony had been established before the war. It was a beautiful area and one of the so-called recreation areas which the occupation forces used for their troops and their families. We drove up the usual narrow, winding gravel road for this weekend and had a most pleasant time in a beautiful European-type Japanese estate, which had been requisitioned for use of senior officers for just such purposes. We took our own maid and driver, of course, although there was a permanent staff for this beautiful estate. It actually was a duplicate of a beautiful English manor house, and the landscaping was breathtaking because, of all the peoples of the world, the Japanese, to me, have the greatest eye for beauty in landscaping and gardening.

Mikimoto's Pearls

My wife and I joined Gen. James Bethea, who had replaced General Martin as the military surgeon in 1946, for a trip to Mikimoto's pearl farms. We went by train to Osaka and to the seashore not too many miles away where the famous Mikimoto pearl farms were located. Mikimoto was an interesting gentleman, who jokingly called himself the Rockefeller of Japan. He, of course, had become tremendously wealthy from his cultured pearls. He had, after many years, found that if he inoculated oysters with a very small bead of calcium carbonate, he could produce pearls when the oysters were recovered after a number of years in his oyster beds. Interestingly enough, these small seeds, as they were called, were obtained from clam shells imported into Japan from the Illinois River in the United States.

It was interesting to watch the women divers go down and fill the baskets with these oysters. Of course, as guests, we were permitted to open some of the oysters and look for the pearls. A pearl is simply the end product of an oyster's reaction to an injury. Naturally, a particle of sand or other material becomes lodged inside of the oyster's shell and irritates the oyster. A "foreign body" reaction occurs, such as would occur if a particle of sand were imbedded in the tissue of the human body, and it is walled off. This "foreign body" reaction is a pearl. Mikimoto, by his artificial inoculation of these pearls, was actually creating pearls as authentic as those which occur naturally. To me, his pearls are most beautiful.

Hokkaido

It was possible to obtain permission to use one of the private cars on the railroad at one's own expense, just as in the United States. My wife and I, with my interpreter, made such an arrangement in order that we might enjoy a trip to northern Hokkaido, which she, of course, had not visited. Although this was to be a vacation trip, as usual, the word was passed through Japanese channels that I was going to Hokkaido. Along the entire route as we passed through the various prefectures or through the principal cities, the Japanese officials would board the train and then ride on to the next stop, and there would be the usual exchange of courtesies and talk. As my wife said, it was like a political campaign tour back home when a major candidate for office goes by train. As he enters each political jurisdiction the various political functionaries board the train and confer as they go along.

In this case, there was business discussed with the various prefectural health and welfare people along the route. The times at which the various groups boarded the train and left extended from before daylight until well after midnight; there was really very little opportunity for relaxation and rest for either of us. I am sure that the Japanese who did pay us these visits along the route did it out of courtesy and did everything within their power to make our trip a pleasurable one.

On our return trip we stopped overnight at a beautiful resort in Hokkaido. The hotel was located on the shores of a lake. Interestingly enough, a new volcano was being born within a few miles of this hotel, and we could watch the new openings in the soil develop before our very eyes. Measurements were being maintained by the Japanese officials as a high plateau in the mountains began to rise literally a measurable amount each day. Fissures in the earth would develop, emitting clouds of smoke and fumes and spewing molten lava.

This resort was also in the area of the "hairy Ainu." This group, of course, is looked on by the Japanese as the original inhabitants or the barbarians, as they are called, of the Japanese islands. Actually, the origin of these people had been the subject of intensive study. They are Caucasians, anthropologically, and apparently moved into the islands by way of Siberia, an unknown number of thousands of years ago. Physically, they look as we do, rather than oriental or Japanese. They are great hunters and have a bear ceremony each year which has been described by others.

The Imperial Family

During the course of my many public appearances at medical or welfare functions, which was part of my job, we had occasion to associate with and to get to know many of the top Japanese. It was my pleasure and good fortune to have had the opportunity of meeting many times and participating in ceremonies with the empress of Japan. She was the honorary head of the Japanese Red Cross, which we were reorganizing. (Prince Shimadzu was the president.) She attended many of the ceremonies. She began to study English, and at one of the receptions she very graciously tried out on me, as she said, her first English expressions during our conversation.

The emperor himself made very few public appearances, but one to which I was also invited was at Keio University, where the emperor appeared and gave a short address. He was a most gracious and gentle man. I was interested in watching the reaction of the masses of Japanese people who lined the way along which the emperor proceeded after he had publicly declared that he was not divine and had become the titular head of the state, rather than the actual absolute ruler which he had been before. The Japanese had lost no respect for the emperor.

One of his brothers, Prince Takamatsu, and his beautiful and charming wife, represented the emperor at the many ceremonies and meetings which I was called on to attend in the welfare field. It was our privilege also to have informal dinners at homes of mutual friends. The prince and his charming wife honored us by attending a dinner in our home.

Another brother of the emperor, Prince Chichibu, and his very lovely wife were also frequent contacts. Princess Chichibu was the daughter of Matsudaira, former ambassador to the United States. She had attended school in Washington, D.C., for a number of years. Because her husband had tuberculosis, from which he subsequently died, she was the imperial household representative and the honorary head of the Japan Antituberculosis Association. In my work with that organization, we had many meetings in which we both participated. It was to me a pleasure and a privilege to have had the opportunity of knowing these very gracious members of the imperial household.

Diplomatic Circles

By virtue of my assignment, I was, as were the other senior officers of General Headquarters, frequently invited to numerous diplomatic social events, as well as

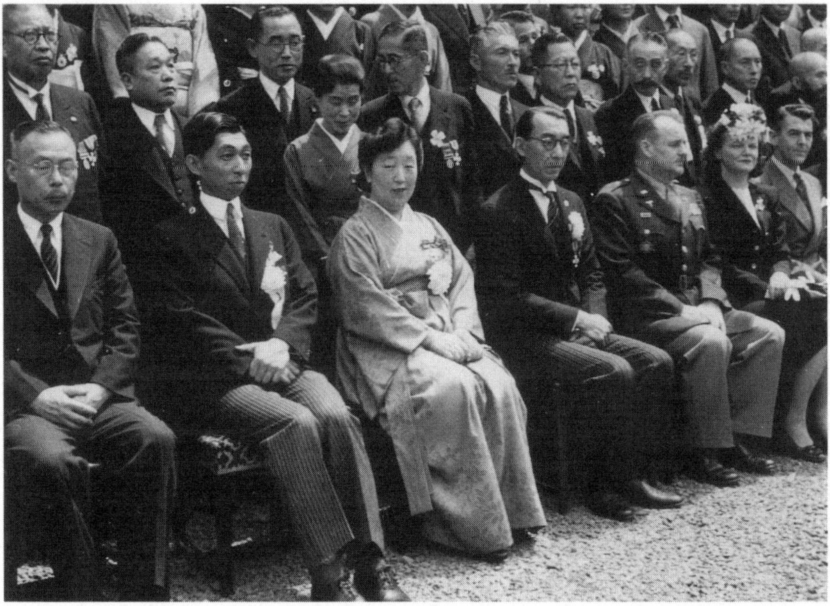

Figure 21. Members of the imperial family attended the first postwar meeting of the Red Cross of Japan following its reorganization. In addition to operating hospitals and clinics and training nurses, the Red Cross Society of Japan began coordinating disaster relief activities of nongovernmental agencies. International Red Cross Hall, Tokyo, circa 10 December 1948. Front row, left to right: unidentified, Prince Takamatsu Nobuhito, Empress Nagako (Honorary Head of the Red Cross of Japan), unidentified, Brig. Gen. C.F. Sams, Virginia M. Ohlson (Public Health Nursing Consultant and later Chief, Nursing Affairs Division, PHW, SCAP), Milton J. Evans (Chief, Welfare Administration Branch, Welfare Division, PHW, SCAP). (Courtesy of the Hoover Institution Archives, Stanford University.)

certain official ones, where we learned to know some very fine people. The British ambassador, Sir Alvery, and his charming wife, Lady Gascoigne, were frequently our hosts at various diplomatic functions. The Spanish ambassador and his wife, the Dutch Minister and his wife, as well as French, Canadian, and Dutch representatives, all became our very good friends. As the occupation neared its end and Japanese Government officials assumed more and more responsibility, and greater freedom was gradually accorded them, there were also numerous social functions at the prime minister's residence and at the official residences of various cabinet ministers.

A Sad Day

When the Korean War began in the summer of 1950, we of the General Headquarters staff, of course, re-entered a period of wartime activities, which we had hoped after the end of World War II in 1945 would not be repeated. Naturally, the social activities were curtailed. Many of us spent a good deal of our time in Korea, and a policy was adopted that as the various officers were rotated to the United States and their families departed with them, families of their replacements would not be brought into Japan during the period of tension. There was a gradual decrease in the number of American families in Japan.

After my son-in-law was missing in action and we learned that our older daughter and her two children would have to move from their living quarters at Letterman Army Hospital in San Francisco, we had a decision to make. We could not bring her and the children to Japan under the circumstances. She, of course, was naturally upset; so we decided that, as her parents, the best way in which we could help her was for my wife to return to the United States and establish a home to which Yvonne and her children could come. So once again, we entered a period of separation, and our household belongings and our personal car, of course, were returned to the United States.

It was a sad day when my wife left Japan after being with me for four years. In my long service as a medic in various parts of the world, our family life in Japan had been a most pleasant period. She left after Christmas in 1950, arriving in the United States in January 1951, just four years after she had joined me in Japan. This separation, of course, was to be shorter than had been our previous separations, which had lasted for a number of years. Eventually, I returned to the United States in summer of 1951.

KOREA

24

1945–1948

Korea is divided by a line drawn on a map during an international conflict. The map showed Korea to be a very small part of the world, an area about which little was known by those who were settling her fate. Because parallels of latitude were easily identifiable on the map, the thirty-eighth parallel became a boundary on the ground dividing this nation into two parts. The purpose of this division was to provide a meeting place for the Russians, who had recently entered the war in Manchuria with the intention of sweeping down the Korean peninsula, and for the Americans, who had been fighting the war, and winning it for some years, with the intention of going into Korea from the south. Somewhere the two military forces would meet. The records show that the thirty-eighth parallel was established for the purpose of accepting military surrender of the Japanese forces alone; it was to be a temporary demarcation. It has now become a permanent line of division between the east and the west, and a part of the iron curtain.

The Occupations of Korea

For forty years the Japanese had been occupying this basically agricultural nation. Korea had been invaded and occupied by the Japanese in the Russian-Japanese War. Korea was a part of the Japanese empire. During the course of this occupation of Korea, the Japanese had a policy that was the reverse of our occupation policy when we occupied Japan in 1945. Our policy was to attempt to carry out certain basic reorganizations, to establish certain patterns, and to train the Japanese as quickly as possible to take over control. We established Japanese governmental organizations and, through our training of the Japanese and our control of activities behind the scenes, eventually reached the point where we felt we could turn over the control of various operations in sequence to the Japanese. At the end of the occupation, they were ready for full control. In the case of the Japanese occupation of Korea, the Japanese literally liquidated the top of the social pyramid; they, themselves, occupied and took over all of the key jobs.

When I first went into Korea on a staff visit in late September 1945, our XXIV Corps, which had been part of the Tenth Army in Okinawa, was moving into Korea to accept the surrender of the Japanese military forces there. This corps was commanded by Gen. John Hodges, an old friend who was born in the little town of Carbondale, Illinois, not far from where I was born and where my father's parents lived. General Hodges met the Russians at the thirty-eighth parallel.

The occupation of Korea by U.S. forces was unilateral and quite different from the Japanese occupation. Only the U.S. troops went into Korea south of the thirty-eighth parallel to liberate this country. No British troops or troops of other nationalities were involved. The responsibility for carrying out the occupation in Korea south of the thirty-eighth parallel was solely that of the United States. This situation more or less paralleled that set up in Europe.—The American commander of the American zone in Germany was responsible to the U.S. Government. The Russian commander of East Germany was responsible to the Russian Government. The French and British commanders likewise were directly responsible to their respective governments. Only in Berlin itself was an attempt made to have a four-power government.

The Russian commander in North Korea was responsible to the Russian Government; the American commander south of the thirty-eighth parallel was responsible only to the U.S. Government. As a result, the nation of Korea for the next five years was to be reoriented in two different ways. The north would become communist; the south would become, we hoped, democratic.

It does not take much study of history to learn that whenever a country is partitioned under such circumstances, and it has been done again and again, reuniting the separate parts after a period of time is seldom done successfully without violence. New generations grow up oriented to different governmental and different cultural philosophies. Violence is usually the result of a struggle for power and domination by the two factions when reunification is attempted.

An agreement had been made on the diplomatic level between the Russians and the Americans and other allies that there would be a five-year period of tutelage. Then a commission would be established under the United Nations auspices (and it was established) which would unify the country. But five years, or even three years, is too long a time for a country to be under different occupation groups where the basic philosophy differs as much as it does between democracy and communism. So the unification has not come about.

The Military Government

General MacArthur as Commanding General of the Far East Command, a U.S. command, rather than in his capacity as SCAP, had the responsibility for the occupation of Korea. He exercised this responsibility through the Commanding General, United States Army Forces in Korea (USAFIK), who, initially, was General Hodges. Military government personnel were sent into Korea as companies and groups, because when the Japanese were sent home there were no

Korean officials left. American officials assumed the functions of government in a direct military government, rather than standing behind the scenes and controlling the government through officials as was done in Japan.

As a chief of a SCAP staff section, technically, I had no business in Korea; however, General Hodges requested of General MacArthur that I, specifically by name, be given an additional "hat" to assume responsibility as his advisor for health and welfare fields for Korea. This role was agreed upon. Therefore, at General Hodges's request, I as an individual, and also my staff, frequently visited Korea in an attempt to assist that very able officer in a very difficult problem.[1]

His problem was to build from scratch some form of government completely staffed by Koreans, which could stand on its own feet in a very few years. Two generations had passed since Koreans had had an opportunity for such responsibility. With the exception of a few individuals who were well advanced in years, such as Rhee Syngman who had been in exile, there were few Koreans who had held high positions in governmental offices before the Japanese occupation began. Forty years is a long time in any man's life.

Out of some 30 million Koreans in both North and South Korea, there were only about 700,000 who made up the top of the social pyramidal structure. I estimate this number to be correct, because about 700,000 Japanese who occupied the top of this pyramid were repatriated by edict out of Korea back to Japan in 1945. They were the governmental officials, the teachers, the doctors, the lawyers, and the business men; the Koreans were the helpers. It is difficult for us to realize what it is like to live in such a situation. For over forty years, the leaders of Korea had been driven into exile or literally liquidated by being killed or put into prison.

The first chief of health and welfare of the military government in Korea was Dr. MacDonald, who was from the Oklahoma State Health Department. He subsequently returned home when the American army was demobilizing. In 1946, I was very fortunate in obtaining the services of Col. Paul Keeney, who had come to the Far East and whom I had asked to be the chief of health and welfare in Korea. I had hoped to have Paul as my deputy on my staff in Japan, but it was simply a case of too few people for too many critical jobs. This position in Korea needed strong leadership. Although it involved personal discomfort and separation from his family, Colonel Keeney did an outstanding job with very limited means.

General Hodges established a military governor as a deputy. The military government staff acted as a national government for South Korea. Military government teams in the eight prefectures of South Korea acted as state or provincial governments. There were health officers, welfare officers, and sanitary engineers on each team, as we had in Japan. They initially exercised direct governmental control until Koreans could be found and tried in various positions and ultimately trained to take over complete responsibility for their own government. The sovereign government of the Republic of Korea was established in 1948, and the occupation terminated south of the thirty-eighth parallel.[2]

Kaesong

My first trip to the thirty-eighth parallel, just north of Seoul, was to Kaesong. The thirty-eighth parallel actually divided this town. I found thousands of Japanese refugees moving south, traveling on foot through bypasses to get around the Russian outposts and trying to enter South Korea and the American zone en route to Japan. As far as the Americans were concerned, the border was open for free movement of people, Korean or Japanese, but not as far as the Russians were concerned. Both the Japanese who were trying to come south and the Koreans who were trying to come south had to use devious methods to get across the border. They were congregated in large numbers in Kaesong and at other border crossing points.

They brought with them smallpox and typhus and typhoid. We had to establish processing centers where they could be fed, where the sick could be cared for, and where immunizations could be given and delousing carried out. There were very limited medical means. Most of the doctors, nurses, and professional people, who were Japanese, were sent out of the country. There were only about fifteen hundred Korean doctors for the 23 million people who lived south of the thirty-eighth parallel; there were fewer Korean nurses. About half of the Korean doctors were located in Seoul, which had a population of about 1 million. The other 750 doctors for the remaining 22 million people were dispersed over the rest of South Korea.

There were only 6,000 general hospital beds for the 23 million Koreans. About half of those beds were also located in Seoul. Again, it is hard for us in America to realize what that means: There was one doctor for every 25,000 people in the area outside of Seoul, and one hospital bed for about every 7,000 people. These hospitals had been operated by Japanese doctors. The equipment and Japanese supplies were left behind Many of the Korean doctors were not trained as first class doctors, but were called "associate doctors." Many of them had learned medicine, as it was done in our own country fifty years ago, by simply accompanying a doctor and reading his limited number of texts and learning by apprenticeship.

Additional examples of the difficulty faced by the military government in Korea in 1945 in developing replacements for the Japanese can be illustrated in fields other than medicine. On my first trip from Seoul to Pusan by rail, the locomotive engineer was a young Korean boy. He was driving the engine for the first time outside of the roundhouse area. The Japanese had been the engineers on the trains as well as the conductors and the pullman porters in the sleeping cars; the Koreans had been the roundhouse hostlers for cleaning the locomotives and cars. In one small pharmaceutical company in Seoul, the business head, of course, had been Japanese and had left. The senior Korean employee, actually a janitor, became the head of the business.

Korea had been a granary for Japan. South Korea, in particular, had a surplus of white rice. The Japanese took the white rice and gave the Koreans small grains, barley and wheat. Actually, from a nutritional standpoint, they were doing the Koreans a favor. Fortunately, Korea had not been bombed or damaged during the war, so there was not the destruction of cities, such as we found in Japan; yet, South Korea was not a complete unit. The hydroelectric power system, which the Japanese had developed in North Korea when Korea and Manchuria were under their control, and the industry such as it was, including the tremendous oil refineries at Wonsan in North Korea, needed integration with the agricultural area in South Korea.

Pusan

On my first trip down to Pusan in 1945, I found many, many thousands of Japanese assembled there waiting for the ferries to take them to Shimonoseki on the Japanese island of Honshu. Some of these Japanese had walked all the way from Manchuria, through North Korea, and slipped across the thirty-eighth parallel; they had walked all the way down or had come by train after our processing centers were established. In this state of confusion, one of the things we must remember is that the Koreans hated the occupying Japanese very sincerely in most cases. We should not have been too surprised to find that many of the Japanese were being attacked and robbed and even killed on the back roads by Koreans. All the former Japanese property had been seized. That still is a bone of contention between Japan and Korea. We must remember there was forty years of bitterness involved.

Koreans were also being repatriated through Pusan to their homeland. Many had come from Japan. Some were coming from China into their liberated country, which actually was an occupied country until a sovereign government could be established. During the repatriation of Koreans in 1945 and 1946, two cases of cholera unfortunately got ashore at Pusan from a group returning by ship from China. Within a few weeks, cholera followed the rail line, literally, and reached Seoul. Some 17,000 cases occurred with over 11,000 deaths.[3] Smallpox, typhoid, diphtheria, and typhus—the wildfire diseases associated with devastation and mass movement of people—were prevalent in Korea as well as in Japan. We had our hands full in trying to control these outbreaks with the limited means available in the way of medical personnel and medical facilities.

The Medical Problems

Our first medical problem was to attempt to provide emergency facilities for handling the epidemics prevalent during the period of mass movement of people; that is, the movement of Japanese from South Korea, and from the north through South Korea, to Japan, as well as the movement of Koreans from China by ship and from Japan for redistribution in Korea. Our second problem was to attempt to build with the limited means available a health and welfare organization in South Korea that could accomplish the most with the extremely limited number of professionally qualified Koreans.

There had been six medical schools in Korea operated by the Japanese basically for Japanese. When we tried to find qualified Koreans to staff these schools after the Japanese doctors left, we were fortunate to find enough for two schools. This situation was a severe handicap. If the problem of building a nationwide medical service is to be solved with very limited native professional people, a start must be made somewhere to train increased numbers to meet requirements over a period of time; otherwise, efforts will be handicapped indefinitely by the limited number of native people to carry out a program.

The same problem existed in all paramedical fields, such as nursing. We started a nursing school at Central Red Cross Hospital in Seoul, which we re-equipped as a model hospital. Severance Hospital and Medical School had been started by American missionaries years before the war. The Americans had been forced to leave in 1940. In 1945, I found the physical plant a mess, filthy dirty. It had to be cleaned up and rehabilitated and re-equipped. Severance also was used as one of the model medical schools. One of the governmental medical schools in Korea had a very fine physical plant, but we were short of teaching staff.

The rounding up of orphans, of which there seemed to be great numbers, and putting them into institutions was a tremendous job in the welfare field. The feeding and handling, processing, delousing, and immunization of the orphans, again, was a major problem.

Dr. Y.S. Lee was made chief of the Ministry of Health and Welfare, as the first Korean trainee for that position. A staff was built up, and by 1948, when it was decided for diplomatic reasons that the Republic of Korea should become a sovereign government and the American military government and American troops withdrawn, a reasonably satisfactory national health and welfare ministry organization had been established and staffed by Koreans, with health departments at the provincial level and a laboratory for producing vaccines. Three medical schools and two schools of nursing were also in operation. A Korean national Red Cross had been organized to replace the branch of the Japanese Red Cross, which had been in existence in Korea before the termination of the war in 1945.

It was far from the progress we would have liked to have made, but I believe it was the best that could be done under the circumstances within the three-year period. I also believe that the Americans responsible for this great progress have not been given the credit they deserve.

25

1950–1951

On Sunday evening, 26 June 1950, we were having a dinner party at my home in Tokyo. The guests included Chief-of-staff, Gen. Ned Almond; Deputy Chief-of-staff for SCAP, Gen. Alonzo P. Fox; Bill Biederlinden of G-1 [personnel—Ed.]; Pinky Wright of G-3 [planning and conduct of operations—Ed.]; and all of General Headquarters. The dinner party was interrupted when we received a telephone call concerning the invasion of the Republic of Korea by the North Korean communist army. This news broke up the party. The problem of evacuating a considerable number of American citizens, most of whom were with the Economic Cooperation Administration and had been in Korea since its establishment as a sovereign republic in 1948, was placed upon General MacArthur. Subsequently, air and naval support of the Republic of Korea forces by U.S. forces was authorized. The communist forces had overrun Seoul and had penetrated deeper into Republic of Korea territory in a drive toward Pusan, the southeastern port city.

The Build Up

Prior to 1948, in the later stages of the occupation of the Republic of Korea, a national military force of approximately 100,000 in number was organized, equipped, and trained primarily for internal security. This force was lightly armed with small arms and light weapons. It was not equipped with supporting heavy weapons, such as artillery and armor, which are essential for defense against external invasion or for attack and, perhaps, invasion of North Korea.

Shortly after the Russians occupied North Korea, in the back pages of the press, announcements were made from time to time that they were organizing an army in North Korea and equipping it not only with light arms but also with supporting artillery and armor. This build up over the five years of Russian occupation of North Korea from the end of World War II to the beginning of the Korean War was publicly known during this period. It raises a question in my mind, and has always raised a question, because the population of North Korea, some 11 million people, could hardly support an army of 400,000 well-equipped and well-trained troops without external assistance. Likewise, a population of 11 million could hardly be expected successfully to attack and overrun their brothers in the Republic of Korea south of the thirty-eighth parallel, which had a population at that time of some 23 million people, if the two halves of Korea were equally armed and equally supported.

In each area of the world, whether it be in Germany or in Korea, or in Southeast Asia, where the communists with Russian support have occupied a portion of a country, they have immediately begun the build up of an army equipped and trained with all the necessary heavy weapons, artillery, and armor for aggressive warfare. We, on the other hand, invariably have followed the policy, for reasons unknown to me, of organizing and training smaller forces for internal security, and they have been so equipped that they could not hold to resist an equal force of adequately trained and equipped communist troops across their borders. It has seemed to me that such a policy can only invite aggressive attack from the communist-held areas when such an attack would seem most opportune to the communists. Certainly, Korea demonstrated what to me has been an unexplainable attitude on our part in supporting the free nations, militarily, when they are faced with well-organized communist armies across their borders.

I recognize the pros and cons of adequately arming the Republic of Korea forces prior to 1950. One group felt that if the Republic of Korea was supported in the establishment of a real army with adequate equipment, with adequate ammunition and supplies, President Rhee Syngman might use this army to invade North Korea in an effort to unify the Republic of Korea. Therefore, we could not afford to support such a risk, which in the opinion of this group, might lead to a third world war. Apparently, such thinking has dominated our military support efforts in other parts of the world as well as in Korea.

In my humble opinion, by such policies we have set up the picture for an invitation to aggression by satellites of the communists without jeopardizing the life of a single Russian soldier. I have listened to many arguments of some of my friends in the diplomatic corps that if we organized adequate military forces in friendly nations facing the communists, we would be charged—as we have been, regardless of what we have done—by the communists with preparing for a war of aggression. It seems to me that with the facts as they have been demonstrated, the communists have unhesitatingly, in each instance, built up real military forces in their satellites; we should be able to counter such propaganda effectively and, at the same time, build up equal or stronger forces among our friends. Having had some contact over the years with the oriental mind, and to me the mind of the Soviet is basically oriental in its scale of values and in its approach to problems, I have noted that respect for strength is the principle deterrent to aggression. If we only weakly support our friends in far places, then the communists feel that we are weak and they have no respect for our positions. This view is one man's opinion.

The Perimeter

When it became apparent that the weakly equipped Republic of Korea army was about to be driven into the sea, General MacArthur was given the responsibility of supporting these forces with U.S. Army ground troops. The Twenty-fourth Division, commanded by my good friend Bill Dean, was sent piecemeal as rapidly as it could be airlifted and sealifted into the combat area. Subsequently, the First Cavalry Division and the Twenty-fifth Division and all available forces from Japan were committed to the Korean War.

We talk in terms of divisions, but it must be remembered that in the interval between the end of World War II and the beginning of the Korean War, there had been a progressive reduction in troop strength in the Far East theater. To carry out this reduction, directed from Washington, D.C., the usual procedure of inactivating battalions within combat teams and inactivating combat teams within divisions had been carried out. The strength of battalions, which normally ranged from 800 to 1,000 soldiers, had been reduced so that battalions were comprised of only about 500 soldiers when they were sent into action. We might talk of divisions, but when the Twenty-fourth Division went into combat, its effective combat strength was only a fraction of that of a full-strength division.

This division had the mission of a delaying action until such time as the other divisions could be committed to action in Korea. By the middle of August, our forces were holding what was called a perimeter around Pusan. The First Marine Regiment and its supporting units and the Second Infantry Division from the United States had arrived and had been committed to action. In addition, the Twenty-fourth and the Twenty-fifth Divisions and the First Cavalry Division from Japan were holding this perimeter, which extended from Mansan just west of Pusan northward to Taegu. The perimeter then turned east to the coast, and this segment of the line was being held by the reorganized and regrouped Republic of Korea forces.

An estimated 6 million civilians had withdrawn into the perimeter as the communists advanced to the southeast. These Korean civilians were living in the river bottoms and in the open fields; the city of Pusan was overflowing with refugees. President Rhee Syngman appealed to General MacArthur as Supreme Commander, United Nations Command, for assistance in caring for these refugees.

The United Nations Security Council, during the absence of the Russian delegate, had resolved to support the Republic of Korea in its attempt to resist the aggression of the communists from the north and had announced its intention of reuniting Korea. The U.S. Government, at the request of the United Nations, had designated General MacArthur with an additional title: Commander-in-chief, United Nations Command. It was the intention of the United Nations to demonstrate to the world that it, as an organization, was capable of defending the principles of freedom and resisting aggression with a United Nations military effort. Appeals were made to the members of the United Nations to furnish troops and supplies to make this truly a United Nations effort. General MacArthur then designated his General Headquarters, Far East Command, which was the military headquarters of the U.S. Government for controlling American troops throughout the Far East, as General Headquarters, United Nations Command for the purposes of prosecuting the Korean War. General Headquarters, SCAP, was not so redesignated, because its basic responsibility was the occupation of Japan and the rehabilitation of that nation under the terms of the surrender.

When the appeal from President Rhee Syngman for food and clothing and assistance for the care of the refugee population was received, I was called in to a conference as chief of Public Health and Welfare, General Headquarters, SCAP, for the purpose of recommending to General MacArthur the action which should be taken. As a result of this conference, I was given an additional assignment: Chief of Health and Welfare, United Nations Command.[1]

The Civilian Health and Welfare Organization

So swift was the invasion by the North Korean communists and so quickly was Seoul, the capital of the Republic of Korea, overrun that only a handful of the top cabinet ministers escaped capture. The medical personnel in Korea who had been largely concentrated in the capital city also fell into the hands of the communists. This situation was equally true of the welfare personnel of the Ministry of Social Affairs.

Knowing the situation in Korea before the invasion of the communists, and knowing the limited number of personnel available in the health and welfare field, I felt that it would be unwise simply to ship tons of medical and welfare supplies into Pusan, unless an organization was established which could see that the supplies were distributed and utilized by the people who required their use. Quantities of medical and welfare supplies have been shipped into various parts of the world and have rested in warehouses; they have not been made available to the people for whom they were intended but have served instead as a means of financial speculation among small groups and frequently have been used for black market purposes. Because the Republic of Korea was a sovereign nation, I, therefore, recommended that negotiations be undertaken through Ambassador Muccio, the American ambassador, with President Rhee Syngman of the Republic of Korea, for an agreement whereby I could take into Korea a group of highly trained health and welfare people to determine the requirements as accurately as possible and to supervise allocation and distribution of the supplies received. This group, which was initially from my own staff in Japan, would work jointly with his cabinet; that is, those members of the cabinet concerned with health and social affairs and related activities. This recommendation was approved and negotiations were carried out. As a result, a Joint Cabinet Committee was established on which the Minister of Social Affairs, the Minister of Finance, Minister of Transportation, Minister of Home Affairs, and other cabinet ministers sat with my corresponding staff members, including myself.[2]

I also asked for volunteers among my staff and the Civil Affairs teams in Japan to accompany me to Korea for the purpose of carrying out this emergency health and welfare program for the civilian population. Our military medical forces, of course, were shorthanded and were taxed to the maximum taking care of battle casualties among our military personnel. I was authorized to establish a health and welfare organization in Korea to carry out these functions. I found myself in the position of commanding this organization in Korea and, at the same time, as chief of Health and Welfare, General Headquarters, United Nations Command, giving myself instructions in the name of General MacArthur, as Supreme Commander, United Nations Command.

The Eighth Army, commanded by Gen. Walton Walker, had established an advance echelon in Korea for prosecuting the war and had retained a rear echelon in Yokohama, Japan. I flew to an airfield in Pusan and then to Taegu, where General Walker had established his advance tactical headquarters. His main advance headquarters was located in the former Korean Fishery School outside of Seoul. I reported to General Walker and discussed the program for which I was responsible. He agreed to give us all possible logistical and other support, because I was acting as a General Headquarters agency and was not under his command; that is, I was not assigned to Eighth Army. His military surgeon, Colonel Davall, was completely occupied with his military medical problems. We subsequently established a small office in Pusan in the headquarters building and immediately began conferring with the cabinet of the Republic of Korea, which was then in Pusan.

Preventing Epidemics

My first problem was to determine how many refugees there were, where they were, and what was the status of requirements for food, clothing, and medical care. It was also necessary to determine what the diseases were in such groups, because a few cases of smallpox or cholera or typhus or typhoid in such a large mass of people will quickly spread under the primitive conditions in which these large masses of people were existing. Widespread epidemics may occur under such circumstances. From my past experience, I knew these diseases were endemic in Korea; I also knew the very limited means available in the form of medical personnel and medical supplies.

The Economic Cooperation Administration had shipped a considerable stock of medical supplies between 1948 and 1950 to supplement those that we had left behind and turned over to the Korean Government when the military forces were withdrawn in 1948. I very quickly learned that these supplies had been captured by the communists, and medical supplies, except in the few hospitals in Pusan, were practically nonexistent. We found that the people, as could be expected, were without bathing facilities, had no means of changing the clothes on their backs, and had become lousy. Typhus, smallpox, typhoid, and diphtheria cases were increasing. There were several million refugees in these mass concentrations which I visited.

Standards of Values

It was very difficult to travel among the refugee camps, particularly behind the Republic of Korea lines in the northeastern portion of the perimeter, because the communists had infiltrated through our thinly held lines, if they could be called lines. They had infiltrated with the refugees, so there were constant attacks on individuals and jeeps and cars moving along roads in the rear areas. One might become the victim of an attack at any time when travelling, particularly after dark, along any of the roads within the perimeter. Many of the small villages in our rear contained communist troops or guerilla forces, which could not, of course, be distinguished by us from friendly forces. On one such trip, Minister Chou, the Minister of Home Affairs, who had control of the national police, lined the road at intervals with police and volunteers who were not facing the road but were facing the crests of the hills which rose sharply on both sides of the road that I was travelling along to visit one of the isolated refugee camps. They were there not to preserve order but, as Chou said, to keep me from being killed or captured by communist guerrillas who were occupying the crests of the hills.

On one of my visits to the forward area near Mansan, occupied by the Twenty-fourth Infantry of the Twenty-fifth Division, I came to a bend in the road from which some of our tanks were firing on one of these villages in rear of our position. The thatch roofs of the mud-walled homes were on fire, and while we waited for this little action to end, the civilians in their white clothes came out with their hands in the air. In watching the interrogation of these prisoners by Republic of Korea soldiers who accompanied this tank unit, a number of these young able-bodied civilians whose white clothing served to disguise their black uniforms as communist soldiers were quickly unveiled as enemy troops who had infiltrated behind our lines and who, on the previous night, had successfully attacked and partially destroyed a convoy of ambulance jeeps which were bringing some of our wounded to the rear.

I asked why the inhabitants of these villages would harbor communist soldiers and attempt to conceal them when the Republic of Korea constabulary or military forces tried to search the villages. Minister Chou gave a very enlightening answer, one which should never be forgotten. Chou said, "You know the oriental well. We must be always on the winning side, otherwise we literally lose our lives. These people are not sure who is going to be the ultimate winner, and at the present time they are trying to protect themselves in the event the communists finally succeed in driving us into the sea by going along with the communist infiltrators and helping to protect them and conceal them." If we could only remember that lesson.

In most parts of the world, particularly in the Far East and the Middle East, that contain such large numbers of underdeveloped nations, the people have learned over thousands of years that if they espouse a cause which ultimately loses, they are literally liquidated. They always turn to the side of the strong and the side of the winner, if they can determine which side that is. They are concerned with survival more than with ideals such as the difference between our version of democracy and the communist version of what they call people's democracy. Certainly, we must remember that if we start a course of action in dealing with these peoples, we must carry it on to a successful conclusion lest they mistake our change of direction as a sign of weakness and ultimate defeat. Vacillation, in their eyes, under such circumstances, can only mean loss of their support for our positions.

In the minds of the great masses of people of the underdeveloped countries, the spirit in which we teach our children—that is, the way you play the game is the important thing, not whether you win or lose—does not apply in their view. To them the important thing is not how you won or how gallantly you might have fought before you lost but, Did you win or lose? I emphasize this point because the standards of values which we hold dear are quite different from the standards of values of the people with whom we are dealing in these parts of the world. We must adapt our concept to an understanding of their standards of values if we hope to gain and hold their support.

Aiding Korea

After we had made our initial determination of requirements for supplies in relation to the limited supplies available in warehouses in Pusan, Taegu, and other places, we immediately dispatched our requirements for food, clothing, and medical supplies to General Headquarters in Tokyo. Very fortunately, my supply people there were able to call on the Japanese governmental sources and our own sources of imported food for diversion of some of these supplies, temporarily, to meet this emergency in Korea. It was indeed fortunate that we had rehabilitated the pharmaceutical and medical supply industry in Japan, because on my instructions we were able to procure all of our needed supplies, including antibiotics, DDT, and other medical supplies and equipment, for Korea from Japanese sources.[3] Their production served as dollar income for the Japanese. It also shortened by many, many months the time for production and delivery which would be required had we been compelled to procure and ship these supplies from the United States.

We established the principle of assembling medical units, which were forty-bed hospitals that could be expanded to two hundred beds, containing the equipment and drugs and other articles which were adaptable to the oriental people. These unit assemblages were necessary together with what we called maintenance units, which were made up of the necessary numbers of expendable drugs, dressings, and equipment for 100,000 people for thirty days. I knew that we would need these because so little in the way of medical installations, such as hospitals, was available in Korea outside of Seoul. We could establish these units in the refugee camp areas and in school buildings or other buildings to serve as hospitals for the care of the sick and to furnish needed medical supplies. We could, through screening the refugee camps, gather together the civilian medical doctors who had come down ahead of our forces as they withdrew into the perimeter and use them to staff these medical facilities. There were actually only parts of two prefectures, or provinces as they were called in Korea, which were within our perimeter, so we had only two prefectural governmental echelons with which to deal. I established the usual teams of my own health and welfare personnel to work at that level, and also in the city of Pusan, to ensure that the organization of health and welfare activities for the control of diseases, provision of medical care, and provision of food, clothing, and such shelter as could be made available was carried on for these homeless refugees.

The Rice Crops

The rice crop normally planted in July would be due for harvest in November. The withdrawal, of course, had occurred during July and the early part of August. In the very rapid withdrawal from Seoul, fighting had occurred actually only in a few places along the principal roads of withdrawal of our forces and of the Republic of Korea forces. General MacArthur's plan was to carry out the invasion of Inchon when he had acquired sufficient troops and equipment and had available the resources for the amphibian lift. In estimating our requirements for the coming winter, I believed that if the breakout of the perimeter, which was to be undertaken simultaneously with the Inchon invasion, were successful, then these homeless refugees could return very quickly to their homes and would be there in sufficient time to harvest the rice crops: this breakout was scheduled for the middle of September. If this were possible, this harvest, which occurs in October and November, would provide sufficient stocks of rice to feed the population through the winter. Our immediate food requirements then would be to sustain the refugee population within the perimeter until the breakout occurred.

It was necessary to see at firsthand whether these villages, which had in many cases been depopulated and which were in the hands of the communists, could be reoccupied by our side. If the few pieces of timber, which are essential for ridge poles and supports, were made available, it only takes a couple of weeks to rebuild a mud and stone house to replace those which had been destroyed in the fighting. By flights over the rear of the enemy positions in small liaison aircraft, I was able to confirm that the crops had not been destroyed to any extent by the fighting and could be harvested, if only we could regain those tremendous rice fields. This gamble paid off.

Averting Catastrophe

We immediately began immunization programs among the refugees for smallpox, typhoid, paratyphoid, and typhus. We also began mass delousing campaigns. We brought in diphtheria toxoid to check an outbreak of diphtheria, which was beginning to spread, and brought under control the wildfire epidemics, which could have become catastrophic.

There are many reasons behind such strenuous efforts. One, of course, is the purely humanitarian desire to prevent mass deaths of people from disease. In this particular situation, there were several other reasons behind this program. We knew that the medical resources in North Korea were very limited. They had very limited stocks of medical supplies and they would be faced with controlling large-scale epidemics. Here was a test of communist versus democratic abilities to protect the people for all the Far East to see. If we could control these diseases among the Korean people on our side and the communists could not, it would be a direct and telling blow to the communist propaganda that living under the communist banner was better than living under the democratic banner, because we could show that literally the chances of dying under the communist banner were far greater than those under the democratic banner.[4]

Another major reason for controlling these diseases is based on military medical history. This history is full of examples of the effect of epidemics on military operations. Many campaigns have been lost because one or another side has been immobilized or literally decimated or even wiped out by an epidemic of disease, causing it to be completely ineffective from a military standpoint. Military medical history shows that until World War I, a soldier's chance of dying from disease in any army was far greater than his chance of dying from a weapon in the hands of an enemy. In fact, his chances of dying from disease in some campaigns had been five hundred times greater than his chances of dying from enemy weapons in battle.

In our own military forces, it was not until World War I that we were able to prevent deaths from disease from exceeding deaths from combat. In that war, they were practically equal. Since that war, particularly in World War II, and in the Korean War, we have been able for the first time in history to bring the deaths from disease among our troops below that produced by weapons in the hands of the enemy. In the Korean War, we knew, or could anticipate, that if we could control the epidemics of disease among the civilian population, then we would also lessen the hazard of the spread of disease to our own troops and those of our United Nations allies. On the other hand, if the communists could not lessen the spread of disease among the civilian population, then they might well have their own troops, who were also in contact, of course, with the civilian population, immobilized or decimated by these same epidemic diseases.

Medical Intelligence

We were constantly on the lookout for information through intelligence channels as to outbreaks of disease in the communist-held portion of Korea. One report which I had received in August was that cholera had broken out among some

Korean troops who had come from China into North Korea and had been moved south by railroad to an area just north of Taegu. I was on the lookout particularly for cholera because, as I have mentioned, two cases killed some 11,000 people out of 17,000 who acquired the disease in the matter of a few weeks in 1946. Cholera can spread very rapidly under such primitive sanitary conditions as existed in Korea, particularly when masses of people are living in the open with no sanitary facilities whatsoever.

This information about cholera among the North Koreans was initially obtained from a North Korean woman medical officer who had been shot in the hip by a machine gun bullet before she was captured. In addition, we had intercepted radio messages from the North Korean military commanders opposite our forces near Chonju asking for DDT from the stocks that the communists had captured in Seoul when they overran that city. The DDT was being requested to control the flies which might serve to spread the cholera vibrio from stools directly to food, if it is not protected. Of course, it was not protected from contamination by flies in such a situation.

We immediately began immunization of the civilian refugees on our side of the line with cholera vaccine. Under such circumstances, we were concerned that they should be protected when, we hoped, they were able to return to their villages after the breakout from the perimeter. If cholera were present in these villages while they were in the hands of the communists, we did not, of course, want such an epidemic to occur among the friendly civilians when they returned. We constantly watched for every source of verification of the presence of cholera among the communists.

Finally, with an interpreter, I interviewed this woman medical doctor. She told me that she was a graduate of Pyongyang, the North Korean capital medical school. She told me that she had been misunderstood: There was no cholera present among the troops in her unit. They thought we had the cholera, because we were immunizing our people against cholera. She had requested cholera vaccine and DDT from her superiors, because they did not want to have their troops infected in their final drive to Pusan, when they entered and overran our perimeter.

This incident showed how both sides in this case were very conscious of the hazard of cholera—a dreaded scourge—particularly in the Orient, and both sides were misinterpreting the intelligence information about the other. As it turned out, cholera did not develop among the people on either side of the communist line during the entire Korean War.

The Critical Days

During the critical days in the latter part of August and the first week of September, the communists were highly confident that they were going to win the war; they were able to penetrate our lines in several places. I was in the position of constantly visiting the areas occupied by our troops in an attempt to clear the lines of refugees. Frequently, I would find as many enemy troops behind certain portions of the line as apparently there were in front.

On the sixth of September, the communists launched several offensives. One was from the north against the eastern portion of the sector, which resulted in complete collapse of that portion of the line held by the hastily reorganized and regrouped Republic of Korea troops. The other was a deep penetration along the boundary between the left flank of the Second Division, which was held by the Ninth Infantry, and the north flank of the Twenty-fifth Division, which was on their left. This drive threatened to cut the single railroad and major supply line from Pusan to Taegu and the divisions to the north. General Walker wisely had ordered his advance tactical headquarters from Taegu to move back to Pusan. I was sitting with him late that evening after the headquarters had moved, when I think, perhaps, we were at the lowest ebb up to that time in the Korean War. Fighting between the First Cavalry Division, which was holding the bend just north of Taegu, was only about five or six miles north of us; as General Walker said, he did not know whether the communists would walk into Taegu from the northeast during the night. He had moved a portion of the Twenty-fourth Division, which had been in reserve, to try and plug the gap that had broken to our east.

During this critical phase of the Korean War, when it was touch and go whether the perimeter would hold until the Inchon landings could be launched, I, of course, made frequent trips back to Tokyo to ensure that our program was moving rapidly from that end, as far as our civilian health and welfare relief activities were concerned. During one of these trips, I learned that the Second Division was en route from the States and that it was short of medical officers, as were all of the other military units.

The policy in the army medical corps at the end of World War II was to try and encourage young doctors to come into the service. In doing so, they were offered what at that time were considered the most desirable benefits; that is, they were offered residency training in specialty fields, because all young docs immediately after World War II wanted to be specialists. None of them had been trained in that basic function of all military medical officers, which is the evacuation and care of the wounded soldier in combat.

Our own shortage of military medical officers in the Far East theater, which General Hume, the theater military surgeon, and I had talked over many times, had made it necessary to limit the number of doctors assigned to our divisions there in peacetime and to concentrate the limited number which was available to him, in the military hospitals. When our troops actually went into combat in 1950, they were very short of medical personnel. When the additional divisions which were scheduled to come from the United States were to move out, they also frequently found themselves with only one or two medical officers out of a complement of what should have been at that time some sixty medical officers as battalion surgeons and as medical officers in the divisional medical battalions, which operated the medical services in rear of the infantry regiments or combat teams.

In an effort to fill these vital jobs, the Surgeon General of the Army was compelled to take young doctors who had come into the regular service under residency programs and ship them to Korea without having had the opportunity of giving them any real training in medical field service. Some of these young lads had been in civilian hospitals, even though commissioned in the regular service. I have in mind a number of young men who had bought their uniforms just before embarking on aircraft for an airlift to Japan. Within a matter of days, they were in the midst of the fight, trying to evacuate and care for wounded in an infantry battalion aid station, the foremost medical installation in combat.

The Arrival of Captain Struthers

My older daughter, Yvonne, had married a young man who was studying medicine in 1946. He had elected to enter the regular army medical corps upon his graduation from medical school in 1949, and had completed his internship at Letterman Army Hospital. He had just started his residency in pathology when he and other young residents were suddenly ordered to Korea on temporary duty to fill vital assignments in our infantry divisions in combat. I was back in Tokyo when "Chuck," Charles M. Struthers, Captain, Medical Corps, U.S. Army, with his fellow residents, arrived at the replacement center at Camp Drake near Tokyo.

My wife and younger daughter had left by boat in August for the United States, where Patsy was to be married to a young man, Dale Dwyer, who was a student in architecture at the University of California. She had met him when she had returned to the United States to enter the university after graduation from high school in Tokyo. I had planned to go on leave to be present at my daughter's wedding at the Presidio of San Francisco Chapel; however, of course, the Korean War necessitated that I remain in the Far East. So my wife and younger daughter had returned to the United States for the wedding.

My older daughter's husband and his young friends, on the other hand, had arrived in Tokyo to engage in the Korean War. Because my wife was gone, I made our quarters available to them as a place where they could spend their free hours while waiting for their new assignments. In my discussions, during the few days I was there, I gave them such advice as I could about the duties of a medical officer with an infantry regiment, because they had been earmarked for such assignments. It was a matter of only a few days until Captain Struthers was assigned to the First Battalion, Ninth Infantry of the Second Division, as battalion surgeon.

This particular situation was one which almost all of the senior officers faced during that war. Most of us had sons or sons-in-law as junior officers in that bitter struggle. In spite of the devotion to duty and honor and country, which is the guiding force of all regular officers worthy of the name, we still are human. During the course of operations when one knows the particular unit to which a young son or son-in-law is assigned is in combat, one has in the back of his mind the constant nagging thought, Will he make it this time? Although you must concentrate all of your conscious efforts in carrying out your own assignment, still, you have this worry that perhaps he will not make it this time. So I was always anxious for news of the course of the operation in which Chuck was participating. Many of the young sons and sons-in-law of my friends, general officers, were killed or wounded in action; yet, their fathers carried on in the best traditions of the service, as to be expected.

In the communist penetration of the Second Division, the communists' principle attack overran the Ninth Infantry to which my young son-in-law was attached. His first real taste of combat was when his aid station was overrun and he was attempting to defend his wounded with a carbine which he had never before fired. He lost some of his men, most of his equipment, and, of course, his personal belongings. When I visited him a few days later, this battalion had been overrun; I found him, a veteran now, unshaven, because he had lost his razor, and anxious to find out more about his job.

In going forward on this particular staff visit, a jeep travelling about a quarter of a mile ahead of me in the rear of the division area, as I was moving forward, was blown up by hand grenades from communist guerrillas and communist troops, which had penetrated behind the front lines of our Second Division. It took a long time for our troops to learn that they could not bind themselves to the roads, which in this country ran through the valleys between precipitous hills and mountains. The communists simply walked along the trails and the ridges up in the mountains; when night came, they could attack from any direction, usually the rear of our troops.

We lost many men by being road bound in the early phases of this bitter war. We had become so used to being hauled around in trucks and vehicles in our peacetime training and in our own land, which has the greatest highway system in the world, that we sometimes forget that other parts of the world do not have such highways and that the roads make us sitting ducks to the enemy, who is willing to leave the roads and walk across country. We should have learned this kind of lesson when the Japanese walked around the road-bound British who were guarding the approaches from the north of Singapore in Malaya. It is a lesson we should keep in mind for the future.

On numerous occasions, I watched our troops digging in to protect their positions in an all-around defense, which, it was ultimately learned, was necessary for survival. Sitting casually a few hundred yards away would be white-clad Koreans. Our troops, unable to identify friend from foe, could not and would not, I think, deliberately shoot up these men who had the appearance of unarmed civilians—even though they eventually learned that most of them were enemy troops wearing black uniforms under their white clothing who would seek to kill our soldiers under cover of darkness by infiltrating through these defensive positions which our troops were digging. Because our troops were holding such tremendous frontages, there was no such thing as a front line. The so-called front lines consisted of comparatively small groups, usually of battalion size, holding a piece of ground and some miles to the north another such position. The communists could move under cover of darkness between and around such positions and they did so freely. In their attacks, when they were frontal attacks, under the human wave concept, they frequently drove thousands of refugees through our lines. Again, our troops were reluctant to fire on such masses of men, women, and children, even though they knew that among them or behind them were advancing communist soldiers.

26

The Breakout

On my frequent trips to Tokyo to keep abreast of the overall planning, I learned the Seventh Division, which had come to Japan from Korea in 1948 and which was occupying the island of Hokkaido, was to be reorganized. Its strength was to be increased by building up the understrength units with Republic of Korea soldiers who were sent to Japan for such training and incorporation. The Third Division, which was coming from the United States, and the First Marine Division together with the Seventh Division, were to constitute the X Corps. Gen. Ned Almond was to be the X Corps commander in addition to his duties as chief-of-staff of the theater.

In our planning for the Inchon landing, I designated Colonel Mallahan my deputy on General Almond's staff to take over relief activities for General Almond when Inchon was captured. Our intelligence had indicated that the communists planned, when they withdrew, to move out all stores of food and medical supplies. Therefore, we obtained a priority on space, and the convoy supporting the Inchon landing had several thousand tons of rice and the usual mobile medical units, which we could use to care for civilian injured and sick when Inchon and Seoul were recaptured.

The I Corps and IX Corps headquarters had only recently been deactivated in Japan; they were re-established in Korea before the breakout. Gen. John B. Coulter commanded the IX Corps; Gen. "Shrimp" (Frank W.) Milburn commanded the I Corps. The I Corps contained the First Cavalry Division. The Twenty-fourth Division was to make the breakout in an attempt to drive toward Seoul to join up with the X Corps forces scheduled to land at Inchon. The IX Corps, made up of the Second Division and of the Twenty-fifth Division, was to drive straight west from their positions running south from Taegu, then make a wide sweep clearing the communists out of South Korea, and then turn northward after reaching the coast of the China Sea.

General Walker had consented to release of the First Marine Regiment, or combat team, to rejoin the First Division. The First Marine Regiment was holding a critical portion of his line and had made the counteroffensive against the communist penetration of the line between the Second Division and the Twenty-fifth Division. He issued his famous stand or die order to our troops in the perimeter.

In discussing informally the critical phase of this holding operation and the attempt to break out at the corner at Taegu, I suggested to General Walker that if the Korean rear were threatened by the capture of Seoul and a doubt placed in their minds as to ultimate victory, the Korean communist soldiers facing our perimeter would suddenly disappear as soldiers; thus, I would as suddenly have a large increase in civilian refugees.

The Front

I went forward to the Fifth and Eighth and Seventh Cavalry Regiments of the First Cavalry Division, commanded by my good friend Gen. "Hap" (Hobart R.) Gay, during the breakout and visited, of course, the front line battalion surgeons. When word had been received that the landing at Inchon had been successful, and Kimpo Airfield on which I had landed many times between 1945 and 1948 was in our hands, I then hopped across the enemy-held territory from Taegu to Kimpo. It was interesting to observe from low altitude the bombing and strafing of our F-80 jets and the old P-51 propeller-driven aircraft in support of our advancing First Cavalry Division.

As soon as the word had apparently spread through the communist forces that the landing at Inchon was successful, they literally melted away, except for a few isolated pockets of resistance. Instead of a communist army in their black uniforms in front of our troops, there was an increase of about a million civilian refugees with their white clothing concealing their military status. Some of these refugees took cover in mountains west of Taegu. Others began the long trek by foot to the north along the mountain chain paralleling the east coast of Korea; ultimately, they were re-equipped and reorganized at the Yalu River crossing cities at Sinuiju and Mapojin. During the fighting in the advance from Inchon to Seoul, Inchon had been badly knocked about. There were many several thousand casualties, as well as communist casualties.

The X Corps headquarters was located at this time at Ascom City. This location was the former principle supply base, which had been built by our XXIV Corps during the American occupation of Korea. It contained a very fine hospital building, barracks, and the usual warehouses. Ascom City itself had been damaged. One of our bombers dropped, apparently, a large-size bomb right through the roof of the rotunda of the former American-built hospital. This building was unusable then for a military hospital. The Fourth Field Hospital, which had been under my control in the Middle East, and which I had last seen in the Vosges Mountains in Europe, was now with the X Corps; it was established in one of the buildings, but not the hospital building, in Ascom City.[1]

Seoul

I entered Seoul from Kimpo with the leading elements of the First Marine Division. The Seventh Division had moved south toward Wonsan. A pontoon bridge had been established across the Han River, which separates the town of Yong-Dong-Po from Seoul. The highway bridge and the railroad bridges over this river had been demolished and the spans dropped into the river by the Koreans in their early withdrawal from Seoul the preceding June. The street fighting in Seoul was severe; many blocks of buildings were on fire, not only from bombing of our supporting air force but also by shelling of our supporting artillery and mortars. A large portion of the fire, as I learned later, was set by the withdrawing communists.

It was a number of weeks after the capture of Seoul before the communists were finally rounded up in Seoul. At any time, particularly at night, if you were unfortunate enough to be silhouetted in a window, you became a target for sniper fire; even mortar fire occurred sporadically in various parts of the city every night.

In Seoul, the Bantu Hotel, which had been used as a headquarters for the XXIV Corps in 1945 to 1948, and subsequently leased as the Economic Cooperation Administration building and billets, had been damaged by a demolition charge placed under one corner by the withdrawing communists. The records in the files had been distributed around the floors. The Chosen Hotel, where I had stayed during my frequent visits during the occupation of Korea, had been only slightly damaged from some twenty-millimeter cannon shells from our strafing aircraft; it was unoccupied and guarded by marines. The communists apparently had withdrawn hastily from the Chosen Hotel, which had been the building used to house their top military staff. They had left the place in a filthy condition; because the toilet bowls could not operate without water, they were particularly offensive. The Seoul city power plant had been sabotaged; consequently, without power, there were no water pumps to operate. So for some time, there was neither light nor water in Seoul.

It was at this point that I met Gen. Frank E. Lowe. He is one of the finest fighting soldiers it has been my pleasure to meet. He had been the national commander of the American Legion when General MacArthur had been chief-of-staff of the U.S. Army between 1930 and 1935. He was a friend of General MacArthur. As time passed, he had been the executive director for the Truman Committee, when President Truman was a Senator. He had been sent to the Far East by President Truman as his eyes and ears to report on the conduct of the Korean War. General Lowe was where the fighting was. He was not an armchair general. He was a major general in the reserves and, as such, had been ordered to active duty for this assignment. When I was in forward areas, I frequently found him in his jeep with its fifty caliber machine guns mounted so that it looked like a small land battleship. He had taken possession of the Chosen Hotel to prevent it from being looted.

The Chosen Hotel, which had been the finest hotel in Seoul, had a very fine stock of liqueurs and wines and, whether we like it or not, soldiers who have been through combat frequently look for and certainly deserve some means of relaxation after the emotional and physical tension of combat. Frequently, if stocks of beverages are located, they are "liberated" by the troops who find them. General Lowe had decided to protect the Korean property and had placed this hotel off limits to all personnel.

General Lowe visited the Bantu Hotel, where we proposed to establish our new headquarters as soon as we could get it cleaned up. He invited me to stay in the Chosen Hotel. General Lowe and his aide and myself were the lone occupants of this hotel for the time being. There was no light except candlelight or Coleman lanterns. There was no water, but we did use "jerry cans" and heated them over fires to get some hot water to wash ourselves, which was a help.

I had intended to stay, in fact I did stay one night, at the American housing area near the outskirts of Seoul. This housing area had been built during the days when the Seventh Division of American troops had been located in Korea prior to 1948. It had been taken over by the Korean people and had been fought over; there were, of course, many bullet and shell holes in the buildings.

Again, the same basic problem, which happens in all such situations, had to be solved in Seoul. First, we had to find out how many civilians we had to look after. How many were sick and wounded as a result of the fighting? What was the status of the hospitals located in Seoul? Where were the stocks of medical supplies that had been captured by the communists in their rapid move into Seoul in June? How many medical people had escaped the communists? What was the food situation? How could we get food into the city? What could be done about providing shelter for those civilians who had lost their homes?

One of the things that the situation in Seoul illustrated is hard for Americans or people of European descent to understand. I saw thousands of bodies of civilian Koreans who had been literally mowed down by the communists near the prison outside of Seoul and at Uijonbu. Among the bodies of the civilians I saw at Uijonbu and at the railroad station were many Korean doctors and nurses whom I had known before 1948. They had been captured by the communists in their rapid overrunning of Seoul in June. The communists had attempted to take some of them north; others they had simply killed.

We found also that Koreans who had been chauffeurs or housemaids even for American personnel between 1945 and 1948 had all been very carefully listed by the communists. When they overran Seoul, these people were rounded up and shot. This literal liquidation of masses of people under such circumstances is foreign to our thinking; but if we remember that it really occurs, it may help us to understand why these people must be sure, if they can, they are on the winner's side. If they take the wrong side and lose, they end up as corpses. Chou, the Minister of Home Affairs, quickly brought back his national police from Pusan to Seoul, and began rounding up communist collaborators who had not gotten away at the time the communists withdrew. Long lines of men were being marched outside of the city at night where they, in turn, were liquidated as collaborators.

Military and Civilian Hospitals

The military plan was for the First Cavalry Division, which began to arrive in a few days, to relieve the First Marine Division, which had driven north to Uijonbu; then the First Cavalry Division would drive north toward Pyongyang. The Eighth Army headquarters was to move into Seoul. The X Corps, when relieved, was to re-embark on its transports, move from the China Sea around to the port of Wonsan in northeast Korea, and make a landing and drive toward Pyongyang from the east, thereby executing a giant pincers movement on the remaining communist forces which might be in North Korea.

An old friend of mine, Col. Vi Gorby, who had been sent to the Far East from Sixth Army headquarters in the United States, was to be the Eighth Army surgeon; instead, he was made X Corps surgeon. His evacuation hospitals were full, not only of wounded American soldiers and marines but also wounded civilians. It was necessary that I get these civilians taken care of in re-equipped and reorganized civilian hospitals as quickly as possible to free his military hospital beds.[2] In addition, there were a good many thousand North Korean prisoners in the old prison area near Inchon. Although Vi had teams from the First Mobile Army Surgical Hospital operating there, it was necessary again to establish a medical service for these civilians, preferably by using Korean medical personnel.[3]

Several hundred Korean doctors had fled from Seoul into the small neighboring villages when it became apparent the communists were withdrawing. Many of them told me that when the communists had entered Seoul in June, they had killed the patients, particularly the Republic of Korea soldiers who had been wounded and were in the Central Red Cross Hospital and Severance Hospital and in the National Hospitals. On visiting these hospitals after we regained Seoul in September, I found that the Severance Medical School and Hospital had been completely destroyed. The Central Red Cross Hospital had been badly damaged by a bomb which had fallen in the courtyard. The two major buildings making up the National Hospital, number one and number two, were undamaged. The City Communicable Disease Hospital was comparatively undamaged. It was occupied by our One Hundred Twenty-first Evacuation Hospital for military personnel. But there was no medical equipment left in the Korean hospitals; the communists had literally stripped everything that could be moved out of these hospitals before they had withdrawn.

Fortunately, in our programming, we were able to fly as well as unload from the ships the units that we had assembled in Japan, and were able quickly to re-equip the hospitals which were left standing. We were then able to move those wounded civilians and Republic of Korea wounded from our X Corps military hospitals into the Korean-staffed hospitals under the supervision of my people.

Just south of Seoul, I found an interesting situation. The Seventh Day Adventist Missionary Hospital was intact. Although the communists had occupied the Mission School, and the buildings had been damaged in the fighting, for some reason this hospital had not been looted. When I visited this hospital I found no patients. There was only one doctor, and the equipment was intact. The hospital was quickly reopened and was used for care of foreign nationals as they began to come in after the fighting moved to the north.

There was a very fine school building, actually a technical school, just to the north of Seoul which had been used by our Thirty-fourth General Hospital, which was an American military hospital, from 1945 to 1948. It had been converted partially into a technical school, but was practically undamaged except for a few cracks in one corner from some bombs that had landed nearby. Because our military forces were looking for hospital buildings for our military medical units, I suggested to Colonel Davall that this might be used for one of his evacuation hospitals, because the other hospital buildings in Seoul were required for the civilian population. This hospital was isolated, and he eventually decided against it because of the hazard of guerrillas attacking his ambulance convoys on the roads.

Water Supplies and Disease Control

My sanitary engineers began to work with the army engineers in getting the electric power operating again and establishing water supplies for the city. This effort took some weeks.

Cleaning up the dead, and burying the dead of both enemy troops and friendly civilians, was another problem. The fly situation, of course, at that time of the year was a major headache. We had shipped in power dusters for spraying DDT. I had difficulty in locating these power dusters but noted that power dusters were being used along the streets by my good friends in the Marine Corps. Col. "Bud" Herring, one of the most gallant medical officers I have known, a naval medical corps officer, who was surgeon of the First Marine Division, graciously offered to trade me some power dusters for some other supplies when they were ready to re-embark. Later, I was to learn that he was giving me back the dusters which I had originally programmed and shipped; but, the dusting got done, which was the important thing for the control of flies and the spread of certain diseases.

Our requirements for blankets, which are really quilts that we procured in Japan, and for medical supplies and other equipment continued. Our medical teams began immunization programs, because we found the usual smallpox, diphtheria, typhoid and typhus occurring among the civilians who had remained behind when the communists withdrew to the north.

The Rice Convoys

We found that the railroad from Inchon to Yong-Dong-Po was capable of being placed in operation very shortly. Sufficient locomotives were found in some tunnels, which were undamaged, to begin operation. We began to move rice supplies from the convoy to Yong-Dong-Po to feed the people in Seoul, because the communists had also removed all of the available rice stocks from Seoul. I obtained a convoy of trucks from General Almond to move rice across the pontoon bridge into Seoul for distribution to the population who had been without food for some days; but, because of the troop movement across this single pontoon bridge over which the First Cavalry Division was being moved to go north to Uijonbu, while the Marine Division was being relieved and returning across the pontoon bridge for re-embarkation, I was told that this would be the only convoy for civilian supplies that I could get across the river pontoon bridge. I was concerned about how I could subsequently move many additional tons of rice across the Han River.

This brought to light an interesting situation. I talked to Chou, and he then took me down to the river where the piers of one of the bridges still stood upright. He said, "We will get the rice across the river the way the communists got supplies across the river when you thought that you had cut their supply lines." He proceeded to show me the means used by the communists in moving supplies, which to us were utterly fantastic. We normally move our supplies by truck, by road, or by railroad; but the communists and the other people in Korea are used to moving things on their backs on A-frames. When the bridges had been destroyed, the communists, as in this case, would build underwater bridges. If the streams were shallow, they would fill sand bags and lay them in the bottom of the streams until they were within a few feet of the top of the water and could not be seen from the air. Then at night, they would proceed to march across this underwater bridge with their supplies of food and ammunition on their backs. In the case of the Han River, they had a rope footbridge which they could pull up out of the water at night. They literally lockstepped thousands of Koreans across this footbridge with food and ammunition; when daylight came, the bridge was not to be seen.

We used this bridge, plus the many small boats which were rounded up, to transport the rice on the backs of men from the railroad sidings in Yong-Dong-Po to the distribution centers in Seoul. It is amazing how much can be done by a mass of humans with very primitive equipment, if there are enough humans. In the Orient and in the Middle East, humans are the cheapest commodity according to their own standards. The rice was moved into Seoul and it was distributed. Eventually, additional bridging was put across the Han, and we were able some months later to move supplies freely through the port of Inchon for the civilian population.

As time passed, the rice harvest began. We were soon able to collect sufficient rice. When the railroads were repaired, we were able to meet the needs of the people of South Korea, so far as rice was concerned.

General Dean

During this time, I learned for certain that Gen. Bill Dean was still alive. In his almost one-man stand at Taegu, he had been reported as missing-in-action and later presumed dead. Because Bill was a good personal friend of mine, of course, I was interested in attempting to find out where he was and if he were alive. I found out through Chou, who brought in a communist professor, Lee, who had been captured by Chou's police dragnet, that General Dean had been captured and had been held in Chonju prison. I talked to a young boy who had also been held by the communists with his father in prison there. He had seen General Dean and had known General Dean when he was military governor of South Korea under General Hodges. Professor Lee, who had also known General Dean before Lee defected to the communists, had talked to General Dean, who had been moved to Seoul from Chonju prison. Lee had attempted to persuade him to broadcast anti-American propaganda. He told me that General Dean, with other American prisoners, had been moved north to Pyongyang prior to our capture of Seoul. This information was sent back through intelligence channels to Tokyo.

27

North Korea

As the First Cavalry Division and the Twenty-fourth Division swept northward, they quickly captured Pyongyang. General MacArthur dropped the Eleventh Airborne combat team north of Pyongyang in an attempt to cut off retreating communists and, particularly, to cut off two trains, which our intelligence people had reported were carrying American prisoners north to the Yalu River. This effort was only partially successful. One train got away. As we would later learn, General Dean was on this train.

The other train was trapped in a tunnel; the prisoners were taken out and massacred by the communists before they themselves fled further to the north. A few of the survivors, particularly one young soldier, stated that he was reasonably certain that General Dean had been moved onto the other train.

Pyongyang

On my first trip to Pyongyang in October 1950, I found the city, which lay on the north bank of a river, had been badly damaged. There were beautiful missionary compounds with schools and fine homes and hospitals. As usual, there was no water.

The water supply of Pyongyang was obtained from a series of wells on sand bars in the river. These wells were necessary because the river froze in the winter. The communists had proceeded to dismantle the generators and pumps and to bury these very critical pieces of equipment. Our sanitary engineers were able to find out from the inevitable squealer that they had been buried, and where, and began to unearth them. Eventually, the generators and the water system were operating again. But all of this took time.

We also found a number of American cars, some of which were dismantled, the parts having been buried. These cars had been left behind by the American civilians who had been hastily evacuated out of Seoul the preceding June, and had been taken north by the communists for their own use.

We found the typical communist state. If one wanted a haircut, then one went to the governmental barber shop. All of the doctors worked for the government. It was a typical totalitarian regime.

The Eighth Army established an advance echelon headquarters in Pyongyang in a missionary compound, as our troops advanced north to Sinuiju. Civilian assistance teams were moved into Pyongyang to begin the work of handling the refugees and the food and medical problem there.

I found a few hospitals still functioning in North Korea. Some of the medical equipment which had been taken from the South Korean hospitals was located, and a few doctors who had been in hiding returned to Pyongyang. There were deep underground shelters, which had been constructed by the communists against air raids; they had apparently worked fairly successfully.

We found the Pyongyang Medical School across the river, south of the city. An institute was located there in which there were a considerable number of experimental animals. We found through interpreters that this was where the communists had made smallpox and typhoid vaccine for use in immunizing the North Korean communist people. This institute had been run under the direction of a Russian woman medical officer. We also found that the Russians had built a very beautiful hospital, which we were told was for Russians only. We found very fine Russian medical equipment in this hospital. We found, of course, a considerable number of homes which the Russians had used. I stayed in a billet that was a former Russian house.

I had previously found out from a North Korean medical officer that they had had very few medical supplies when the North Korean army invaded Seoul. They had known of the fairly large stocks of American supplies, which had been turned over to the Republic of Korea, and which were in storage at Ascom City and around Seoul; they had counted on capturing these supplies for their own use. That is exactly what happened. We found American drugs, including some streptomycin, in the hospitals in North Korea. On investigation, I found some of these drugs had come a long way around. They had entered Red China through Hong Kong, and from Red China had gotten into North Korea. Some had been, of course, smuggled across the border through black market channels, but apparently the main supply of comparatively recent equipment for the communists had come through Hong Kong.

Hamhung

After starting operations in Pyongyang, I went back to Sèoul. Colonel Champaney was to be the head of a newly created United Nations Civil Assistance Command to be assigned to the Eighth Army, which was to replace the initial health and welfare organization I had set up. We took off in two small L-17 liaison aircraft for Hamhung on the northeast coast of Korea. The X Corps, which had re-embarked from Inchon to move to the northeast coast of Korea, had run into difficulties because of extensive mine fields in the Wonsan harbor area. We had been informed that they had finally landed and were establishing their headquarters in Hamhung. We were eager to find out the refugee situation in those comparatively industrialized areas. Wonsan was the site of a tremendous oil refining industry, which the Japanese had built during their long years of occupation. Hamhung was the most industrialized city in North Korea. Both had been targets for our air attacks.

We took off early in the morning and flew across the mountains to Hamhung. We saw fairly large concentrations of civilians in white moving into some of the villages and towns which had not been occupied by our advancing troops. These, obviously, were remnants of the North Korean army en route, as we learned later, to Mapojin and Manchuria for re-equipment and reorganization to re-enter the war later as North Korean troops.

We landed in a street of Hamhung. We found the railroad yards and stations and many of the buildings had been badly damaged or destroyed by air attack. It was not long until a crowd of North Koreans gathered around our small aircraft. Because of the long years of missionary work in Korea prior to World War II, some Korean who had been missionary trained and spoke some English could usually be located. We asked where the American army headquarters was. We were told by an English-speaking Korean there were no Americans in Hamhung, only the communists.

The Republic of Korea Capital Division had swept up the east coast of Korea and was well beyond Hamhung on its way to the Yalu River. Apparently, the movement of this unit had been so rapid, with so little opposition, the communists had closed in behind it—much as the divided waters of the biblical Red Sea episode. We found ourselves, therefore, in the middle of an enemy-held city and thought it advisable to get out quickly before we became prisoners.

We did not have enough gasoline to get back to Seoul, so we flew down the east coast to Wonsan, where the X Corps, presumably, was laying off the port. We saw the ships in the convoy, and, fortunately, some landing craft coming in to shore. We landed at the beat-up airfield near Wonsan, which was located adjacent to the burned-out oil refineries. The advanced echelon of the X Corps headquarters was coming ashore at Wonsan. It was to be some days before they established themselves in Hamhung.

The Eastern Coastal Area

This narrow eastern coastal area is physically separated from the western part of Korea by a very high rugged range of mountains, which can be traversed only by a very few roads. These roads could easily be held as defiles by a group of determined enemy against any attempted movement by our troops; so they were. It was unsafe to leave any of the principle cities because chances of being ambushed were practically one hundred percent. In fact, small parties entered Hamhung and Wonsan from time to time doing a little sabotage and occasionally killing troops.

In Wonsan and subsequently in other visits to Hamhung and Kilju, after our troops had occupied those areas, I found the same situation as I had found on the west side of North Korea. One hospital in Wonsan, run by the Methodist missionaries, remained in the burned-out area. The Catholic hospital was intact. One very fine hospital building, which the few remaining Korean doctors told me had been taken over by the Russians, had been badly damaged by aerial bombing.

The Occupation of North Korea

During the few months of our occupation in North Korea, I found many cases of smallpox, typhus—the dreaded louse-borne scourge—typhoid, and diphtheria. Although I was told that the people had been immunized against smallpox and typhoid by the communists, they obviously were not protected. We were able to obtain samples of their vaccines, which had been in the institute in Pyongyang. They were found to be practically worthless. I knew, therefore, that the infected people in these cities represented small bonfires, which could during the coming winter spread into a forest fire of epidemic disease if we could not immediately get to work to begin immunizing, delousing, and getting this thing under control, as we had done in South Korea. We flew in our vaccines and our DDT and blankets and food and began our programs in North Korea.[1]

When the final remnants of the North Korean army had been defeated, General MacArthur had received instructions to make a token occupation of all of the provinces of North Korea. The instructions from the United Nations through the U.S. Joint Chiefs of Staff to General MacArthur were that he was to hold elections for governors and for the mayors of local communities. The United Nations proposed to keep North Korea under its direct supervision for a time until it felt North Korea could be united politically with the Republic of Korea. This proposal, of course, was quite different from the concept of Rhee Syngman, who proposed the immediate extension of control of his own government to the provinces of North Korea.

The Constitution of the Republic of Korea, when that Republic had been set up as a sovereign nation and approved by the United Nations, provided for the form of national government in which the Diet or Parliament was made up of elected representatives from all of the provinces. The Diet elected the prime minister, who appointed his cabinet as a coalition cabinet. The Home Minister, then, recommended to the prime minister who should be governors of the various provinces. The governors, as in Japan, executed national laws in their respective provinces. The mayors were also appointed. They, in turn, executed the national laws and the local laws in their cities or towns. Following the elections in which this parliamentary system was set up, one hundred seats were left vacant in the Republic of Korea Diet for representatives from North Korea. The United Nations Commission, which had been appointed to supervise the political unification of North Korea in 1945, was never permitted by the communists to enter North Korea to hold free elections to elect these one hundred delegates.

Rhee Syngman, in my opinion, quite properly felt that the election should be for representatives from the North Korean provinces to the Republic of Korea

Diet, and not for governors or mayors, because they are not elected under the Korean Constitution. It was the responsibility of his government, again under supervision of the United Nations Commission, to see that the authority of his national government should quickly be established in North Korea; but, the directives from the United Nations were quite to the contrary.

It was the military plan for the American troops to be withdrawn from North Korea and for the Republic of Korea troops to man the Yalu River border as soon as the elections were held. Because the North Korean resistance had completely collapsed and the fighting had terminated for all practical purposes, except for guerrilla activity and ambushing of individuals and convoys on roads, General MacArthur in complying with his directives immediately dispersed various columns of troops to make this token occupation. There was no need then for the X Corps to drive westward through the narrow defiles of the rugged mountain chain to join the Eighth Army at Pyongyang. The X Corps began its token occupation of the provinces along the east coast, while the Eighth Army advanced to make its token occupation of the provinces west of the mountain ranges. These mountain ranges are rugged and heavily timbered north of the thirty-eighth parallel. They are almost uninhabited, except for a few isolated villages housing lumber workers and for bears, who look upon the mountains as their natural domain.

28

The New War

The movement to make a token occupation of the principle cities and capitals of the provinces of North Korea was under way in late October 1950. It soon became apparent that this occupation by United Nations forces north of the thirty-eighth parallel was not to be completed without further fighting. A Republic of Korea battalion moved north through Kangye toward Mapojin and disappeared. The Eighth Cavalry Regiment of the First Cavalry Division, which was moving to the northwest, was suddenly overrun by a Chinese Communist cavalry division mounted on Mongolian ponies. A column of the First Cavalry Division, advancing directly west to Sinuiju at the mouth of the Yalu River dividing Manchuria and North Korea, came within sight of the town. The sudden attack on the Eighth Cavalry by Chinese Communists caused the First Cavalry Division to halt its advance.

The Chinese Communists had massed many armies along the Manchurian border. Reports had come in of the capture of occasional Chinese volunteers. When the Eighth Cavalry was overrun and the Korean battalion had disappeared, the survivors indicated they were being fought by organized Chinese forces, which obviously had entered North Korea; a new war was under way.

The Industrial Power Complex

Why might this occur? North Korea is very mountainous. It is a potential source of a large amount of hydroelectric power. We had been told by the Japanese in 1945 that, after taking over Manchuria in 1931, they no longer considered the Yalu River a boundary between Japanese-held Korea and Manchuria; it was a source of electrical power. They had undertaken tremendous industrial development in Manchuria, building steel mills, opening coal mines, and expanding their industrial empire. As a source of electrical power in this Manchurian, Korean, and eventually Chinese industrial area, North Korea was the heart of the industrial power complex.

The Japanese had constructed gigantic dams at Chonju and Huichon and a series of dams and power plants, called the Suiho, along the Yalu River. The power lines from these tremendous power plants served Manchuria and even ran northward to Vladivostok.

When Korea was artificially divided at the thirty-eighth parallel, the electrical power to South Korea was immediately shut down by the communists, who controlled the powerhouses and reservoirs north of that parallel. It is reasonable, therefore, to assume that the Chinese Communists, recognizing their dependence upon this North Korean area for their hydroelectric power, which had been built up by the Japanese, could not afford to let us take over control. According to their standards, they could expect that we would automatically shut off all power to Manchuria, and even to Vladivostok, as they had shut it off to South Korea. Some thought is required as to the motive or motives of the Chinese Communist Republic in starting a new war with the aim of regaining control of the power source of the industrial complex of Manchuria.

The Western Perimeter

As soon as it was apparent that organized Chinese troops had slipped across the Yalu River in large numbers and were concealed in the area north and west of Anju, which threatened the rear and flank of the Eighth Army, General Walker quite wisely drew in the "fingers of the hand" and established a perimeter north of Pyongyang, generally through Anju, where the west coast of Korea turns towards the northwest.

Our troops to the north had only relatively small supplies of ammunition. The destroyed railroads running north from Seoul to Pyongyang had to be rebuilt. A new port and line of supply was opened, but it was necessary then for a delay to occur while winter clothing and ammunition and other military stocks, including food, were moved north to support our troops which had been withdrawn to the perimeter north of Anju.

The Advance

On one of my trips back to Seoul, I visited the Second Division and found my young son-in-law in a rest area, still with the First Battalion of the Ninth Infantry. Because the original plan was for our troops, including the Second Division, to be withdrawn from North Korea, the Second Division had, without too much fighting, gone into reserve south of Seoul. He was wondering, as were the other young medical officers, whether he was to be returned to his family. They were still living at Letterman Hospital in San Francisco, where my daughter and their young son and newly born daughter were awaiting his return from what was intended to be a five-month tour of temporary duty.

During this short trip, he was given a pass to Seoul. At the Chosen Hotel, we heated a "jerry can" of water. He had a bath and a good sleep in a bed. Then, as I had to take off from the airfield again, I sent him back in my jeep to his unit.

After this unexpected entry of the Chinese Communists, the Second Division, instead of being released for movement back to Europe, was hastily ordered north for the build up to renew our offensive and to quickly end the Chinese

Communist phase of the war. The Second Division was moved into the line north of Anju. The day after Thanksgiving, 24 November 1950, the Ninth Infantry of the Second Division advanced north very cautiously toward Kangye. The Twenty-fifth Division on its left and the Twenty-fourth Division, which was in line further to the west, moved respectively to the northwest. The Twenty-fourth moved very slowly toward the west. The Republic of Korea troops were on the right of the Second Division moving directly north.

This cautious advance began, and little or no resistance was encountered. The latter was characteristic of communist tactics. Once having established contact, before they themselves launched a new offensive, they might withdraw from such contact for what they call "a night's march," which may be up to fifteen miles or more. We had experienced such a complete vacuum in front of our positions a number of times before. Each time the communists had closed this vacuum rapidly during the night and launched an attack.

The patrols of the X Corps, which were separated by the precipitous mountain range from the Eighth Army, had never been able to establish contact with patrols of the Eighth Army, because of the ambushes and large numbers of North Korean soldiers infiltrating northward on foot.—Some of these troops had been rearmed and sent back into this rugged mountainous terrain.—The X Corps was directed to move from the Chosen Reservoir toward the northwest to join with the Eighth Army in the Kangye area. The First Marine Division led this advance. The Third Division, which was in the Wonsan area, was to hold that area. The Seventh Division, which had begun its token occupation of northeast Korea, one regiment of which had actually reached the Yalu River north of Kilju, was to support the First Marine Division.

In the meantime, my wife had returned to Japan. On a trip to Tokyo, I had learned that my daughter had been informed that her husband, together with his medical resident friends, was to be relieved and would return home by Christmas. But this was not to be.

I went north again after returning to Korea. I had gone to Seoul and had then flown to Pyongyang and north to Anju, where the I Corps and the IX Corps headquarters were very close together. There had been reports of large numbers of refugees having recently infiltrated our lines and then having disappeared. This pattern was an old communist tactic: to infiltrate their soldiers along with women and children, go into hiding, and then strike us from the rear as well as the front.

While I was in Pyongyang, we had also received reports that hundreds of young men from Pyongyang, who presumably were civilians, had disappeared during the night and marched to the east. Later on, we had seen smoke clouds coming from various peaks. The communists had learned that by setting these tremendous smudges, the smoke clouds would conceal the movement of their troops from our aircraft; so we knew there was considerable communist activity east of Pyongyang.

The Onslaught

On the nights of the twenty-sixth and twenty-seventh of November 1950, the communists struck with full force, overrunning the Ninth Infantry of the Second Division and penetrating the position of the Twenty-fifth Division. The sudden onslaught of the Chinese Communists caused the Republic of Korea troops, to the right of the Second Division, to completely collapse; consequently, the communists poured southward and southwestward around our exposed right flank. They also penetrated the positions of our other divisions. Because the entire rear of the Eighth Army was threatened, the First Cavalry Division, which had been in reserve, was moved rapidly to the south and east to block this enveloping movement of the Chinese Communists, thereby permitting an orderly withdrawal of Eighth Army troops to the south to the vicinity of Pyongyang.

While I was in the Twenty-fifth Division area during this attack, I tried to get over into the Second Division area but found the communists had a road block north of Anju. I knew the Ninth Infantry was in trouble and, of course, had the ever present and recurring worry about the boy. I knew they were cut off.

Over the months that followed, I was able to piece bits of information together. After the initial overrunning, they had fought until daylight around his aid station. The Ninth Infantry had been withdrawn southward to join the Twenty-third and Thirty-eighth Infantries and eventually had gotten to a position north of Kunuri, where the remnants of that regiment were to hold while the rest of the division went through a defile. This operation has been well described in a book by the able author Marshall.[1] The boy, I was reasonably certain, was dead. As time passed, this was found to be true. He was killed in action by a hand grenade as the Chinese overran his aid station.[2]

The Missing-in-Action

Officially, the Second Division was declared to be wiped out as an effective combat unit. The stragglers were gathered together and moved south of Seoul. They were a mere handful but included my good friend Sladen Bradley, the assistant division commander, and Dutch Kramer, the division commander. When I saw them shortly afterward, they, like everyone else, were in more or less a state of shock. The regimental commander of the Ninth Infantry had also escaped.

The policy was that all those missing-in-action would be kept on that status unless at least five people had seen their bodies. After the Ninth Infantry regimental commander's jeep driver was shot in the head, the regimental commander thought he was dead, only to find later that withdrawing troops in his rear had found his driver still alive and had brought him back. He was reluctant to declare anybody killed-in-action unless it was verified by a number of witnesses; so some five thousand young men were carried as missing-in-action for about four years.

We knew that about only three thousand American prisoners who had been captured since the beginning of the war remained alive in North Korean prison camps. We had agents who could count, but they could not identify these people by name. We also had some word from Americans who were released in small groups by the communists as to the status of various individuals; but, the idea, which seemed to have been held back in Washington, D.C., that all of these dead young Americans were alive and in the hands of communists we knew to be untrue.

Evacuating the Wounded

I stayed in Anju until all American troops had been withdrawn, with the exception of the Thirty-fifth Infantry, which was the covering force, the last unit to be withdrawn. All medical units had been moved southward, and the final problem was to get the last wounded from the Thirty-fifth Division area down to an airfield just south of Anju, where they were to be evacuated to the south. Because the medical units, including the divisional medical service of the Twenty-fifth Division, had been moved to the south, I did what I could to assist in moving the last of the wounded by truck and by jeep ambulance to this airfield.

As the Thirty-fifth Division began its final withdrawal south of Anju, I got out during the night on one of the last C-46 aircraft to leave that airfield. It was a dismal feeling. The weather was extremely cold. The countryside was practically deserted. No one knew where the communists were. We knew they were behind us as well as in front. Again, as in every fluid military situation, we knew not where was friend or foe.

I would like to salute the young flight nurse of the air force who was on this last plane, which was overloaded with American wounded and a few wounded Turks from the Turkish brigade, which had also been chopped up when it was attached to the Second Division. She did a magnificent job on that last flight out of Anju.

The Withdrawal

After the evacuation of Pyongyang began our further withdrawal to the rear, I flew in an old DC staff plane over the mountains to Hamhung for another trip. The new plan there was to withdraw from Hamhung by sea, and some of my personnel were there. General Almond was quite perturbed, because he felt that he could have held on indefinitely at Wonsan and Hamhung and would have been a thorn in the communists' side. He could have been supplied by sea; but, it was the policy of the Joint Chiefs of Staff, at least as their orders so stated, that the withdrawal would be made.

The Seventh Division had come to the rescue of the First Marine Division in the Chosen Reservoir area but had had the lead battalions of two of its regimental combat teams literally chopped up. There were some six hundred wounded American soldiers who were being moved by truck to a small plateau at Hagari, at the south end of the lake, when they were again attacked. Many of the survivors crawled out on the ice on the lake.

Col. Vi Gorby had a number of his evacuation hospitals at Hamhung. Finally, an airlift was established to Chosen Reservoir. Initially, the wounded were brought out in light planes. After the airfield was extended, C-46s and C-47s could get in, and the flow of wounded became a flood. Some of these men had frozen feet and frozen hands. One of the rare cases I saw was a soldier who had a partial evisceration of his intestine from a bayonet wound. These were frozen solid while lying outside of his abdominal cavity. The final evacuation of the Third Division, the Seventh Division, and First Marine Division was completed by Christmas Eve, 24 December 1950.

Approximately 100,000 civilian refugees were taken off on LSTs and other craft. There were also several hundred thousand refugees who went south with the Eighth Army on the western coastal area of Korea at the same time as they withdrew south of Pyongyang. I talked with many of these refugees. My question was, Why do you go south with us? We presumably are your enemies. The answer, although phrased in many ways, was, in effect, "Yes, we have been under communist training and indoctrination for five years. We have seen the communists take from us. We have seen our people killed who attempted to bring food into the cities which you occupied. The communists would rather see us starve than let food come to us. You have brought in food to us. You have given us medical care. You have attempted to save the lives of our children."[3]

This lesson is one for all of us to keep in mind in this cold war of many years' duration for the battle of men and of men's minds. Demonstration of the value of the human life is far more important than all the words spoken.

We left behind the medical supplies, the blankets, and the equipment for hospitals. We left behind some other things. We left behind agents who were, of course, Koreans. One of the essential elements of information that I asked G-2 [U.S. Army intelligence—Ed.] to have the agents report on was the presence of epidemics.

We had seen the small bonfires of typhus, typhoid, diphtheria, and smallpox present in the communities that we had occupied in North Korea. We had not gotten very far in our protective programs for immunization and delousing. We knew that it was quite likely, under the communist regime, that these bonfires would blow into a wildfire which would sweep the country.[4] We knew from military history that if this occurred, epidemics of typhus, typhoid, and smallpox could immobilize a large portion of the communist forces and could affect, of course, their military operations. It was essential that we knew if this situation began to develop.

Leaving Seoul

I made another trip back to Seoul in January 1951, when we evacuated Seoul for the second time. This evacuation was disheartening. Again, we left behind our medical supplies and equipment, which we had used to re-equip the hospitals, hoping this time the communists would not carry it off. It was a tragic thing to see the civilians take to the roads in the dead of winter, because the winters are very severe with fahrenheit temperatures of thirty degrees below zero. All of the outgoing trains were jammed with civilian refugees when the final phases of the evacuation were completed. It was a bitter sight to see the crowds who could not be accommodated on the remaining trains, knowing that families would be separated, some to fall into the hands of the communists and others to go south.

Eventually, the line was held south of Seoul, roughly south of Suwon, extending to Chonju and to the east coast. In the meantime, General Walker was killed in a jeep accident, and Gen. Matthew Ridgeway came to take command of the Eighth Army. After reorganization and arrival of additional troops, Operation "Killer" was begun. It was a new advance again to the north in the spring of 1951.

29

A Complication

The United Nations continued to send instructions through the U.S. Government to a committee made up of representatives of the Defense Department, the State Department, and the Economic Cooperation Agency, which passed these directives through the Joint Chiefs of Staff to the commander-in-chief, United Nations Command. One of the directives required that we should make the United Nations Civil Assistance Command into a real United Nations unit. The member nations by agreement began recruiting health and welfare personnel through national organizations from various countries. The United Nations was also receiving token supplies from various countries. By agreement within the United Nations, these supplies, whether they came from governments or from voluntary organizations within the respective nations, were to be pooled; they were to lose their identity as separate donations. Personnel and supplies were to be moved to Japan, where they came under control of the United Nations Command; they were to become, in effect, personnel of the United Nations and supplies of the United Nations for relief of Korea.[1]

Prior to the new war in December 1950, the United Nations had set up an Agent General: initially, Kingsbury Smith. The United Nations also sent out a group to set up a governing body for control of the North Korean provinces after elections were held until Korea could be politically reunited. We were to prepare to turn over to the United Nations what I considered our field organization for the assistance of the Republic of Korea. All of this was predicated upon the end of the North Korean opposition and the end of the token occupation of North Korea. Eventually, of course, we were to turn over all responsibility to this United Nations group.

When the Chinese Communists started the war, these instructions were changed. We were to continue as a military organization assisting the Republic of Korea. I eventually had teams for all of the provinces and the principle cities in Korea. There were sanitary engineers, welfare people, and health officers from many nations: Mexico, Sweden, France, Canada, Britain, Denmark, and the United States.

There was one difficult period during this uncertain phase of the Korean War. Various national Red Cross societies—the British Red Cross, the Dutch, the Canadian, and others—had recruited health and welfare people from their societies. They arrived in Tokyo in their Red Cross uniforms. Under our instructions from the United Nations, they were to become United Nations Command health and welfare personnel; however, they refused to do so after their arrival. They had been instructed by their respective national Red Cross societies that they were to retain their identity as Red Cross personnel and that they were to distribute Red Cross supplies, as distinct from United Nations supplies. This interesting situation became a matter of public controversy, particularly in the European press, where it became a political problem. General MacArthur and I, personally, were attacked in Parliament in England and by the various national societies.

The International Committee of the Red Cross, which is a Swiss organization under the Geneva Conventions, is responsible for seeing about the welfare of prisoners-of-war and also about the welfare of the civilian population in occupied countries. A representative of this International Committee of the Red Cross, a legal expert, came to Tokyo with his documentation claiming that he had the responsibility for taking over all relief activities in Korea, which the United Nations had directed General MacArthur to assume, and for which I had been designated to direct for him in the civilian assistance field.

In addition, the League of Red Cross Societies, which was made up of national Red Cross societies, felt that they should, in this case, undertake relief activities for the liberated people of the Republic of Korea and for the occupied area of North Korea when it came under United Nations jurisdiction. There was a battle between the two organizations at a meeting in Switzerland, in which we had no direct concern, except that they both claimed jurisdiction over our activities in Korea. On the other hand, the national Red Cross societies, which had responded to the invitation of the United Nations to their governments, had furnished personnel and supplies; they maintained that they had responsibility.

The United Nations decided to enter the picture and, for the first time, decided to go into the relief business. The United Nations had issued very detailed instructions to us that any relief in Korea for the assistance of the Republic of Korea, and for relief in the area north of the thirty-eighth parallel when we occupied it, was to be a United Nations responsibility. Because we in General Headquarters of the United Nations Command were acting under instructions of the United Nations, transmitted through the U.S. Government Committee to the Joint Chiefs of Staff and then to General MacArthur, we, as his staff, were compelled to carry out their instructions for him.

The widely publicized controversy resulted from three organizations which were actually having their disagreements in Europe and New York, transferring their inability to agree through the public press by attacking General MacArthur and myself for, as they said, refusing to allow the Red Cross to operate in Korea. Actually, they refused to release supplies which they had donated to the United Nations until they were permitted to establish separate channels for distribution through their Red Cross personnel.

After one particularly vicious attack in the British press on General MacArthur, I prepared a simple statement of the facts as I have outlined them above as a press release for General MacArthur, in order quickly to lay the cards on the table. Following the press release, there was a subsequent embarrassment among those officials in Europe who were using us as whipping boys, because it brought out in the open the fact that they had refused to release either their personnel or their supplies in accordance with their agreement with the United Nations. They had hoped to get around this agreement by attacking us in the Far East for failing to give in to their demands, which were contrary to their agreement with the United Nations.

Eventually, the problem was solved in that they complied with their agreement. Their personnel became United Nations personnel, just as we had, although I was also an officer in the U.S. Army. The supplies eventually were released and pooled with other United Nations governmental and privately sponsored donations for relief based on need, and not because of affiliations with a Red Cross chapter or with some religious unit.

In connection with this controversy, a representative of the American Red Cross Society visited the theater. He had been unable to win his battle in New York with the United Nations for a separate Red Cross channel into Korea. He had gone to Korea and had visited President Rhee Syngman with a proposal that he demand the Red Cross channels be separate from the United Nations relief channels. The Korean president, of course, called me in and outlined the proposal he had received from the American Red Cross representative and asked what I thought about it. I explained what the instructions were, which we had received, as to the handling of all relief supplies on a pooled basis. The Korean president decided not to make an appeal to the president of the United States.

Such complications, of course, occur in any large-scale operation. I simply mentioned these to clear up what had become a controversial and perhaps misunderstood situation, which may well develop again in the future in the rapidly evolving international relief situation.

30

A Korean Episode

Through the intelligence agents, we received reports of epidemics sweeping various villages and cities in North Korea during January and February 1951. These agents were laymen, and they could not identify what the diseases were. They reported considerable unrest among the people, who were dying by the thousands, and emphasized that no medical steps were being taken by the communists to alleviate the suffering of these people.

As our troops began their advance northward for the second time in Operation "Killer," and Seoul was recaptured, we found thousands of civilians, who had been under the control of the communists during these months, ill with typhus, smallpox, and some typhoid. Many died. In addition, our troops captured many thousands of Chinese and North Korean prisoners who were ill with typhus, smallpox, and typhoid. I interrogated many of these prisoners myself and learned from them that not only had they been sick while they were in combat but also sometimes a half or a third of their particular units were ill with these diseases.[1]

The picture began to build up, from an intelligence standpoint, as we had anticipated it might. Epidemics were sweeping the communist-held areas; they were sweeping not only the civilian population but also their military forces. Our intelligence map showed that fairly large concentrations of communist troops were not in immediate contact with our forces but were held in the north, in the areas of Pyongyang, Hamhung, and Wonsan. There was much speculation why this fairly large concentration was held there.

Our fleet was constantly bombarding the supply lines along the east coast, particularly at Wonsan and Hamhung and at other places along the northeast coast. They were attempting, through threatened action of a possible reinvasion through amphibious operations, to hold there the large Chinese Communist forces, which had attacked our X Corps in the Chosen Reservoir area and had moved into Wonsan and Hamhung after our evacuation. Our air force thought that perhaps these troops were held north of the combat lines because the air force had succeeded in cutting the supply lines. Other intelligence sources showed that the communists moved their supplies on man-back and pack animals through devious ways. Although many truck convoys were destroyed by our ever active air force, there was doubt as to their real effect in cutting these other supply lines, because the Chinese Communist troops which were in combat seemed to have adequate supplies of food and ammunition. Their needs are very small compared to ours.

"The Black Death"

I was back in Tokyo when a message was received through intelligence sources of a new outbreak of disease: what was called the "Black Death." The "Black Death" was translated as the plague. We knew plague was endemic in Manchuria.

I had seen plague in the Middle East—the rat disease transmitted by fleas from the dead bodies of rats to humans. In its original form, it is called bubonic plague, because the lymph glands swell and break down and ulcerate, particularly those draining an area in which a flea has transmitted the plague from rats. In its passage through the human body, the organism may involve the lungs; then it becomes pneumonic plague. It is then capable of being transmitted by droplets from one person to another, as in an influenza epidemic; it can sweep through a population like wildfire. The mortality is terrifically high.

This report by an agent who claimed to have seen these cases, which were attacking not only the Chinese Communists but also the civilian population, indicated that this disease might have been brought into Korea by the Chinese Communists. It was important to find out if this were true, because of its potential impact on the course of our military operations as we advanced northward. The plague had great capabilities of knocking out additional large numbers of their troops, as well as the civilian population, particularly when added to the epidemics of smallpox and typhus, which we knew were sweeping these two elements of the communists.

As we moved northward, our troops would also be exposed to plague, if it were present, either among enemy troops or among the civilian population with which our troops would come in contact. We had vaccines for bubonic plague; but, normally, we did not immunize our troops, except in the presence of an epidemic, because the duration of immunity conferred by the vaccines that were available at that time was very limited. If we were to be threatened with an epidemic of plague, the production of vaccine in the amounts needed, not only for our troops and those of the Republic of Korea and the token forces from other countries which were present in the combat area but also for the protection of the civilian population of some 23 million people, would be a tremendous program. It would take time; we had to get it under way, if it were needed.

Confirming Intelligence

Because we had no medical agents in North Korea, and because I could not rely too well upon the professional training of the North Korean doctors and their diagnoses, or the so-called doctors of the Chinese Communist forces, it was necessary for us accurately to determine whether this disease were really plague. Not too many of our American doctors had seen the pneumonic form of bubonic plague; so far as I knew, there were none who had who were in the Far East at that time. I had seen such an epidemic at Said, Egypt.[2] I felt that it was necessary for me to determine not only whether these cases were actually plague but also to confirm the impact of the reported epidemics of typhus, smallpox, and typhoid.

The agent who had made this report also reported a number of communist hospitals in the Wonsan area as being filled with these cases, so I felt that Wonsan was the area in which we should attempt to see these cases. I had been in the area a number of times during our brief occupation and was fairly familiar with the terrain. As far as the communists were concerned, their so-called hospitals in the areas indicated were largely villages from which they had removed the civilian populations. They had simply moved thousands of military personnel who were sick and wounded into the mud huts where they either got well or they died. The question was, How could I see these cases?

I first considered being dropped in, because I was a qualified paratrooper.[3] The dropping of agents is fairly common and, of course, occurred during the Korean War. The questions, however, were, Should I safely land in this rugged terrain, could I reach one of the hospitals or villages known as a hospital? If I had doubt as to the clinical diagnosis, how could I get out one of these patients, or at least some blood for laboratory confirmation? Then, of course, probably the least important but still a consideration was, How would I eventually get out? Travelling through this rugged terrain as an occidental among orientals in the dead of winter was a very difficult task indeed. Although I might infiltrate through our lines several hundred miles to the south, again, I might not make it and time was essential. The important thing was to be able to get in and get out with the information and, if possible, also to get out with the necessary material for laboratory confirmation of this reported epidemic. So it seemed that being dropped in by parachute was not the solution.

I appealed to my friends in G-2 [U.S. Army intelligence—Ed.] in special operations and in the navy to see whether I could get ashore in a one-man amphibious operation, or at least a small group. This approach was finally decided upon as the best. The navy had a small ship or craft. In the army, it would be a landing craft tank (LCT): one of these small craft in which we load tanks and personnel and it goes ashore and opens up its nose and a tank rolls out. The craft does not have bulkheads. The navy called this a ship, and on this ship they had established a laboratory which had some very competent people and facilities for laboratory diagnosis and study.

The Plan

It was decided that I should go secretly to Korea from Tokyo and board this LCT, which the navy was eager to use. It was lying in the harbor at Pusan. We would then proceed northward to Wonsan to join the fleet there and attempt to get ashore from that general locality.[4] A young naval line officer, a lieutenant junior grade, by the name of Drake, was assigned to his project.[5] A Korean naval officer who also was an outstanding guerrilla fighter, by the name of Commander E. Yun, was also to go along.[6] I obtained orders to Pusan on a routine staff visit to Eighth Army as a so-called cover.

My wife had returned to the United States, because my older daughter had to move off of the military reservation at Letterman after her husband was declared missing-in-action. My daughter had no place to live, so my wife returned to establish a home for our older daughter and the grandchildren. Having written the usual letters under such circumstances, which were to be mailed only if I failed to come back from this trip, and which I left with my deputy, I proceeded to Pusan. No one on my staff knew the purpose of my visit to Eighth Army, which I visited frequently. Without contacting anyone in the Eighth Army, of course, I boarded the LCT. A young Lieutenant Miller was in command. After dark, we slipped the moorings and proceeded out to sea for the trip to Wonsan.

Getting Ashore

It was the first of March. This time of year the seas can be very rough. As we proceeded northward, the little craft began to buck and roll; mal de mer began to affect more and more of the crew. Finally, because of the terrific strain on this little ship, which had no bulkheads that could be closed if she broke in two, the skipper decided to return to Pusan to wait for more favorable weather. Fortunately, I do not become seasick or airsick. Because of my ability to withstand the rigors of the sea, I was facetiously made an honorary "Admiral of the Navy" by this small group of very fine young men. We returned to Pusan and tried again the next night. This time, after a rough passage, we succeeded in approaching Wonsan harbor.

As daylight occurred, lookouts reported occasional floating mines, which had broken loose from Wonsan harbor and were drifting in the sea. We attempted and did sink a few of these by rifle fire. They were somewhat of a hazard, because had we accidently hit one of the horns of one these old-type floating mines, our ship without bulkheads would, of course, have immediately sunk. We eventually arrived in the Wonsan harbor area where our minesweepers were still trying to clear the mines. A narrow channel had been swept in which our cruisers and a battleship would go to shell Wonsan each evening. One of the ships served as a headquarters for communications with various agents ashore who had some radio contact.

For twelve days we tried to find various means of getting ashore. The communists were worried about an amphibious landing there in conjunction with our advance to the north.—Eighth Army and X Corps, which had been placed under command of Eighth Army, had been moving north since February.—Any small boat or other ship that approached the shore was immediately placed under fire. The beaches were mined as well as the waters. Gun emplacements and barbed wire, as part of the overall beach defense and network, made it very difficult to find a spot where one could land undetected.

There were some small islands in the harbor, one serving as the base for agents who got ashore. (They were, of course, Koreans in fishing boats.) We went ashore and found that typhus and smallpox had swept the population of this small island. I saw many cases of typhus there among the survivors. The population had been reduced to about ten percent of its normal number as a result of these epidemics.

We sent various groups of Koreans ashore at various points by various means. Some ten groups were placed ashore. Unfortunately, they were all captured, with the exception of two members of one team who succeeded in avoiding capture and reported by small hand radio the fate of the other groups. Unfortunately, in the torturing which preceded the death or execution of the captured agents, some apparently yielded to such fantastic pressure as the oriental mind can devise in torture; so the communists were aware of the fact that I was trying to get into Korea from that location.

We could approach the coast at any point with the little LCT and go ashore. Finally, a plan was developed. We boarded a destroyer and moved out to sea, which we did after dark. We approached the shore south of Wonsan opposite one of the villages called Chilbo-ri. The destroyer was to remain some twenty miles off the coast so that it would not be detected from the shore. We then boarded a whale boat, a small motor-driven open boat, and proceeded toward the shore. We towed an inflated four-man rubber raft. As we approached the shore, radio contact apparently was established with the surviving agents. We were advised as to the point at which we should attempt to go ashore through the heavy surf in the dead of winter. We were warned about the mine fields and the shore patrols maintained by the communists but were advised to come ashore.

The Korean agent in the boat, who was in contact with the presumed friendly agents, found that these agents could not respond properly to certain code words, which could be known only by our own people. The agents tried to talk us ashore. As we learned later, they were not our agents but were communists who were using one of the captured walkie-talkie radios; they had laid a trap for us. We, therefore, had to give up the attempt that particular night and return to the destroyer which, in turn, rejoined the ships in the narrow channel in Wonsan by daylight.

There was some disposition on the part of the navy then to stop any further efforts to get ashore, because we had lost so many agents. Apparently, the communists were so well aware of our attempts that the navy considered the chances of my getting ashore and getting the information out successfully were negligible. I insisted, however, that we make at least one more try. Lieutenant Clark and Commander Yun, for whom I have the greatest admiration and respect, also volunteered for another attempt.[7]

On the following night, we again moved out of Wonsan harbor and proceeded to a point some twenty miles offshore from Chilbo-ri. We again embarked in a small whale boat with our rubber raft in tow and approached the shore. This time radio contact was successfully established with the two surviving agents who had previously warned us of the trap. They had broken in on the same radio channels used by the communists who had tried to talk us into the trap the preceding night.

As we approached the shore, it was indeed an awesome sight. The very high and rugged mountains, which come within a mile or so of the shore, were covered with snow. A convoy of trucks with headlights ablaze could be seen traveling southward along a highway which parallels the shore. As we approached the shore in our rubber raft, into which we had transferred ourselves, our ever vigilant aircraft, which had not been let in on our secret, began to bomb and strafe this motor convoy. The bomb explosions and flashes were almost continuous. We knew that we now had an additional hazard in that the occupants of the trucks would undoubtedly abandon their vehicles and scatter throughout the neighborhood at least until the attack was over. In addition to the military patrols, which we expected to encounter, we knew that we might well accidentaly run into some of these communist troops who were so dispersed. It was with some trepidation that we finally approached the beach, only to be warned by our radio contact, who could apparently see us, that we were approaching a mined area of the beach and should move a little farther to the south, which we did using small paddles. We were, of course, drenched with icy spray.

"Operation SAMS"

We were in our normal combat uniforms. In the dark, the Chinese quilted combat jacket and our own combat jackets, and their dog or rabbit fur headgear and our headgear, were indistinguishable; so we were not too concerned with being identified as Americans, if we could steer clear of communists at a distance of forty or fifty feet. We had, of course, removed, our military insignia. We were armed with the usual pistols and hand grenades. I had in my pockets under my jacket some culture tubes and the necessary needles and syringes. I had also included in my own personal armament a number of syrettes of morphine.

The purpose of the morphine was twofold. First, I felt that if I could not obtain blood serum from a patient without discovery as to who I was, it might be necessary to put the patient into a condition through the use of intravenous morphine, which reacts very quickly; so, we could get this patient out and aboard our rubber raft and take him aboard one of the ships. We could then, in his quiet state, make our laboratory determinations. The other purpose of the morphine syrettes was a little more drastic. We had agreed that if we fell into communist hands, the fate that would await us would be such that it was better not to remain alive too long. Intravenous morphine in adequate dosage can terminate life very quickly and without the pain of torture.

We were met at the beach by a small group of Korean agents, which included the two with whom we had been dealing. We were guided through a mine field to an underground tunnel, which they had very cleverly constructed and had camouflaged into a cave. In such business, one is not always sure who can be trusted. Certainly, as we crawled through the mouth of the narrow tunnel, the idea naturally came to mind that we might be crawling into our own tombs. I kept my own pistol, which had been cocked with the safety off, in my hand for a last-minute attempt to regain freedom if we found ourselves in such a situation.

In this cave, I was able to interrogate the agents who had actually seen the patients. In the meantime, Clark and Yun and several of the other agents had approached the village of Chilbo-ri, which was just a few yards from this cleverly concealed entrance to the cave, and had quietly eliminated a military patrol.[8] We could not use firearms under the circumstances without revealing our presence. We were then able to determine that these cases were not bubonic plague but were a particularly virulent form of smallpox known as hemorrhagic smallpox: The "Black Death" was in fact as fatal as the bubonic plague but was, of course, a different disease.[9]

I had hoped to go across the highway to another village and tried to induce the agents to go with me and spend, if necessary, another day or two; however, because of the dispersion of the personnel of the convoy, they considered such a plan too great a hazard. They told me that no one could move over the roads or even over trails without the danger of interrogation by military or police patrols. If the necessary documents were not available to prove that one had authority to make such a move, one was immediately jailed—and that would be the end of us. I was, therefore, unable to visit the other villages which served as hospitals. I was able to confirm that the epidemics of typhus, typhoid, and smallpox had been the basic cause for the immobilization of the Chinese divisions that were held well in rear of contact with our troops. I was also able to confirm that there was great unrest in the country because the communists had done nothing to relieve the suffering of the people.

The original plan had been that the whale boat was to lie offshore until shortly before daylight; then, if we had not appeared, it was to return to the destroyer and to approach the shore again the following night. In this case, because we were unable to go beyond Chilbo-ri village, the so-called hospital, but we had obtained the information that was needed, and I felt confident in my clinical diagnosis of the cases, it was not necessary to attempt to take a patient out of the area for further laboratory study.[10] We returned eventually to our rubber raft, which had been concealed. After some difficulty in trying to get out through the ice cold surf, we succeeded in contacting the whale boat and returned to the destroyer by daylight.

Concluding the Mission

We were not only cold and wet but also extremely fatigued, because the tension under such circumstances is exceedingly great. My good friends in the navy decided that a little spirits from a medicinal standpoint might serve a useful purpose, and I took the medical responsibility for so prescribing it to "ward off the pneumonia" and relieve tension.

A radio message was sent to General Headquarters in Tokyo giving a brief statement as to the findings. The LCT then began its journey back to Pusan, without our having had to use the very fine laboratory facilities available on this little craft. Because no useful purpose could be served by my returning the same way in which I had arrived, I was transferred in a small boat to an ammunition ship that was to return to Sasebo, which was being used as one of the naval bases. I climbed the usual Jacob's ladder up the side of this rolling ship.—I was not sure whether I would have sufficient strength to reach the deck.—I was very cordially received by the commander of the ship, who gave me a room which I strongly suspect was probably his own room. I slept the clock-around as this ship proceeded from Wonsan back to Sasebo, Japan.

At Sasebo, I boarded an amphibious craft and was flown to Iwakuni, where I was transferred to an air force C-47 staff plane and returned to Tokyo. A detailed report was made to the Chief of Intelligence and to the Chief-of-staff, Lt. Gen. Tom (Doyle O.) Hickey, and through him to General MacArthur.

The Aftermath

We subsequently learned that the communists were so incensed that I had succeeded in getting ashore and avoiding their trap that they executed some twenty-five people in the little village of Chilbo-ri, who they suspected of having collaborated with us and our agents. They had lost considerable face in the fact that we had succeeded in our mission.

I might mention that according to my contacts with American medical officers who had been held prisoner during this time, they had been told by their communist captors that they knew we were trying to get ashore. The communists themselves thought they had the plague, and they boasted about what they would do when they had captured me. I was to be taken to Pyongyang, where I would have sufficient pressure placed on me to reveal such military secrets as I might know. I was to be an example of their ability to counter our intelligence activities.

After this Korean episode, *Newsweek* magazine in one of its columns mentioned the fact that an epidemiological ship had been off the coast of North Korea and conjectured as to its purpose. This news broke the highly classified status of this episode. As a result, a public announcement was released on approval of the Defense Department in which part of the information was released in connection with the fact that I had been in North Korea and was to receive a decoration.—This episode was considered of such sufficient importance that I was awarded the Distinguished Service Cross; Lieutenant Clark was awarded the Navy Cross, the comparable naval decoration; and Commander Yun of the Korean Navy was awarded a comparable decoration.—A limited amount of information was also released to the press, which caused considerable publicity, apparently not only in the United States but also in other countries.[11]

The communists then, in typical communist fashion—being highly chagrined that they had not succeeded in capturing us and also as an alibi to the North Korean people for their failure to look after either military or civilian sick or to control epidemics—charged us, in the spring of 1951, with having started biological warfare, or bacterial warfare.[12] They ignored the fact that we knew these small bonfires of epidemic diseases were present in North Korea the preceding fall and that unless they were controlled, as we controlled them in the population of South Korea, they would become a forest fire. Unfortunately, such charges, being sensational in character, received wide acceptance among the uninformed throughout Western Europe and other parts of the world.

I think the facts, as I have presented them, clearly puncture this balloon of fallacy. The communists finally began to move medical personnel into North Korea after it was too late. Some satellite countries sent medical units into North Korea at the end of the war. The extent of this disaster for the communists is indicated by the confirmed reports that the initial population of 11 million people in North Korea was reduced to approximately 3 million. They have once again demonstrated that their promises cannot be fulfilled because they could not control the epidemics.

The impact of disease on military operations is a repetition of history over and over again. As long as we retain our leadership and capacity and capabilities of controlling such epidemics under the most difficult conditions, not only among our troops but also among the civilian populations in the countries in which we may be operating, we shall always have the advantage.

After the return to Tokyo on 15 March 1951, the Supreme Commander and Eighth Army commander were well aware of the situation among the communist troops. The senior military commanders have presented testimony before Congress, and subsequently in articles, that they felt they could have continued north and recaptured North Korea had they been permitted to do so. One of the major considerations was the effect of disease on the enemy; it was a major factor in their calculations of the ability to move north and reconquer North Korea without too great a difficulty. This advance northward, however, was not permitted; as a result of intergovernmental decisions, it was halted by order.

31

The Relief of General MacArthur

Early in November 1950, I had received a personal letter from a very good friend of mine in Washington, D.C., who had asked if I would object if steps were initiated leading to my selection for the assignment as Surgeon General of the Army.—Surgeon General Bliss was due to complete his tour in June 1951.—My reply had been that I would take no personal steps to attempt to secure such an assignment; but if it were offered to me, I would accept it and do the best I could within my capabilities to carry out the duties of such an office.

In the latter part of March 1951, a medical group arrived from the United States, including some individuals from the American Medical Association. The president of that organization, Dr. Elmer Henderson, who was a good friend of mine, and Gen. James S. Simmons, whom I had repeatedly invited to Japan to review our public health activities and to give us his very valued recommendations and comments, were in the group.[1] Other members were Harry Armstrong, who was then the Surgeon General of the Air Force, and Al Schwictenberg, my classmate and good friend who was then with the Defense Department. Dr. Henderson told me that he had received a message in a radio telephone conversation with a friend in Washington, D.C., that my nomination for selection as Surgeon General of the Army to succeed General Bliss had been approved by the president; consequently, he had a small celebration in the Imperial Hotel. My good friend Gen. Erskine Hume, who was the military theater surgeon, and many other friends participated.

This group then proceeded on their way for a short visit to the hospitals in Korea. General Simmons remained behind. Then came a series of interesting events. The story was not made clear until my return to the United States some months later.

In the middle of April 1951, General MacArthur received a message that, upon a decision by the president, he was being relieved. Some three days later, General Simmons received a message from friends in Washington, D.C., that the president had been so incensed at General MacArthur that he had torn up my nomination because of my close association with General MacArthur, which of course was the president's prerogative. I, therefore, felt free of any further obligation to remain on in the service after the completion of my assignment in the Far East.[2]

General MacArthur

Those of us who had been very closely associated for many years with General MacArthur felt particularly bitter about his relief. Gen. Courtney Whitney and Gen. Charles Willoughby and others asked to be relieved of their assignments at the time he was relieved. His departure from Japan was a memorable event in the minds of all of us. When we told him goodbye at the airport at Haneda, many eyes were filled with tears. It was a sad day for the United States and for our people as a whole.

The relief of General MacArthur was more than the relief of a military commander who had displeased the civilian head of the United States: General MacArthur was a symbol to the peoples of the Far East of the interest of the United States in that part of the world. Our friends in the Far East had been well aware of our close ties with Western Europe, and had felt that in the event of a showdown between the communist world and the United States, we were likely to abandon them. This particular episode tended to confirm such a feeling.

The shock to the Japanese people was tremendous. Repercussions among very high level Japanese and Koreans with whom I had contact were such that they felt that the relief of General MacArthur meant that we were turning our backs upon that part of the world. This attitude could be well understood in view of the fact that the United Nations had announced, and it had been well disseminated throughout the Far East, that the objective of the United Nations forces in Korea was to defeat the aggressor and reunite Korea.

Before the relief of General MacArthur, the discussions in the press, as reflected in the news reports which were also disseminated widely throughout the Far East, had begun to raise a doubt in the minds of our Asian friends. The discussions in the press in America and Britain about hesitancy of accomplishing this mission, and demands on the part of some of our allies, specifically the British, that we should not go north of the thirty-eighth parallel again was an obvious manifestation of fear of the possible consequences of such action. Naturally, in the minds of the Orientals, this meant that a basic change in policy was taking place. They were worried lest we would withdraw from that part of the world and again center our entire activities in Europe.

Winners and Losers

In the minds of most of the peoples of underdeveloped nations in the world, the people have learned that they must be on the side of a winner if they are to survive. To them, you either win or you lose; how you played the game is of secondary importance. In the minds of many of these people, we lost in Korea: We failed to win, as we had stated we intended to win.

This view should give us some thought. We might delude ourselves in our own rationalization that in failing to carry out our announced objective of driving the aggressor out of Korea and uniting that divided country, it was better to stop at the thirty-eighth parallel and ignore our original stated objective. We could, therefore, feel that we had succeeded in terminating an unprofitable war, which in the minds of some top officials was the wrong war in the wrong place at the wrong time; but not so in the minds of the Orientals. Those Orientals who raised the question in conversations with me very definitely felt that we were the losers.

Thought must also be given to efforts that we have made in the past, and might make in the future, to persuade these peoples, particularly of the smaller newly created nations, to stand up against communist indoctrination and communist infiltration and, in some cases, communist armed aggression, literally at the risk of their lives. We should not be too surprised to find that there might now be some hesitation about their going to such extremes, because there is considerable doubt about our backing them up in a future struggle. The Orientals are intelligent people.

The course of our action in Korea has not been something in which we can take great pride, so far as our ultimate solution to that situation is concerned. I know, personally, many of the senior commanders who were quite bitter, as well as many of the junior commanders, who felt that they had been let down by the people at home. I, personally, felt very strongly and was extremely bitter toward the leaders of America and the people of America for "letting us down" by selling us out for a presumed political advantage with our Western European allies. Not only was there a sacrifice of human life and suffering, but also a loss of prestige. Some of us had spent some years in trying to build up United States prestige in the eyes of friends in the Far East.

32

The Twenty-second of April Offensive

General Ridgeway, who replaced General MacArthur as Supreme Commander, was in my opinion one of our outstanding combat soldiers. I had known him for many years, and I had great admiration and respect for him. General Van Fleet had arrived to take over command of the Eighth Army, which General Ridgeway had relinquished. I had known him as a battalion commander in the Twenty-ninth Infantry at Fort Benning years before. He, in turn, was a very able fighter. Having been required to halt the advance of the United Nations Command at the thirty-eighth parallel, he had disposed his troops in depth over this tremendous front.

A Final Duty in Korea

I had an additional confidential and informal assignment which occupied a considerable portion of my time in Korea: It was an attempt to determine why our percentages of missing-in-action, wounded-in-action, and killed-in-action were so far out of line with past experience during this first year of the war. The weapons used and the type of terrain could not account for this great discrepancy in the high incidence of missing. I had spent considerable time with the infantry battalions, which I felt were the very foundation stones of the failure or success of a medical evacuation system. I had found, of course, that the young medical officers, who had not had any training whatsoever in their duties and responsibilities for evacuation and care of wounded soldiers on the battlefield, were doing the best they could; but the wounded who were not being recovered and who fell into the hands of the enemy were the ones who were largely responsible for the comparatively high number of missing-in-action. This finding was made the basis of a subsequent report at the request of the theater surgeon, General Hume, to the new Surgeon General of the Army, Gen. George Armstrong.[1]

We knew that the Chinese Communists were building up for another offensive in an attempt to drive us into the sea. When it became apparent that the communists were likely to launch their offensive in April, I again went to Korea with the intent of being present in one of the infantry battalion aid stations at the time the communists launched the attack. So we went forward to the First Battalion of the

Twenty-third Infantry of the Second Division, which had been newly reorganized and placed into combat again. This battalion was at the eastern tip of the Huichon Reservoir. The Seventh Division was on the right. When the communists, following their usual practice of having broken contact with us, suddenly launched their attack, they succeeded in penetrating the line in numerous places. They penetrated through a Korean position just east of the Seventh Division. They penetrated between the battalion of the Second Division and the Seventh Division on our right. They also penetrated through a Korean division to our east. They made a wide penetration between the First Marine Division on the left of the Second Division and the Twenty-fourth Division still further to the west.

Again, we went through a period of considerable fluidity. The communists were pouring through the gaps in the line and attacking units in the rear. I attempted to go by vehicle from east to west to visit the aid stations. The First Battalion, being pretty well cut off temporarily, was subsequently reinforced by deployment of the remainder of the regiment and the Thirty-eighth and the Ninth Infantry, which had been deployed in depth. I was able, subsequently, to go along the southern shore of Huichon Reservoir to the marine division area and found I could go no further to the west because the communists had infiltrated and moved through this gap. One of the mobile surgical hospitals, which was moving into a location in the marine division area, was ordered to withdraw, because there was nothing between them and the enemy but some open terrain, with no combat troops remaining in front.

I later returned to the X Corps, where I succeeded in getting a lift over the enemy lines in a liaison aircraft to the I Corps. There I found that General Milburn was having a difficult time. The communists had overrun a British brigade and had penetrated to a position just south and west of his command post. In visiting the Twenty-fifth Division, I found my good friend Sladen Bradley, who had been assistant division commander of the Second Division during the time that unit was in the north, and who was now in command of the Twenty-fifth Division. He had enemy troops on both sides. The enemy had broken through one position in his front, which he was trying to regain. The First Cavalry Division, which had been in reserve, had been moved quickly to the northeast to attempt to plug the hole east of the Twenty-fourth Division. During this battle, which lasted for a number of days, the communist offensive was finally stopped because of the military wisdom of Eighth Army commander General Van Fleet, in deploying his troops in depth rather than attempting to hold the line very thinly over a very wide front.

On my return, when checking out through Eighth Army on my final return to Tokyo, General Van Fleet told me that he was quite sure that now with the communists literally chopped to pieces in his immediate front, and knowing the difficulties they were having with their troops in the rear because of the widespread epidemics, he felt that he could successfully carry his drive to the Yalu River. I agreed with him. But he was not permitted to do so. So we have lost the war in Korea, in the eyes of our friends in the Far East.

Completing a Mission

Since the occupation of Japan was about to be terminated and preliminary negotiations had been completed for the peace treaty, which was to be signed in September 1951, I felt that I had then completed my mission as far as Chief of Public Health and Welfare of General Headquarters, Supreme Commander for the Allied Powers in Japan, was concerned. I requested that I be returned to the United States and that I be voluntarily retired from the military service.[2]

The Japanese had felt that, while we had made great progress in the health and welfare fields, they desired a group of advisors in those fields to continue on after the occupation. John D. Rockefeller, Jr., who was a cultural advisor to Foster Dulles in the negotiations prior to the signing of the peace treaty, and I had had a number of talks. I had also talked with Mr. Dulles as to the health and welfare program in Japan. In my discussions with Mr. Rockefeller, an agreement had been reached that he would attempt to have the State Department take over the responsibility of placing some fourteen key individuals, representing the various fields that were included in public health and welfare, as advisors. These individuals would become attachés at the American Embassy and could serve as technical advisors to the Ministry of Health and Welfare at the request of the Japanese Government. The same applied to certain other fields, such as natural resources and information and education.

At the time, apparently, it was the policy to have such technical advisors on the staff of the American ambassador to various nations. I, therefore, recommended to the new Supreme Commander, General Ridgeway, that, in view of the approaching peace treaty, the Public Health and Welfare Section of General Headquarters be abolished and that the fourteen selected individuals be attached to the military surgeon's office as a division, pending the completion of arrangements after the signing of the peace treaty for these individuals to be taken over by the State Department as advisors to the Japanese Government.[3]

COMING HOME

Return to the United States

When word was announced in a press release by the public information officer of General Headquarters that I was returning to the United States to retire from the service, the Japanese leaders with whom I had been working so many years came as individuals and as groups to express their appreciation for the work which we had done in attempting to establish or re-establish health and welfare activities in the rebuilding of that nation during the preceding six years. Various professional groups, such as the Japan Medical Association, the Japan Pharmaceutical Association, the governmental groups, including the prime minister, and the family of the Imperial household, sent tokens of their gratitude. I have among my treasures many scrolls, including one from the Diet, expressing such appreciation. Deservedly or not, I do feel some pride in such expressions. To me, they represent a tribute to all of the health and welfare staff rather than to me as an individual.

Leaving Japan

In my last meeting with the prime minister, at his request, we discussed at some length the significance of the relief of General MacArthur and also the future attitude of the Japanese Government regarding the continuation of the programs in the health and welfare field that had been undertaken and established, most of which were now embodied in Japanese law. I had great admiration and respect for Prime Minister Yoshida.

It was most difficult to go through the period of deactivating my own organization that I had built up. This particular group in the Public Health and Welfare Section of General Headquarters had, through the years, become such a highly selected and close-knit group that it was difficult to bid them goodbye. I can say, and re-emphasize, that I believe this particular group, in its ability and competence to achieve great things in the health and welfare field, has had no equal so far in the history of medicine. It was a pity to see such a fine group disperse to the four corners of the world.

After my wife had left Japan, we had, of course, shipped our household goods from the home in which we had been living, and I had moved back into the Imperial Hotel. When I was not in Korea, I again lived in this gloomy cavern, although it was quite different in atmosphere and physical appearance, furnishings, and service than it had been on that day in 1945 when I had first gone to live there.

I finally departed late at night on a Northwest Airlines plane from Haneda Airport. Because my baggage, of course, was limited to the usual forty pounds, I had given away most of my personal belongings and was able to carry back to the States only a few treasured gifts. I returned by way of Alaska. I was reunited with my family—this time in Atherton, a residential area south of San Francisco, where my wife had bought a home for us, our older daughter, and two grandchildren.

I was ordered to Washington, D.C., to report to the Surgeon General, which I did. My good friend George Armstrong had been selected and assigned as Surgeon General of the Army Medical Corps.[1] I was also requested by the medical policy council of the Defense Department to make a report on the findings and recommendations on the handling of casualties among our troops, which I did as requested by General Hume.

The Medical Field Service School

I had counted on embarking on a new career in civilian medicine in California, and on my return from Washington, D.C., was granted leave while my request for voluntary retirement was being considered by the Department of the Army.[2] I was eventually informed that this request for voluntary retirement would not be approved. Instead, I was ordered as assistant commandant to the Medical Field Service School at Fort Sam Houston, Texas.[3] Gen. Ed Noyes was commander of the Brooks Army Medical Center of which the school was a part. Gen. Joe Martin was the commandant of the school. The assistant commandant at one of our military schools is comparable in position to that of dean of a school in our civilian universities; the commandant is in a position comparable to that of the president of a university. The assistant commandant is primarily concerned with the faculty and the curriculum and the teaching and handling of the students; the commandant is concerned with the overall operation of the school, its physical plant, and all of the many administrative and other activities essential to the operation of any large installation.

We, accordingly, leased our home and moved to San Antonio, Texas. I found that the school in the intervening years had again become didactic and academic.[4] Being acutely aware of the difficulties of our young medics who were in combat and who had not received training in medical field service, I again, with the cooperation of the staff and faculty and all concerned, was able to initiate for the third time a series of demonstrations, which would visually impress on the students the responsibilities, the organization, and the function of the army medical service in combat.[5] Once again, the attitude of the student body, which had been somewhat rebellious under the academic classroom type of teaching, changed as it had in 1943. There was a war on, so there was a great interest in these demonstrations and field exercises in which they felt they were receiving actual training in duties to which they would shortly be assigned with combat units in Korea.

There were some thirty-six different types of courses at the school, not only for medical officers but also for nurses and various types of technicians. Our program involved training some 22,000 individuals.

I had not been stationed in Texas before. I was most happy to find there many of my older friends who had been general officers and with whom I had served in the past. These officers were retired in most cases and were living in the immediate vicinity. In addition, among the people of Texas, I met many fine individuals. Some who knew of my pleasure in hunting were kind enough to invite me to their ranches, where I could enjoy this favorite sport.

Governor's Island

After two years of this duty, I was assigned to the First Army, which was stationed in New York at Governor's Island, where I was responsible to the army commander, Lieutenant General Burroughs, who was one of our fine combat leaders, for the medical service in army medical installations in New England, New York, and New Jersey. We lived on this very old post in very old quarters. It was a return to the type of army life that we had enjoyed so much in peacetime early in our career.[6]

In this area, there was great demand for senior army officers, as well as air force and naval officers, to be included in the guest lists of the endless social and organizational functions in New York City and neighboring areas. From a social standpoint, the nights were filled with social engagements, it seemed sometimes. In addition to renewing acquaintances with military friends who had retired and were engaged in business in New York or Boston, our new civilian friends there made this a worthwhile and enjoyable experience. From a professional standpoint, as part of my responsibilities, I established contact again with many of my professional colleagues and met many new friends in the outstanding medical installations in New York, Boston, and Philadelphia.

The Study of Korean War Casualties

During this period from 1953 to 1955, a board was established at the direction of the assistant secretary of health and medicine of the Defense Department, to review the Korean War experience. I was made a member of this board. After a year-and-a-half of work, the conclusion of the board, which was finally rendered in the spring of 1955, substantiated my early findings in 1950 and 1951, as to the reasons behind the changes in casualty figures, which were of such great concern at that time.[7]

History repeats itself, and I am quite sure that the lessons learned will be forgotten. We will go through the same experience again, if we are unfortunate enough to enter another war. Time passes, people get older, new individuals come in, past lessons are forgotten. We always have to learn the same lessons over and over the hard way. So it has been throughout our national life in the case of every war which we have entered.

Going Home

In the fall of 1954, a policy was announced that voluntary retirements would again be authorized. I was eager to get back to California, where we had retained our home and where my two daughters and the grandchildren were living. Eventually, the Defense Department declared the "missing-in-action" actually dead. Our older daughter had been re-established in a home in San Leandro, California. Our younger daughter and her husband had moved to Sacramento. My wife and I were both eager to go back to California, after so many years of separation during the two wars and after so many years of living in foreign countries. I had, in my career as a medic, held all of the various types of major assignments that I could receive.

In April 1955, my good friend Gen. Silas Hays was selected as Surgeon General. Si informed me that if I would remain on, as he desired that I should, I would be returned to the Far East to take over as theater surgeon, relieving Gen. Earl Standlee. I had, however, spent ten years overseas, and I felt that I had stayed on in the service long enough, having completed thirty-three years in the military service, of which twenty-six years had been in the medical corps. I had served twice as head of the army medical service in an overseas theater. A third such assignment would offer no new challenge and would only serve to prevent some other medic junior to me from gaining the valuable experience he would receive if I blocked his advancement by remaining on until forced to retire for age some seven years later.

I submitted my request for voluntary retirement, which was approved. I ended a career as an army medic on the thirty-first of July 1955, at which time we left New York and returned to California, our home. Since that time, I have been fortunate in being able to continue my professional activities, because a doctor never really retires from his profession, nor even fades away.

What has been, then, the total result of this career as an army medic? To me, the highlight of such a career has been the accomplishment of what I believe was constructive work, actually in a non-military field, in helping to rebuild a destroyed nation and to establish health and welfare programs which, on a nationwide basis, are among the most modern in the world today. In the course of doing so, I hope to have influenced the thinking of many peoples in the underdeveloped countries so that they can know that, literally, their lives are worth saving and that this very essence of our concept of democracy is more desirable than the promises of the dictatorships of the welfare or socialist state, where the individual is nothing and the welfare of the state is of primary importance.

Notes

The archival sources for the following notes are the Hoover Institution Archives at Stanford University, Stanford, California, the National Archives and Records Administration, Suitland, Maryland, and the Rockefeller Archive Center, North Tarrytown, New York. The archives and collections are abbreviated as follows:

CFS	Crawford F. Sams Collection (79066)
HIA	Hoover Institution Archives
RG 331	Allied Operational and Occupation Headquarters, WWII Public Health and Welfare Section Collection
NARA	National Archives and Records Administration
JZB	John Z. Bowers Collection
RF	Rockefeller Foundation Collection
RAC	Rockefeller Archive Center

The official reports of the Public Health and Welfare (PHW) Section, Supreme Commander for the Allied Powers (SCAP), contain numerical and documentary information. Repositories for the documents cited in the following notes include the Library of Congress, Washington, D.C., and the National Archives and Records Administration, Suitland, Maryland.

Introduction

1. Crawford F. Sams, Memorandum for General Maxwell, 18 July 1945, CFS, Box 4, HIA; Crawford F. Sams, "Medic," 1958, 329–34, CFS, Box 1, HIA.

2. Shortly before Sams concluded his mission in Japan, Simmons wrote to Sams that the "civilian public health program organized by you in Japan has never been duplicated in the history of the world." James S. Simmons to Crawford F. Sams, 23 April 1951, CFS, Box 4, HIA. See also the comment regarding the "unmatched" achievements in public health during the occupation of Japan, which is attributed to Simmons, in Harry Emerson Wildes, "Post-War Public Health Developments," *Contemporary Japan* 21 (1951): 583; James S. Simmons to Robert F. Pitts, 7 August 1953, CFS, Box 5, HIA.

3. Michio Hashimoto to Zabelle Zakarian, 17 February 1997.

4. The more recent literature on the occupation of Japan by western scholars largely overlooks public health and welfare reforms. For example, in *The Legacy of the Occupation—Japan*, Herbert Passin writes, "Occupation reforms are often better evaluated not in terms of their immediate effects, but as the starting point of a long causational chain." This work, which was written between 1967 and 1968, omits public health and welfare as a category of reform. Herbert Passin, *The Legacy of the Occupation—Japan*. New York:

East Asian Institute, Columbia University, 1968, 34. Edwin O. Reischauer's discussion of occupation reforms in *The Japanese* also neglects the topic, though he notes that Japanese men and women now have longer life expectancies than Americans and that Japanese children born after the war are, on the average, physically larger than prewar generations. Edwin O. Reischauer, *The Japanese*. Cambridge: Harvard University Press, 1981, 23, 103–9, 230. Nor does Ardath Burks mention provisions for public health and welfare in discussing the Japanese Constitution of 1947 as a legal and political framework for reform in *Japan: A Post Industrial Power*. Ardath W. Burks, *Japan: A Post Industrial Power*, 2d ed. Boulder: Westview Press, 1984, 120–27. Only one reference to public health reforms appears in recent literature on postwar social change: John W. Bennett notes that "health and sanitation was an especially successful program of the Occupation period" and Japan's low infant mortality rates have reflected favorably on its level and pattern of industrialization in subsequent international comparisons. John W. Bennett, "Japanese Economic Growth: Background for Social Change," in *Aspects of Social Change in Modern Japan*, ed. Robert P. Dore, 411–53. Princeton: Princeton University Press, 1967, 416.

5. James Atlas, "Choosing a Life," *New York Times Book Review*, January 13, 1991, sec. 7, 23.

6. Crawford F. Sams, "Medic," 57.

7. Crawford F. Sams, "Medic," 3, 19–20.

8. Crawford F. Sams, "Medic," 64.

9. Crawford F. Sams, "Medic," 19, 77.

10. Crawford F. Sams, "Medic," 268.

11. Public Health and Welfare Section, *Mission and Accomplishments of the Occupation in the Public Health and Welfare Fields*. Tokyo: Supreme Commander for the Allied Powers, December 1949, 1.

12. W.R. Hodgson, "Rehabilitation for Peace," *Contemporary Japan* 21 (1952): 10. Lt. Col. W.R. Hodgson represented the British Commonwealth on the Allied Council for Japan and was head of the Australian Mission to SCAP in Tokyo from 1949 to 1952. He became Australia's ambassador to Japan in 1952.

13. Crawford F. Sams, "American Public Health Administration Meets the Problems of the Orient," *American Journal of Public Health* 42 (May 1952): 565.

14. Harry Harootunian, "Ideology as Conflict," in *Conflict in Modern Japanese History: The Neglected Tradition*, ed. Tetsuo Najita and J. Victor Koschmann, 25–61. Princeton: Princeton University Press, 1982, 26. Although the historical circumstances of the occupation of Japan differ from those of the Meiji Restoration, readers who are interested in the role of European and American technical experts in Japan during periods of institutional reform may find part IV of "Medic" a companion to *An American Scientist in Early Meiji Japan: The Autobiographical Notes of Thomas C. Mendenhall*. In reforming the infrastructure of the fields of public health and welfare in Japan during a time of institutional transition, and in his practical and pragmatic approach to problems in these fields, Sams's contributions and methods parallel those of Thomas C. Mendenhall in the field of physical sciences. Mendenhall was an American physicist who became the first professor of physics at Tokyo University in 1878. He belonged to an earlier group of European and American technical experts known in Japan as *oyatoi*. See Richard Rubinger, ed., *An American Scientist in Early Meiji Japan: The Autobiographical Notes of Thomas C. Mendenhall*. Honolulu: University of Hawaii Press, 1989.

15. See Crawford F. Sams to John Z. Bowers, 21 August 1981, JZB, Box 1, Crawford F. Sams Folder, RAC. John Z. Bowers served as deputy director of the Atomic Energy Commission from 1947 to 1950, and first met Sams in Tokyo in 1949. In 1981, while Dr. Bowers was working with the Rockefeller Foundation, he wrote a history of the Atomic Bomb Casualty Commission at the request of the National Research Council. In the

course of his research on the ABCC, he interviewed Crawford Sams on 5 October 1981.
16. Crawford F. Sams to Zabelle Zakarian, 8 October 1991.

Preface

1. See, for example, Peter Packer to Crawford F. Sams, 30 June 1952, CFS, Box 4, HIA.
2. In a letter to a potential collaborator, written shortly after the occupation, Sams mentioned two such books but did not embrace their heroic claims: "There are some who think that the work in Japan constitutes one of the so-called "monumental" pieces of work in medical history. You will find references along that line in books that have been written such as Russell Bryant's book on Japan; Gunther's book, "The Riddle of MacArthur," and various others. However, such an evaluation is one for historians to make in a better perspective than we have at this early date." Crawford F. Sams to Peter Packer, 19 July 1952, CFS, Box 4, HIA.
3. See, for example, James Stevens Simmons to Walter Kahoe, 26 November 1952, CFS, Box 5, HIA; James Stevens Simmons to Crawford F. Sams, 5 August 1953, CFS, Box 5, HIA.
4. One reason Sams waited until he retired to write "Medic" had to do with his expressed desire to write about his experiences "without censorship or suppression." Anything he wrote while in the military service was subject to censorship and could not be published without approval of the Department of the Army. Given this constraint, the army's denial of Sams's requests for voluntary retirement in 1951, and again in July 1952, only frustrated the possibility of providing "source material" for "those who through the passage of time will have a better perspective in evaluating its final worth." Crawford F. Sams to Peter Packer, 19 July 1952.
The cold war broadened the possibility of censorship. In the summer of 1952, the U.S. Department of Defense refused to sanction the script of a motion picture depicting an epidemiological intelligence mission that Sams had led in North Korea in 1951. (For a discussion of Sams's mission, see chapter 30.) Although Sams did not write the script and the film companies could independently produce it, the Department of Defense disapproved it in part because of the potential for the film's misuse by "the Russians" to support allegations of germ warfare by the United Nations forces. Robert D. Burhams to Crawford F. Sams, 11 August 1952, CFS, Box 4, HIA.
At the same time, suggestions that Sams record his professional experiences before such information became lost took on fresh meaning. Requests from army historians who were reconstructing a record of activities in the Middle East during World War II, in which Sams had participated, had demonstrated to Sams the possibility of losing or misplacing official records "in the short space of ten years." By waiting until he retired to write "Medic," Sams may have lost an opportunity for short-lived celebrity; but he had gained "a measure of freedom" to write what he hoped would contribute to an "impersonal evaluation of whatever ... [he] may have contributed to ... [his] fellow humans." Crawford F. Sams to Peter Packer, 19 July 1952.

The Move

1. The conventions for naming naval ships would indicate the Sturgeon was a submarine: battleships are named after states (for example, the U.S.S. *Missouri*); cruisers, after cities; destroyers, after people; submarines, after fish. In this instance, however, the Sturgeon was a nickname for the U.S.S. *General S.D. Sturgis*. Based upon the number of

passengers and Sams's account of its naval escort, this ship was probably a passenger vessel with communications equipment aboard, not a destroyer. See Maj. John C. Greer, Memorandum No. 2, "Passenger List and Officer Stateroom Assignments," U.S.S. *General S.D. Sturgis*, 26 August 1945, CFS, Box 4, HIA.

2. Stateroom assignments on the ship were made according to rank. Among the army officers with whom then Colonel Sams shared stateroom fourteen was Col. Ashley Oughterson, who subsequently headed the Joint Commission to study the health effects of radiation on survivors of the atomic bombs. (See chapter 16 on the Atomic Bomb Casualty Commission.) Maj. John C. Greer, 26 August 1945. See M. Susan Lindee, *Suffering Made Real: American Science and the Survivors at Hiroshima*. Chicago: The University of Chicago Press, 1994, 23–24, regarding the Joint Commission.

Chapter 1: The Perimeter

1. No exception was made for hospitals. Occupation forces found hospitals in a physically deteriorated state and noted that "Large quantities of heating and central cooking equipment had been removed for scrap metal." Public Health and Welfare Section, *Mission and Accomplishments*, 18.

2. The Geneva Conventions are a series of agreements among nations that embody a humanitarian code for the treatment of armed forces at war, the consideration for personnel responsible for them, the treatment of prisoners of war, and the protection of civilians. Convention I, which is associated with the founding of the International Red Cross in Geneva, Switzerland, in 1864, deals with the care of the sick, wounded, and dead in battle. It calls for the respect of wounded soldiers and the neutrality of hospitals bearing the Red Cross sign. This convention was extended to naval warfare in 1907, and subsequently became known as Convention II. Convention III pertains to the treatment of prisoners of war. It was first agreed upon in 1929, in response to the treatment and repatriation of war prisoners in World War I. Convention IV deals with the protection of civilians. It was adopted in 1949, in response to the effects of technological warfare on civilian populations during World War II.

3. With regard to the restoration of hospital services for foreign nationals at Seibo Hospital in Tokyo, see the discussion of hospitals in chapter 2.

4. The cargo of the seven planes, which was turned over to the International Red Cross at Hiroshima on 6 September 1945, consisted of twelve tons of medical supplies taken from First Cavalry Division stocks. These were the first relief supplies provided to the Japanese civilian population by the occupation forces. Brig. Gen. H.E. Eastwood, Memorandum on Civilian Relief Supplies, 18 October 1945, RG 331, Box 9350–56, NARA.

In a study of the Atomic Bomb Casualty Commission (ABCC), Lindee notes that the leaders of two ad hoc medical teams, which were formed to study the health effects of radiation on atomic bomb survivors, namely, Col. Ashley Oughterson of the army and Dr. Stafford Warren of the Manhattan Project, accompanied a "special survey to Hiroshima around 5 September," under the direction of Gen. Thomas Farrell of the Manhattan Project. These two groups along with an ad hoc naval team, headed by Dr. Shields Warren, and two groups of Japanese scientists later constituted the Joint Commission, which was the predecessor to the ABCC. M. Susan Lindee, *Suffering Made Real*, 23–34. This "special survey" may have been the transport that Sams had arranged for the IRCC supplies and the American medical scientists. See also chapter 16 on the ABCC.

5. The first "SCAPIN" to address public health, sanitation, hospitals, medical supplies, food distribution, port quarantine, and vital statistics on a programmatic basis was issued three weeks after surrender on 22 September 1945. It ordered specific actions and information relating to disease surveillance and control: (1) an immediate survey of dis-

ease prevalence by prefecture; (2) a report of the number of public health personnel available in each prefecture; and (3) steps to control communicable diseases affecting civilian health, with special emphasis on the control of venereal diseases, which at that time were not reportable diseases in Japan. Lt. Col. Harold Fair, SCAPIN 48, "Public Health Measures," 22 September 1945, RG 331, Box 9350–56, NARA. Shortly after the organization of SCAP on 2 October 1945 (see chapter 3), this directive was followed by SCAPIN 98, which required the preservation of "all vital statistical records" and the collection of additional information: a report on the numbers of people, by prefecture and city, in need of relief supplies and medical care or hospitalization; copies of laws pertaining to welfare and social insurance; and documentation on the production, manufacture, and consumption of narcotics. Col. H.W. Allen, SCAPIN 98, "Information on Japanese Public Health," 6 October 1945, RG 331, Box 9350–56, NARA.

Chapter 2: Tokyo

1. In deciding how to restore hospital services to foreign nationals in Japan, Sams was able to draw upon his experience in the European theater in arriving at a solution. In December 1944, while serving as chief of the Program Branch of the Logistics Division of the U.S. War Department, Sams went on a two-month mission to the European theater to assess requirements for hospitals and medical personnel, given the plans for the occupation of Germany, the redeployment of military forces from Europe to the Far East, and the relative shortage then of U.S. medical and nursing personnel. He toured U.S. military hospitals, prisoner-of-war camps, and displaced persons camps to determine whether additional American personnel should be brought in to provide medical services for these populations. He found that, in the case of German prisoners-of-war, and in the case of a camp of Poles, Czechs, and other European people who had been taken into Germany as forced labor, which had been overrun by Americans, the encamped people, for psychological reasons, preferred to be treated by doctors and nurses of their own nationality and were happier if they received "treatment of the kind to which they are accustomed from their own medical people." This psychological factor presented an alternative to using American medical personnel to treat displaced persons; that is, was to provide the medical equipment but allow the medical personnel within the camps to care for their own people, thereby relieving American staff to care for American battle casualties. Sams described this possible solution as one which he would find "useful later on." Crawford F. Sams, "Medic," 302–3, 309–10.
2. See the discussion of the demilitarization of hospitals in chapter 15.
3. See the discussion of the model hospital administration program in chapter 15.

Chapter 3: The Decision: SCAP

1. The Public Health and Welfare Section was initially comprised of thirteen divisions. By January 1950, these were consolidated into ten divisions: Administrative, which included interpreter and translator services; Supply, which included pharmaceutical education and supplies; Preventive Medicine, which included Dental Affairs; Medical Services (formerly Hospital Administration); Nursing Affairs; Veterinary Affairs; Health and Welfare Statistics (formerly Vital Statistics); Welfare; Social Security; and Narcotic Control. General Headquarters, *Selected Data on the Occupation of Japan*. Tokyo: Supreme Commander for the Allied Powers, June 1950, 192–94.
2. This decision to use the structure of the Japanese Government and reform it as necessary, instead of abolishing it, differs from the U.S. policy for the occupation of

Germany. Hugh Borton, *Japan's Modern Century: From Perry to 1970*, 2d ed. New York: Ronald Press, (1955) 1970, 446–47.

3. This plan was initiated with respect to health and welfare by SCAPIN 48, which required working through the various levels of government to restore public water supplies and sewerage systems, to distribute food and medical supplies, and to reopen or operate civilian hospitals and public health laboratories. Lt. Col. Harold Fair, 22 September 1945.

4. Sams's use of various figures for the total population of Japan may appear haphazard and inconsistent, but the size of the population was changing rapidly. By 1951, it exceeded 84 million, largely as result of repatriation of over 6 million people and, to a lesser extent, a natural increase (annual births minus annual deaths) by 1947. Crawford F. Sams, "Medic," 440; Ministry of Health and Welfare (*Kōseishō*), *Health and Welfare Services in Japan*. Tokyo: Japanese Government, March 1986, 72.

Chapter 4: First Reconnaissance of Japan

1. Although the Japanese Government has subsequently taken steps to transfer the ownership and operation of the national railroads to the private sector, Sams's statement was accurate at the time and in the context in which he wrote it.

2. One of the earliest of these directives was SCAPIN 93, which ordered the abrogation of the Religious Body Law (Shukyō Dantai Hō) of 8 April 1939, as well as numerous other laws and agencies through which prewar militarists restricted freedom of thought, religion, assembly, and speech. Col. H.W. Allen, SCAPIN 93, "Removal of Restrictions on Political, Civil, and Religious Liberties," 4 October 1945, RG 331, Box 9350–56, NARA.

3. Edwin O. Reischauer made similar points about patterns of social life and sexual norms among married Japanese men and women and about the role of geisha. See Edwin O. Reischauer, *The Japanese*, 204–7.

Chapter 5: Food Relief and Nutrition

1. During the eighteenth century, Japan's population growth was fairly stable, and its one-staple agricultural economy sustained a population of 30 million people. By the late nineteenth century, this equilibrium was upset, and Japan faced the dilemma of how to feed a growing population when there was little way to expand its highly productive rice cultivation on the limited arable land. By the early twentieth century, this dilemma was viewed in terms of a food deficit, which in Japan had reached nearly 20 percent of its food supply. For brief comparative discussions of agricultural development in relation to population growth in feudal Japan, see Edwin O. Reischauer, *The Japanese*, 16–19, 70–74; George B. Samson, *Japan in World History*. Tokyo: Charles E. Tuttle, 1984, 19–30.

2. The basis, object, and level of this concern are evident in "secret" memoranda, to which Sams then had access but which may not yet have been declassified at the time he wrote "Medic." These memoranda indicate U.S. military officials had initially feared a breakdown of the Japanese Government's supply and distribution system in the event of a low harvest or poor distribution of food. The chance of such a breakdown, which might imperil occupation forces and their mission, was thought to be "sufficiently strong." The fear of this contingency presented a basis for a change in policy toward the Japanese and warranted a reserve of medical supplies and food to serve 7 million civilians for 30 days in such an emergency:

> the policy not to provide any supplies for enemy population in Japan this winter is premised on effective operation of the Japanese government. Breakdown of the gov-

ernment in its machinery for supply and distribution may make it necessary for the Army to act in order to avoid acute distress and epidemics. ...

A breakdown if it did occur would be most likely to do so during the 2d or early part of the 3d quarter of 1946. ...

An emergency situation endangering the health of our troops and our occupational mission would exist if during the course of one month ten percent of the Japanese population needed to receive emergency supplies.

Brig. Gen. H.E. Eastwood, 18 October 1945; Brig. Gen. H.E. Eastwood, Memorandum on Civilian Relief Supplies, 22 October 1945, RG 331, Box 9350–56, NARA.

This concern about rice riots highlights the dynamics and interdependency of military security and civilian public health and welfare during the early years of the occupation. Although the PHW Section's mission was to safeguard the security and health of occupation forces and their mission in Japan by preventing widespread disease and unrest, the security and health of the occupation forces was measured in relation to civilian distress and epidemics. (For an example of the relationship between disease and social unrest and the fears it engendered, see the discussion of typhus fever in chapter 8, including note 6.)

3. Sams planned as well as directed the release of emergency relief supplies. Before he departed for the Philippines in July 1945, he had prepared plans for military and civilian medical care and civilian relief, which included programmed grain supplies, based upon wartime assumptions of a ground invasion of Japan. He had prepared these plans for the Pacific theater as chief of the Planning Branch of the Logistics Division of the U.S. War Department in Washington, D.C., a position he held from February to July 1945. Crawford F. Sams, "Medic," 328–33.

4. In addition to the task of trying to change a culture-bound nutritional pattern, the relative unfamiliarity of these foods to the Japanese people presents another contrast with the setting of the occupation of Germany.

5. Prime Minister Yoshida Shigeru became the first prime minister to serve under the postwar Constitution. He was prime minister from 1946 to 1954.

Chapter 6: The Reorganization of Health and Welfare

1. The Diet passed the new Constitution of Japan on 24 August 1946. When it became effective on 3 May 1947, the Constitution reversed the precedence of the state and society over the individual citizen, instituting a new legal framework for democracy. It introduced a number of political reforms ranging from vesting sovereignty in the people, rather than the emperor (Article 1), to reforming the family system and assuring freedom of compulsion in marriage (Article 24). Article 21 guaranteed freedoms of speech, press, and political organization. Article 15 extended the eligibility to vote to women; it also lowered the voting age from 25 to 20 years of age. Reform of the Civil Code (Article 17) made it possible for citizens to bring suit against the government. These and all subsequent references to the Constitution of Japan are from Hugh Borton, *Japan's Modern Century*, Appendix IV.

The formalities of its promulgation, depicted in figures 11 and 12, were more worldly compared with the time, place, and manner of promulgating the Meiji Constitution, which Robert J. Smith has described as follows: "The ceremony was held in 1889, on February 11, which is *kigensetsu*, the mythical date of the founding of the Japanese state upon the accession of the first emperor, Jimmu. They chose as the locale the imperial palace, where in a brief declaration to the small assemblage of government officials, men of affairs, and diplomatic representatives, the emperor granted a constitution to his people." Robert J. Smith, *Japanese Society: Tradition, Self, and the Social Order.* New York: Cambridge University Press, 1983, 24.

2. Article 41 of the Constitution established the Diet as "the highest organ of state power" and "the sole law-making organ of the State." Articles 92 and 94 empowered local governments to enact ordinances consistent with national law.

3. Articles 67 and 68 of the Constitution specify the manner in which the prime minister and cabinet are chosen: The Diet selects the prime minister; the prime minister appoints the cabinet. A majority of the ministers of state must be members of the Diet.

4. Article 93 of the Constitution gave voters the right directly to elect prefectural governors, mayors, and local assembly representatives, thereby abolishing their appointment by the national government.

5. This distinction between national and federal forms of government is important for determining which levels of government decide and implement provisions for health and welfare. Unlike the delegation of all residual powers to the states under the U.S. Constitution, prefectural and local governments in Japan could not assume authority for health and welfare under a national form of government; hence, Article 25 of the Japanese Constitution establishes the promotion and extension of public health, along with social welfare and social insurance, as a legitimate function of government in a manner consistent with the national form of government:

> All people have the right to maintain the minimum standards of wholesome and cultured living.
> In all spheres of life, the State shall use its endeavors for the promotion and extension of social welfare and security, and of public health.

Note the choice of *shall*, not *should*. Hugh Borton, *Japan's Modern Century*, 495.

In an interview with this editor, Sams indicated that he drafted Article 25 of the Constitution. Interview with Crawford F. Sams, Atherton, California, 28 October 1991.

6. Local governments in Japan depend upon revenues from the national treasury for about seventy percent of their revenues. National revenues are allocated through a system of loans, grants, subsidies, and tax revenues, which are collected and distributed by the national government. Certain subsidies tend to be used as a spoils system between the party in power and their affiliates in local government, thus reinforcing the fiscal dependency of local governments. For a discussion of local finance in postwar Japan, see Kurt Steiner, *Local Government in Japan.* Stanford: Stanford University Press, 1965, 263–99.

7. The House of Representatives of the Diet has the power to dissolve the cabinet by passing a no confidence resolution or rejecting a confidence resolution. See Article 69 of the Japanese Constitution.

8. In January 1938, the Ministry of Home Affairs transferred authority for health administration, social welfare, social insurance, and labor affairs to the newly established Ministry of Health and Social Affairs. Local and prefectural administrative bodies were preserved, so public health and sanitation remained a police function at the local level; accordingly, the authorities responsible for licensing prostitution and controlling public disorder were also responsible for public health and sanitation.

The founding of the Ministry of Health and Social Affairs, as well as the Institute of Public Health, coincided with the rise of reactionary imperialism in Japan. Two political forces steered the administration of health and welfare and the application of public health knowledge during this period: the suppression of progressive movements; and the redirection of science and technology for military purposes. The National Mobilization Law of 1938 and the National Health Insurance System, which extended medical insurance to the entire population in 1938, were directed toward assuring adequate military and industrial personnel. Militarists supported the training of medical personnel, but not for serving civilian populations. Consequently, the Ministry of Health and Social Affairs underwent several reorganizations beginning in April 1938. Welfare and social insurance related to the care of sick and wounded soldiers or their families dominated its functions between 1938 and 1945; hence, it became known as the "Ministry of Welfare." For a summary of the development and organization of governmental health and welfare functions in Japan from 1853 to 1945, see Public Health and Welfare Section, *Public Health and Welfare in Japan*. Tokyo: General Headquarters, SCAP, 1948, 1–4. See also Michio Hashimoto, *Development of Social Consciousness in the History of Public Health in Japan*. Tokyo: History of Science Society of Japan, 1964.

9. The reorganization of the public health and welfare system occurred slowly, as relief programs and the control of epidemics dominated the PHW Section's activities during the first year of the occupation. The preliminary structure and functions of the Ministry of Health and Welfare and the prefectural health and welfare offices were outlined in SCAPIN 945, which was issued in the months prior to the enactment of the Constitution. The preliminary organization attempted to decentralize the functional activities. Activities dealing with the public were to be conducted as far as possible at the prefectural and local levels; the national government would administer policy, decide technical matters, and coordinate functions. The existing health centers were allowed to continue operations and were not reorganized until 5 September 1947, when the Diet enacted the Health Center Law. Brig. Gen. B.M. Fitch, SCAPIN 945, "Reorganization of Governmental Public Health and Welfare Activities," 11 May 1946, RG 331, Box 9350–56, NARA; Public Health and Welfare Section, *Public Health and Welfare in Japan*, 12–15, 74–77. See also Crawford F. Sams, "American Public Health Administration," 557–63; Public Health and Welfare Division, *Public Health and Welfare in Japan: Final Summary 1951–52*, 2 vols. Tokyo: Supreme Commander for the Allied Powers, 1952, vol. 1, 5–6, 21–23.

10. Model health centers provided an "awakening to public health" for their staff as well as the populations they served. Dr. Hashimoto Masami, on the occasion of his retirement from the Institute of Public Health in Tokyo on 25 September 1982, recalled his experience as a medical officer at the Toyonaka Health Center in Osaka Prefecture between 1948 and 1952:

> [These] five years at the model health center were really a highly challenging and exciting period for me under an extremely severe, but hopeful social milieu then. . . . There were then some 50 full time staffs [sic] [members] (7 medical officers, 15 public health nurses, and others), and we made all efforts day and night as a health team aimed at the promotion of health education based on [the] daily life of the people in the community. . . .
> . . . However, through such an integrated team approach of [the] whole health center staff. . . I was really awakened [to] the essentials of public health.

Masami Hashimoto, "Fourty [sic] Years of My Public Health Study," *Bulletin of the Institute of Public Health* (Tokyo) 33 (1984): 2–4.

11. The PHW Section used various media to promote public health and welfare programs, including daily fifteen-minute radio programs, articles in women's magazines, films, and courses offered at the health centers. In addition, one of the more popular and entertaining strategies for communicating with people and demonstrating disease control and hygienic practices was the Public Health Train. This traveling exhibit highlighted the breadth and scope of public health and welfare reforms, reinforcing the basic public health services provided by the newly reorganized health centers. Comprised of three converted

railway coaches, it contained "exhibits, charts, diagrams, pictures and models dealing with nutrition, tuberculosis, venereal diseases and other communicable diseases, parasitic diseases, public health nursing, dental hygiene, social security, environmental sanitation and veterinary activities." The train itself not only exemplified the aim and dynamics of public health reforms but also captured the astonishingly open and popular spirit in which they were being implemented. Between November 1947 and August 1948, it toured thirty-three cities throughout Japan. Local officials often collaborated by welcoming its arrival with music and fanfare, and local health center staff set up tents near the station stops, where they provided nutrition and dental hygiene consultations, showed health education films and cartoons, screened visitors for venereal diseases and tuberculosis, and offered BCG inoculations. Approximately 900,000 persons visited the train, with as many as 4,600 people on a single day, before its tour concluded in September 1948. Public Health and Welfare Section, *Public Health and Welfare in Japan*, 77; Welfare Ministry [of Japan], Report on the Public Health Train, 21 September 1948 and 30 September 1948. RG 331, Box 9373–75, NARA.

12. Public Health and Welfare Division, *Public Health and Welfare in Japan*, 5–6.

13. The Institute of Public Health offered one-year programs for graduates of medical schools and pharmacy schools beginning in April 1939. Shorter courses for veterinarians began in September 1939. Courses for nurses began in December 1940, and a program in nutrition education began in April 1941. Eight fields of study constituted its original departments: statistics; demography; epidemiology; physiological hygiene; nutrition and biochemistry; microbiology; sanitary engineering; and architectural hygiene engineering and housing. Institute of Public Health. *Announcement of the Institute of Public Health*. Tokyo: Institute of Public Health, 1985, 1.

14. Nurses constituted a high proportion of the complement of health center personnel. Courses for nurses resumed in April 1947; medical officers, in June 1947; pharmacists and veterinarians, in January 1948; and nutritionists and engineers, in May 1948. Public Health and Welfare Section, *Public Health and Welfare in Japan*, 74. Regarding the renewed interest of the Rockefeller Foundation in the Institute of Public Health during the occupation "to support the SCAP program" as well as Sam's "enthusiastic" reaction to this interest, especially the possibility of obtaining on loan from the Rockefeller Foundation a full-time director for the institute, see Marshall C. Balfour to George K. Strode, 31 January 1947, RF, RG 1.1, Series 609, Box 3, Folder 18, RAC; Crawford F. Sams to Marshall C. Balfour, 14 March 1947, RF, RG 1.1, Series 609, Box 3, Folder 18, RAC.

15. Most short courses at the Institute of Public Health were three-months long. A small number of medical officers, nursing instructors, and veterinarians completed longer courses, six- or twelve-months long. By 1952, sanitarians (886) were the largest category of trainees. Next were nurses (743), medical officers (660), veterinarians (629), statisticians (561), nutritionists (482), pharmacists (270), laboratory specialists (268), sanitary engineers (183), and health educators (104). Public Health and Welfare Division, *Public Health and Welfare in Japan*, 22.

16. In 1951, the International Health Division of the Rockefeller Foundation provided a grant of $3,000, which enabled the Institute of Public Health to subscribe to sixty journals and add about two hundred books to the library. Public Health and Welfare Division, *Public Health and Welfare in Japan*, 23.

17. For a discussion of the training of sanitary engineers and sanitarians and the organization of sanitary teams, see chapter 9.

18. See Crawford F. Sams to Marshall C. Balfour, 14 March 1947, 2. For a study of the competition and institutional loyalities surrounding financial support, control, and affiliation of the Institute of Infectious Diseases in the period leading up to World War I, see James R. Bartholomew, *The Formation of Science in Japan*. Yale University Press, 1989.

Chapter 7: Statistics: A Health and Welfare Tool

1. Leonard Phelps, then with the U.S. Census Bureau, became chief of the Statistics Division in May 1946. He was preceded by Dr. F.E. Linder, also of the U.S. Census Bureau, who conducted a study of the *koseki* system and the census-, vital statistic- and disease-reporting system in Japan in relation to the task of establishing modern public health and welfare statistic-reporting systems in Japan. Linder's study provided the baseline for the reforms that ensued. Eiji Marui, "The U.S. and Japanese Experience with Vital Statistics Reform in the Early Occupation Days," Tokyo, 1988, 17–25.

2. The ascertainment of disease and death within a defined geographic location, and its related population, is a basic element of epidemiological analysis used in public health administration as well as research.

3. Vital and health statistics were needed to assess public health and welfare conditions in relation to medical supplies; hence, two of the earliest SCAPIN concerning public health, namely, SCAPIN 48 and SCAPIN 98, required preservation, reporting, and analysis of vital and health statistics. Lt. Col. Harold Fair, SCAPIN 48, 22 September 1945; Col. H.W. Allen, SCAPIN 98, 6 October 1945. See note 5 to chapter 1, above.

4. For a study of how the PHW Section planned and negotiated the reform of the vital statistic- and disease-reporting system, without nullifying the cultural heritage of the *koseki* system, see Eiji Marui, "The U.S. and Japanese Experience."

5. The ten reportable diseases at the start of the occupation were as follows: cholera; typhoid fever; dysentery; typhus; smallpox; diphtheria; plague; scarlet fever; paratyphoid fever; and epidemic meningitis. Public Health and Welfare Section, *Public Health and Welfare in Japan*, 2. Venereal diseases were the first diseases made reportable by the occupation forces: syphilis; gonorrhea; and chancroid. Crawford F. Sams, "Japan's New Public Health Program, Part Two," *Military Government Journal* 2 (January-February 1949): 7. For a table of the thirty-five reportable diseases, see Public Health and Welfare Division, *Public Health and Welfare in Japan*, 9.

6. Reformation of the vital statistic-reporting system to achieve a high level of completeness of the data was an element of the public health infrastructure which supported the research of the Atomic Bomb Casualty Commission. For example, accurate data on stillbirths and infant mortality were important for studies of genetic effects of radiation exposure and reproductive outcomes. See M. Susan Lindee, *Suffering Made Real*, 169–74.

7. One means of achieving a high level of completeness was to match registrations of vital events from the alternative systems of registration: Reports from the *koseki* registration system and reports by midwives and physicians were compared to the vital statistics reported to the local health centers to refine ascertainment. Public Health and Welfare Section, *Mission and Accomplishments*, 16.

8. Referring to the attempts to reverse many occupation reforms after 1952, Marui Eiji calls the disease and vital statistic-reporting system "a success that endured." Eiji Marui, "The U.S. and Japanese Experience," 41.

Chapter 8: The Preventive Medicine Program, Part I: Controlling Wildfire Diseases

1. Discussions of the preventive medicine program can also be found in reports of the PHW Section, SCAP. For references on the incidence of and methods of controlling the specific diseases mentioned in this chapter, see Public Health and Welfare Section, *Mis-*

sion and Accomplishments, 2–16; General Headquarters, *Selected Data*, 31; Public Health and Welfare Division, *Public Health and Welfare in Japan*, 5–9.

2. This policy with regard to supplies for the Japanese civilian population was initially set by the Joint Chiefs of Staff in its Basic Directive to General MacArthur, as Supreme Commander of the military government, dated 3 November 1945; it was later adopted by the Far East Commission. The directive allowed imports

> . . . only to supplement local resources and only to the extent supplementation is needed to prevent such widespread disease or civil unrest as would endanger the occupying forces or interfere with military operations.

Such imports were also limited to "minimum quantities of food, fuel, medical and sanitary supplies." Requests for "additional imports to accomplish the objectives of . . . [the] occupation" were to be channeled through the Joint Chiefs of Staff. This directive also required the distribution of supplies to be "fair and equitable." Joint Chiefs of Staff, "Basic Directive for Post-Surrender Military Government in Japan Proper," 3 November 1945, published in Government Section, *Political Reorganization of Japan: September 1945 to September 1948*, 2 vols. Tokyo: Supreme Commander for the Allied Powers, 1949, vol. 2, 436.

In practice, this directive posed a dilemma:

> In planning to provide adequate medical supplies and equipment to meet the needs of the civil [sic] population, the problem of utmost importance that confronted SCAP was (1) should all needed supplies be imported at the expense of the American taxpayer, or (2) should every effort be made to increase and stimulate indigenous Japanese production, and import only those materials, preferably in raw form, which would not be available in Japanese supply. It was decided that the latter course would be followed and immediate steps were taken to rehabilitate the Japanese medical supply and equipment industry.

Given the magnitude of the disease control problems, the exacting terms of this directive led to the economically far-reaching precedent to rehabilitate the Japanese medical supply and equipment industry. Public Health and Welfare Section, *Mission and Accomplishments*, 32.

3. Flaws in the vaccination technique became apparent during March and April 1946; revaccination in accordance with corrective instructions was required by 25 May 1946. Brig. Gen. B.M. Fitch, SCAPIN 921, "Vaccination Against Smallpox," 4 May 1946, RG 331, Box 9350–56, NARA; Lt. Col. J.W. Mann, Memorandum on Information of General Application Pertaining to SCAPIN 921, 4 May 1946, RG 331, Box 9350–56, NARA.

4. The U.S. Army Typhus Commission was established by presidential directive and dispatched to the Middle East theater where the largest outbreak of typhus occurred during World War II. The commission set up laboratories to produce vaccine, trained personnel in laboratory techniques, and studied various methods of controlling the disease. Its members included eminent medical scientists who were officers of the U.S. Army, Navy, and Public Health Service, including Drs. John Cushing, Speck Wheeler, Albert Sabin, and Fred Soper. Crawford F. Sams, "Medic," 256–57.

5. Requirements for civilian medical and relief supplies were re-evaluated when the plans changed from invasion to occupation. A shipment of emergency supplies from the United States was cancelled on 24 September 1945, with the exception of 6,270 tons of medical supplies, which included 960 tons of typhus control supplies. Brig. Gen. H.E. Eastwood, 18 October 1945; Brig. Gen. H.E. Eastwood, 22 October 1945. SCAP issued

instructions for the control of typhus on 21 November and 29 November 1945. Col. H.W. Allen, SCAPIN 331, "Prevention and Control of Typhus Fever in Japan," 21 November 1945, RG 331, Box 9350–56, NARA; Col. H.W. Allen, SCAPIN 368, "Prevention and Control of Typhus Fever in Japan," 29 November 1945, RG 331, Box 9350–56 NARA.

6. While serving as theater surgeon of the U.S. Army Forces in the Middle East, Sams witnessed a situation in Egypt in the winter of 1942–43, in which thousands of people died of typhus and the ruling cabinet was overturned as consequences of the government's misallocation of the very limited supply of vaccine. This experience provided an object lesson concerning the relationship between disease and social unrest, which he later applied in Japan: "When wildfire epidemics are sweeping nations, they become the most powerful element in human experience, and the government who fails to take all steps within its capabilities [to control the epidemics] is very likely to be overturned." Crawford F. Sams, "Medic," 258–59.

7. Various techniques to control typhus were field-tested for their effectiveness in Egypt in 1942–43, under the direction of the Typhus Commission. This research linked the knowledge that was developed in the laboratory with epidemiological analyses and environmental methods to control the spread of disease among masses of people; thus, in recalling the work of the Typhus Commission over a decade later, Sams wrote, "It was in Egypt that we learned how to control typhus." Crawford F. Sams, "Medic," 191, 257–60.

8. Typhus reached epidemic proportions by December 1945; the epidemic peaked in March 1946, which was two months earlier than in previous years. The epidemic was controlled by a combination of case finding, vaccination, dusting with DDT, and health promotion using radio broadcasts, newspapers, posters, and pamphlets. The number of cases declined from 31,141 in 1946 to 1,141 in 1947. Only 121 cases occurred in 1949. Public Health and Welfare Section, *Mission and Accomplishments*, 3–4.

9. During the early months of the occupation, when typhus was reaching epidemic proportions, the active ingredients of DDT could not be manufactured in Japan without importing "certain critical materials"; hence, DDT concentrate was imported "for disease control purposes." Production of DDT in Japan was not authorized until May 1946. Col. H.W. Allen, SCAPIN 106, "Manufacture of DDT in Japan," 8 October 1945, RG 331, Box 9350–56, NARA; Brig. Gen. B.M. Fitch, SCAPIN 922, "Manufacture of DDT in Japan," 4 May 1946, RG 331, Box 9350–56, NARA.

10. See Brig. Gen. B.M. Fitch, SCAPIN 791, "Medical Supplies for Repatriation Program," 3 March 1946, RG 331, Box 9350–56, NARA.

11. The medical processing of unprecedented numbers of repatriates to and from areas with high communicable disease rates, and the potential international consequences of deficiencies in processing, necessitated "stringent" measures. The demands of reestablishing port quarantine stations under these conditions made this basic public health function a "high priority undertaking." See Public Health and Welfare Section, *Mission and Accomplishments*, 13–14.

12. Under the supervision of the American medical officers trained by the U.S. Public Health Service, a series of problems received critical attention early in the program: inequitable distribution of supplies; lax supervision and insufficient personnel at the centers; lack of vaccine and medical supplies; and poor sanitary conditions on the ships. See Col. H.W. Allen, SCAPIN 561, "Inequitable Distribution of Supplies to Reception Centers," 7 January 1946, RG 331, Box 9350–56, NARA; Brig. Gen. B.M. Fitch, SCAPIN 731, "Deficiencies Noted at Reception Centers in Japan," 12 February 1946, RG 331, Box 9350–56, NARA; Brig. Gen. B.M. Fitch, SCAPIN 781, "Unsatisfactory Conditions Aboard Repatriation Vessels," 1 March 1946, RG 331, Box 9350–56, NARA.

Chapter 9: The Preventive Medicine Program, Part II: Environmental Sanitation and Viral Diseases

1. The death rate from enteric diseases ("gastroenteritis") decreased in Japan from 221.4 deaths per 100,000 population in 1930 to 159.2 in 1940. By 1940, it ranked below tuberculosis and pneumonia (and bronchitis), which were then the two leading causes of death; however, during the last two years of the war, when Japan was being severely bombed and sanitary conditions were deteriorating, the incidence of enteric diseases increased. Approximately 96,500 cases of dysentery, with over 20,000 deaths, and approximately 58,000 cases of typhoid and 10,000 cases of paratyphoid fever were reported in 1945. That year, enteric diseases displaced pneumonia (and bronchitis) as the second leading cause of death. Ministry of Health and Welfare (Kōseishō), *Health and Welfare Services in Japan*, 73; Public Health and Welfare Section, *Mission and Accomplishments*, 5–7; Harry Emerson Wildes, "Post-War Public Health Developments," 584, 591; Crawford F. Sams, "American Public Health Administration," 564.

2. At the start of the occupation, six cities had sewage treatment plants. Only about 25 percent of the population was served by municipal water supplies; the remaining 75 percent obtained their drinking water from wells, streams, or springs. Public Health and Welfare Section, *Mission and Accomplishments*, 12–13.

3. SCAPIN 93, issued two days after the formation of SCAP, ordered the abolition of organizations and agencies involved in restricting freedom of thought, religion, assembly, and speech, including "all secret police organs." Col. H.W. Allen, 4 October 1945.

4. Training of sanitation personnel was initially conducted at regional training schools and later at the Institute of Public Health in Tokyo. Sanitarians (and sanitary engineers) constituted the largest category of public health personnel trained at the Institute of Public Health following its reopening and reorganization as a training institute in April 1947: A total of 886 sanitarians and 183 sanitary engineers had completed a three-month course by 1952. Public Health and Welfare Section, *Mission and Accomplishments*, 13; Public Health and Welfare Division, *Public Health and Welfare in Japan*, 22.

5. Following a conference in Kyoto in April 1946, SCAP directed the appointment of full-time Insect and Rodent Control Officers in each prefectural health office to organize, train, and manage sanitary personnel and activities at the prefectural and local levels. Public health and sanitary officers of the military governmental companies in each prefecture provided technical advice. SCAP also removed earlier sanctions against domestic production of DDT and supplied the teams with materials and equipment for controlling insects and trapping rodents. Brig. Gen. B.M. Fitch, SCAPIN 920, "Appointment of Insect and Rodent Control Officers," 4 May 1946, RG 331, Box 9350–56, NARA; Lt. Col. J.W. Mann, Memorandum on Information of General Application Pertaining to SCAPIN 920, 4 May 1946, RG 331, Box 9350–56, NARA; Brig. Gen. B.M. Fitch, SCAPIN 922, 4 May 1946.

6. See chapter 6 for a description of the health center system.

7. Efforts to improve sanitation and water supplies were a labor-intensive effort, and a model health center in each prefecture provided training for health center personnel who were unable to complete courses at the Institute of Public Health. Many of these sanitary inspectors and assistant inspectors were probably trained locally, as their numbers exceed the number of sanitarians who had completed courses at the Institute of Public Health by 1952. Crawford F. Sams, "American Public Health Administration," 562.

8. The use of 1945 as an index year can be criticized for indicating relatively greater declines in death and disease rates than would earlier years, because of the increased rates of death and disease during the last year of the war and immediately after the war, despite disruptions in reporting.—As Sams has noted, the filth and louse-borne diseases spread

rapidly under the conditions of the war and its aftermath. Nonetheless, the morbidity rate for dysenteries in 1948 was then the lowest rate in Japanese history. Crawford F. Sams, "Japan's New Public Health Program, Part One," *Military Government Journal* 1 (September-October 1948): 10; Ministry of Health and Welfare (*Kōseishō*), *Health and Welfare Services*, 73.

9. In 1951, the incidence rate for dysentery reached 110.3 cases per 100,000 population in Japan; the death rate was 17.6 deaths per 100,000 population, which was still below prewar death rates. Public Health and Welfare Division, *Public Health and Welfare in Japan*, 9.

10. The immunization program began in September 1947. On 1 July 1948, the Diet enacted the Preventive Vaccination Law, which required typhoid and paratyphoid immunizations for all persons between 3 and 60 years of age. Public Health and Welfare Section, *Mission and Accomplishments*, 6–7; Crawford F. Sams, "Japan's New Public Health Program, Part One," 13–14.

11. In 1951, the incidence rate for typhoid fever was 4.6 cases per 100,000 population in Japan; the death rate was 0.4 deaths per 100,000 population; the incidence rate for paratyphoid fever was 1.5 cases per 100,000 population; the death rate was 0.1 deaths per 100,000 population. Public Health and Welfare Division, *Public Health and Welfare in Japan*, 9.

12. As with the reversal of dysentery rates after cutting back the sanitary teams, this epidemic was attributed to incomplete mosquito control, which was hampered by budget constraints in early 1948. Public Health and Welfare Section, *Mission and Accomplishments*, 7.

13. The PHW Section's reports on the preventive medicine program mention Japanese B encephalitis but not poliomyelitis. Research interest in polio reflected an American preoccupation with this disease during the early postwar period as well as hopes for its prevention. As Paul Starr notes, the March of Dimes campaign of the National Foundation for Infantile Paralysis was "the single most popular medical cause [in the United States] in the postwar period." Paul Starr, *The Social Transformation of American Medicine*. New York: Basic Books, 1982, 346–47.

14. Interest in the inverse correlation of Japanese B encephalitis and poliomyelitis incidence in Japan continued after the occupation; it was a topic of correspondence between Sams and Dr. Carl Taylor. See Crawford F. Sams to Carl E. Taylor, 12 November 1952, CFS, Box 5, HIA.

15. In 1951, the incidence rate for poliomyelitis was 5.0 cases per 100,000 population in Japan; the death rate was 0.7 deaths per 100,000 population. Public Health and Welfare Division, *Public Health and Welfare in Japan*, 9.

Chapter 10: The Preventive Medicine Program, Part III: Treatment and Prevention

1. Crawford F. Sams, "American Public Health Administration," 564.
2. General Headquarters, *Selected Data*, 31.
3. The *Nippon Times* reported 64 deaths and from 700 to 900 reactions of varying severity following the immunization of 7,500 children in November 1948. In addition to suspending vaccine production, the laboratory in question was closed. Sams was reported to have requested prosecution of the laboratory workers and inspectors because of their indifference toward the consequences of their negligence. "Gen. Sams Asks Action in Faulty Serum Case," *Nippon Times*, 5 January 1949; "Immunizations for Japanese Halted Following 64 Deaths," *Nippon Times*, 5 January 1949.

4. The death rate from diphtheria also decreased to 1.1 deaths per 100,000 population in Japan in 1951. Public Health and Welfare Division, *Public Health and Welfare in Japan*, 9.

5. In 1951, the incidence of pneumonia was 195.3 cases per 100,000 population in Japan; the death rate had dropped to 60.5 deaths per 100,000 population. Public Health and Welfare Division, *Public Health and Welfare in Japan*, 9.

6. Sams defended the "unorthodox" methods used to control venereal diseases among American soldiers in the Middle East during World War II, while he served as theater surgeon in the Middle East theater; but he did not disclose the methods. In his unpublished manuscript, Sams went only so far as to note a visit by Thomas B. Turner, who was the venereal disease consultant to the Surgeon General of the Army during and immediately after World War II:

> The measures which were used for venereal disease control in the Middle East by the Army Medical Corps were successful although they differed markedly from those used in the United States and also those which I have used in other theaters. They were methods which were adaptable, unique, and could be carried out in that Middle East Theater when no other methods could be successfully used. I will not go into detail.... Tommie [sic] Turner came, he saw, and returned to the United States and, I hope, did not disclose the methods used; but they were successful, although unorthodox as far as United States policy in the United States is concerned.

Crawford F. Sams, "Medic," 272–73.

7. It is unclear whether the rates of newly diagnosed cases of venereal disease in 1946 are incidence rates or period prevalence rates. In 1951, "case rates" for three venereal diseases in Japan were reported as follows: a rate of 91.4 cases of syphilis per 100,000 population; a rate of 212.5 cases of gonorrhea; and a rate of 18.9 cases of chancroid. Public Health and Welfare Division, *Public Health and Welfare in Japan*, 9.

8. The toll of tuberculosis on the civilian population of Japan prior to and during World War II bespeaks a tragedy as harsh as the war itself. Tuberculosis was among the leading causes of death in Japan since at least 1900, and tuberculosis morbidity probably contributed to deaths by other causes. Japanese sources report tuberculosis death rates ranged from 230.2 to 212.9 deaths per 100,000 population between 1910 and 1940. SCAP's reports indicate that from the time of the Russo-Japanese War (1904–5) through World War II, tuberculosis death rates among civilians were higher in Japan than in any industrialized nation, except, perhaps, the Soviet Union. Crawford F. Sams, "American Public Health Administration," 563; Ministry of Health and Welfare (*Kōseishō*), *Health and Welfare Services*, 73; Public Health and Welfare Section, *Mission and Accomplishments*, 37.

9. Despite the ratio of beds to active cases, the PHW Section reported that tuberculosis sanitaria in Japan had an occupancy rate of only 25 percent in 1945, "mainly due to active cases leaving these institutions to seek food." Public Health and Welfare Section, *Mission and Accomplishments*, 7–8.

10. In 1950, tuberculosis was still the leading cause of death in Japan, but the death rate had decreased to 146.4 deaths per 100,000 population, which was lower than that reported in 1900. By 1960, tuberculosis was no longer a leading cause of death in Japan. Ministry of Health and Welfare (*Kōseishō*), *Health and Welfare Services*, 73.

Chapter 11: The Veterinarians

1. Sams's view of the role of veterinarians in protecting human health is reflected not only by the establishment of Veterinary Affairs as one of the initial divisions of the PHW

Section, but also by the aims of SCAPIN 214, which outlined three veterinary concerns related to the mission of the PHW Section: the control of "animal diseases that might seriously affect [human] health"; the control of animal diseases that might impair food supplies; and the inspection of milk and meat products for human consumption. Dated 30 October 1945, SCAPIN 214 requested periodic reports on fourteen diseases of animals, including anthrax, rabies, and bovine tuberculosis; annual reports on the preparation and use of veterinary sera, vaccines, and biologicals; and monthly reports on meat and milk inspections. Col. H.W. Allen, SCAPIN 214, "Information on Japanese Animal Disease Control," 30 October 1945, RG 331, Box 9350–56, NARA.

2. SCAPIN 48 included a request for the number of veterinary personnel available in each prefecture. See Lt. Col. Harold Fair, 22 September 1945. For notes on the training of veterinarians at the Institute of Public Health before and during the occupation, see notes 13, 14, and 15 to chapter 6, above.

3. In 1951, over 1 million slaughtered animals were inspected in Japan; 184,000 milk inspections were conducted; and nearly 3 million inspections of food establishments were conducted. Public Health and Welfare Division, *Public Health and Welfare in Japan*, 6.

4. This policy not to subsist off of resources needed by the Japanese population follows from a directive of the State, War, and Navy Coordinating Committee (SWNCC) to General MacArthur, dated 1 October 1945: "The only responsibility on our part for the Japanese standard of living is the purely negative one prohibiting us from requiring for the Occupation Forces goods or services to an extent which would cause starvation, widespread disease and acute physical distress." Quoted in Harry Emerson Wildes, "Post-War Public Health Developments," 575–76.

Chapter 12: Medicine and Dentistry

1. For an account of medical education in American universities prior to reforms during the early 1900s, see Paul Starr, *The Social Transformation of American Medicine*, 112–16.

2. See Sams's discussion of the separation of the professions of medicine, dentistry, and pharmacy in chapter 13.

3. Sams's approach was to use the American Medical Association's method of reforming American medical schools in 1904. These reforms, which were initiated by the profession in the absence of federal intervention, were designed to raise standards of medical education in accordance with the Johns Hopkins model of medical education as a graduate-level study rooted in science and clinical hospital practice. See Paul Starr, *The Social Transformation of American Medicine*, 115–23.

4. This group of doctors included the more progressive representatives of the leading medical schools in Japan at the time. Public Health and Welfare Section, *Mission and Accomplishments*, 17.

5. Despite Sams's misgivings about the internship requirement, it apparently served its purpose until the time when most of the practicing doctors were expected to be graduates of medical schools of the same caliber of education. In 1968, the internship requirement was opposed by students and abolished, making it one reform instituted by the PHW Section that was not sustained. See Eiji Marui, "The U.S. and Japanese Experience," 2. See also Interview Notes, 5 October 1981, JZB, Box 2, RAC.

6. Sams's decision reflected his cognizance of the opposing tendencies of the academic orientation of medical specialties and the practical orientation of "old-line" medical practitioners in the United States. See Paul Starr, *The Social Transformation of American Medicine*, 123.

7. For Sams's view of the Japan Medical Association (JMA) before and after its

democratization, see Crawford F. Sams, "Japan's New Public Health Program, Part Two," 9. Since its reform, the JMA has vigorously opposed the Ministry of Health and Welfare (MHW) on proposals that affected medical practice and physicians' incomes. The first major issue was the proposal, initiated by SCAP's PHW Section, to separate medical treatment from the preparation and sale of medicine by physicians. A second issue involved ongoing reforms of the health insurance system. In opposing the MHW on these issues, the JMA has, at various times, amalgamated conservative and socialist physicians and solidified its political effectiveness. For a case study of the JMA, see William E. Steslicke, *Doctors in Politics: The Political Life of the Japan Medical Association*. New York: Praeger, 1973.

8. In addition to overcoming the compartmentalization of medical knowledge, Sams's purpose in translating contemporary medical journals and disseminating them to Japanese doctors was to reduce the variance between the state of medical education and practice in Japan at end of the war and the norms of modern medical science abroad. As Nishimura notes, the zeal with which the Japanese physician-translators undertook the task of translating the *Journal of the American Medical Association* (*JAMA*) resembled that of Japanese doctors who translated Dutch medical treatises in the eighteenth century. Despite the rising price of the journal, its circulation continued, affirming what its Japanese advertisers hailed as the profession's aspiration: "To recover from backwardness caused by the War, and to catch up to the international standards as swiftly as possible." For a description of the first issue of the Japanese edition of *JAMA*, see Sey Nishimura, "The US Medical Occupation of Japan and History of the Japanese-Language Edition of *JAMA*," *Journal of the American Medical Association* 274 (August 2, 1995): 437–38. Nishimura's reference to SCAP's Civil Censorship Detachment "censors" implies the issue involved censorship or non-disclosure of the content of medical research reports. See also chapter 14 regarding the translation of nursing texts and manuals.

9. According to Sams, this complication involved a legal technicality concerning a copyright issue, which was beyond the PHW Section's jurisdiction, and which frustrated Sams's efforts to provide wider access to current medical knowledge. Nishimura's reference to SCAP's Civil Censorship Detachment "censors" implies the issue involved censorship or non-disclosure of the content of medical research reports. See Sey Nishimura, "The US Medical Occupation of Japan," 436–37.

10. For a discussion of popular and folk medicines in the United States during the early nineteenth century, see Paul Starr, *The Social Transformation of American Medicine*, 47–54. For a lively account of the rivalry between students of traditional medicine of Chinese origin and students of Jennerian vaccination in Japan circa 1855–58, see Yukichi Fukuzawa, *The Autobiography of Yukichi Fukuzawa* [*Fukuō Jiden*], trans. Eiichi Kyooka. New York: Columbia University Press, (1899) 1966, 91–92.

Chapter 13: Pharmacy and the Pharmaceutical Industry

1. The Pharmaceutical Affairs Law of 29 July 1948 regulates education and licensure of pharmacists. It also regulates the manufacture, preparation, sale, and distribution of drugs, medical devices, and cosmetics according to standards recommended by a National Board of Pharmacy to the Ministry of Welfare. Public Health and Welfare Section, *Mission and Accomplishments*, 33.

2. By June 1945, the distribution of medical supplies to the civilian population had been suspended. Public Health and Welfare Section, *Mission and Accomplishments*, 31–33.

3. The Japanese military initially resisted the release of medical supplies for civilian use; hence, on 19 September 1945, representatives of the Japan's Ministry of Welfare requested assistance from SCAP in securing them for this purpose. Their request was followed by SCAPIN 48, which ordered, in broad terms, the distribution of what were

previously army and navy medical supplies in accordance with the plans of the military government. Shortly after the formation of SCAP, SCAPIN 97 directed the release and distribution of these supplies for civilian use through the Ministry of Welfare. Lt. Col. Harold Fair, 22 September 1945; Col. H.W. Allen, SCAPIN 97, "Release of Surplus Japanese Army and Navy Medical Supplies for Civilian Use," 6 October 1945, RG 331, Box 9350–56, NARA.

4. See the discussion in chapter 10 regarding the production of diphtheria toxoid and the incident leading to the establishment of nationwide controls over standards of assay.

5. This policy was set by the Joint Chiefs of Staff in its directive to General MacArthur. See note 2 to chapter 8, above.

6. See note 9 to chapter 8, above.

7. The production of X-ray film was needed in Japan particularly for diagnosing tuberculosis. Public Health and Welfare Section, *Mission and Accomplishments*, 9.

Chapter 14: Nursing

1. There were large differences in the numbers of nurses reported by Japanese and occupation sources owing to differences in nomenclature and the absence of a uniform curriculum in nursing schools prior to the occupation. Harry Emerson Wildes, "Post-War Public Health Developments," 580.

2. For Sams's description of the customs of caring for patients in hospitals and the inter-relationship between nurses and hospital administrators in improving standards of bedside nursing care, see chapter 15.

3. For Sams's description of St. Luke's Hospital at the start of the occupation, see the discussion of hospitals in chapter 2.

4. Maj. Grace Alt was succeeded by Virginia M. Ohlson as chief of the Nursing Affairs Division in April 1949. Virginia M. Ohlson to Z. Zakarian, 10 March 1997.

5. The recommendations of the Council of Nursing Education, which was formed in March 1946, became the basis for the reorganization of nursing education in Japan. For highlights of other developments in the nursing profession, see Public Health and Welfare Section, *Mission and Accomplishments*, 20–21.

6. The Council of Nursing Education had recommended one additional year of training for public health nurses and midwives, but this recommendation was not approved because of limited training facilities. Harry Emerson Wildes, "Post-War Public Health Developments," 580. For notes on the training of public health nurses and nursing instructors at the Institute of Public Health before and during the occupation, see notes 13, 14, and 15 to chapter 6, above.

Chapter 15: Hospitals

1. SCAPIN 48, dated 22 September 1945, ordered the reopening of civilian hospitals "as rapidly as conditions permit or require" and the use of suitable schools or other buildings as emergency facilities where hospital space was inadequate. Lt. Col. Harold Fair, 22 September 1945. With regard to the occupancy of tuberculosis sanitaria, see note 9 to chapter 10, above.

2. Regarding the removal of heating and cooking equipment in hospitals during the war, see note 1 to chapter 1, above.

3. In designating all former Japanese army, navy, and veterans hospitals as civilian facilities under the supervision of the Ministry of Health and Social Affairs, SCAPIN 273 and SCAPIN 304 each prohibited the "restriction of hospital care and medical treatment to veterans and their families." Col. H.W. Allen, SCAPIN 273, "Relief Board for Veterans,"

13 November 1945, RG 331, Box 9350–56, NARA; Col. H.W. Allen, SCAPIN 304, "Imperial Japanese Army and Navy Hospitals," 19 November 1945, RG 331, Box 9350–56, NARA.

4. In 1949, a total of 299 directors and managers of public and private hospitals completed training. Public Health and Welfare Section, *Mission and Accomplishments*, 20.

5. The reorientation of hospital administrators to a new concept of patient care, which involved normative and cognitive dimensions, was an educational task with which Sams had experience as a teacher and as a student of psychology. As an instructor at an army medical field service school in the 1930s and early 1940s, Sams had developed techniques to integrate professional medical instruction with field maneuvers, which he described as follows:

> Under the premise well known in education, that most people learn and retain best that which they have learned through visual perception rather than auditory perception alone, constant emphasis has been placed on *showing* students rather than *talking* to them in classrooms, particularly those things such as organizations and equipment which they have never before seen and of which they have no previous visual images.

Crawford F. Sams to James P. Cooney, 4 May 1953, CFS, Box 5, HIA. The device of a model hospital, like the demonstration schools, model health centers, demonstration studies of new drugs, and even the public health train, provided such visual images, which were not limited by language. Later, in response to an inquiry by an American student of health education who was interested in the methods used during the occupation, Sams summarized this approach as follows: "My thesis is that if you can demonstrate something to people it is far more effective than just talking about it." Crawford F. Sams to Rosella Linskie, 2 November 1953, CFS, Box 5, HIA.

Chapter 16: The Atomic Bomb Casualty Commission

1. From its inception, the ABCC's research mission was "to undertake a long range, continuing study of the biological and medical effects of the atomic bombs on man." James Forrestal to The President, 18 November 1946, RG 331, Box 9350–56, NARA. As chief of the PHW Section, Sams was formally responsible to the Supreme Commander for advice on "all matters concerning the public health and welfare of the civil [sic] population of Japan"; yet, neither the PHW Section's mission to safeguard the security and health of occupation forces, nor the limited but unknown duration of the occupation was originally intended to facilitate long-range programmatic research of the type anticipated for studies of the effects of the atomic bombs on people. Nor was there a research division as such within the PHW Section; most of its research projects were initially organized within the Consultants Division, which was dissolved by 1950, or linked to specific disease control programs of its Preventive Medicine Division. General Headquarters, *Selected Data*, 192–94. Regarding the formal divisions of the PHW Section, see note 1 to chapter 3, above. Regarding the initial movement of Red Cross supplies and American scientists into Hiroshima, see the discussion of First Instructions in chapter 1.

2. Dr. Stafford Warren headed the medical team of the Manhattan Project. Dr. Shields Warren headed the naval medical team; later, he became Director of the Division of Biology and Medicine of the U.S. Atomic Energy Commission (AEC), the agency which provided the early funding for the ABCC. See note 4 to chapter 1, above.

3. President Truman approved the formation of the ABCC in concept on 26 November 1946; the AEC provided the initial funding in late 1947. For a discussion of the founding of the ABCC, see M. Susan Lindee, *Suffering Made Real*, 23–37.

4. William J. Schull, a scientist who worked at the ABCC during the occupation, later described the relationship between the PHW Section and the ABCC in similar terms. William J. Schull to Zabelle Zakarian, 12 March 1997. Beyond the movement of scientists and supplies from the United States, the PHW Section's administrative direction and technical supervision—from redefining the Ministry of Health and Social Affairs's functions to re-establishing a new health center system; reorganizing the system of vital statistics; reviving the medical supply system; reforming medical, nursing, and pharmaceutical education; and reinstituting welfare and social insurance—served to rebuild the health and social service infrastructure upon which medical research depends. Eventually, a number of PHW Section staff also went to work at the ABCC, including Dorothy Toom (medical-surgical nursing consultant, Nursing Affairs Division), Virginia M. Ohlson (public health nursing consultant and chief, Nursing Affairs Division), and Milton J. Evans (chief, Welfare Administration Branch, Welfare Division). Interview with Virginia M. Ohlson, 16 March 1997.

5. With regard to the interest of the Japanese professionals, Lindee notes that before the American ad hoc medical teams had arrived in Hiroshima, Japanese medical scientists had initiated studies of survivors suffering from "A-bomb sickness." These "parallel efforts" not only continued "throughout the Occupation" but also served to justify the need for studies by American scientists, based in part upon the views of some who then believed that "the Japanese could not independently conduct a scientific study of the survivors." Other American scientists expressed the need to bring Japanese scientists "back into the sphere of science," from which they had become isolated during the war; yet, U.S. military policies of censorship regarding classified "atomic secrets" formed "a barrier" to full collaboration and cooperation between the Japanese and Americans. By violating scientific norms, such policies served to provoke the resentment of Japanese scientists and to kindle their view of occupation policies as coercive and authoritarian, regardless of the source of such policies. M. Susan Lindee, *Suffering Made Real*, 17–32, 44–51; Sey Nishimura, "Censorship of the Atomic Bomb Casualty Reports in Occupied Japan," *Journal of the American Medical Association* 274 (August 16, 1995): 520–22.

As for the possibility of expelling the ABCC after the occupation, this scenario may have anticipated a level of criticism of the ABCC (and SCAP) that one might expect in a sovereign state following its occupation, and in the absence of political censorship by SCAP. For example, in August 1952, following the anniversaries of the atomic bombings and the end of the occupation, Milton J. Evans, who had served as chief of the Welfare Administration Branch of the Welfare Division, PHW Section, SCAP, before working as an administrator with the ABCC, informed the National Academy of Sciences that the ABCC was "coming in for a share of adverse publicity," particularly with regard to the policy on whether the ABCC should treat its human research subjects. Milton J. Evans to G.D. Meid, 13 August 1952, Atomic Bomb Casualty Commission Files, Papers of John C. Burger, Rockefeller Archives, quoted by M. Susan Lindee, *Suffering Made Real*, 123. For an account of SCAP's prepublication and postpublication censorship policies from 1945 to 1947, which were designed "to prevent destructive criticism and attacks against the Occupation forces by the Japanese media," see Sey Nishimura, "Censorship of Medical Journals in Occupied Japan, *Journal of the American Medical Association* 274 (August 9, 1995): 454–56.

6. Such a deliberate effort to avoid claims of imposing a high caliber U.S. organization upon the Japanese may have masked an underlying uncertainty and fear should the occupation's overall political mission miscarry. Consequently, the continuity of legal reforms and the stability of democratic governmental institutions after April 1952 would be the measure of the occupation's success.

Short of establishing a new medical research institute, which would have had to have been a governmental agency, Sams then had three choices: the Institute of Public Health; the National Institute of Health; and National Hygienic Laboratory. See Notes entitled "Sams and SW Agree, 4 June 1947," JZB, Box 2, RAC. See also the discussion of the National Institute of Health in chapter 6.

This strategy of including the National Institute of Health of Japan in the research being conducted by the ABCC involved "the creation of new vested interests," a method which Ward notes was used in connection with a large proportion of the reform programs that survived the occupation. Robert E. Ward, "Reflections on the Allied Occupation and Planned Political Change in Japan," in *Political Development in Modern Japan*, ed. Robert E. Ward, 477–535. Princeton: Princeton University Press, 1968, 527–28.

7. This "counterpart" relationship mimicked the parallel organization of SCAP sections and the functions of the Japanese Government; it also formalized an interdependency, which is reflected in a brief summary of the history, organization, and programs of the ABCC that was submitted to Sams in May 1951—that is, in the period leading up to the signing of the peace treaty with Japan on 8 September 1951—by Dr. John C. Bugher, Deputy Director of the AEC, on behalf of Dr. Grant Taylor, who was then Director of the ABCC. In a statement that projected the end of the occupation, and which might serve to strike an accord between the on-going research of the ABCC and the new vested interests of governmental health agencies, Bugher wrote: "Continuity of cooperation with the established Japanese public health agencies is assumed following the termination of the Occupation." He concluded by stating that the program "must involve the close cooperation and collaboration of the Japanese medical agencies with the American institutions." John C. Bugher, "Atomic Bomb Casualty Commission," 3 May 1951, RG 331, Box 9350–56, NARA; John C. Bugher to Crawford F. Sams, 3 May 1951, RG 331, Box 9350–56, NARA. See also Notes regarding "Proposed Clause for Japan Peace Treaty," JZB, Box 2, RAC. With regard to the parallel structure of SCAP and the ministries of the Japanese Government, see the discussion of The Public Health and Welfare Section in chapter 3.

8. What Sams saw as an organizational structure to ensure the continuity and acceptance of the ABCC in Japan after the occupation, the ABCC saw as a burdensome and "unproductive institutional alliance dictated by SCAP policy." Following the occupation, this alliance was expanded to include scientists from Japanese universities. For an account of ABCC's frustrations with this early institutional arrangement involving scientists from the National Institute of Health of Japan, see M. Susan Lindee, *Suffering Made Real*, 51–54.

9. The provision of "free medical care" for the ABCC's human research subjects would have exceeded the norms of medical research practices at that time. Lindee argues that the issue of whether the ABCC should provide medical treatment to the survivors who were participating in the ABCC's studies involved deeply unsettling meanings of responsibility for acts of war. See M. Susan Lindee, *Suffering Made Real*, 117–42.

In seeking explanations of how such decisions were initially made, certain factors binding upon SCAP should not be overlooked. Most important, perhaps, was the policy with regard to civilian medical supplies and relief that was set by the Joint Chiefs of Staff in its directive to General MacArthur, as Supreme Commander of the military government. This policy not only required "fair and equitable" distribution of supplies but also advised against "direct provision" of supplies to the civilian population, except as required by "military necessity":

> In order to limit direct provision and distribution of supplies by you to the civilian population, you should assure that the Japanese do not necessarily involve the occupying forces in such responsibility. . . .

... When military necessity requires, civilian supplies may be made the subject of direct relief issue by you or by supply agencies under your supervision or control.

Joint Chiefs of Staff, "Basic Directive for Post-Surrender Military Government in Japan Proper," 436–37. See also note 2 to chapter 8, above.

Accordingly, the ABCC observed a similar policy of examination and referral in the case of its Japanese employees, who, of course, were not research subjects. In June 1948, after consulting Japanese labor officials and SCAP, the ABCC began a program of periodic health examinations for its Japanese employees after one of its physicians was suspected of having tuberculosis. The "main purpose" of these examinations was "to protect American personnel by detection and isolation of sick Japanese co-workers." A second aim was to teach "the value of routine physical examinations" by identifying conditions "requiring" medical attention.

Although the Japanese Government was responsible for the examination of Japanese nationals employed by the occupation forces, the ABCC undertook these examinations in part because various groups among the occupation forces were "suspicious of the accuracy" of government-sponsored examinations and laboratory tests performed by Japanese laboratories. The ABCC depended upon the employees' cooperation in seeking treatment from Japanese doctors, because the ABCC was "not in a position to treat patients." Lt. R. Anderson, Memorandum on Health Examination for Japanese Employees of ABCC, 12 June 1948, RG 331, Box 9350–56, NARA; Capt. R. Anderson, Memorandum on Health Examination Program and Medical Facilities in ABCC, 7 September 1948, RG 331, Box 9350–56, NARA.

10. In late 1950, the AEC began to reassess its financial support of the ABCC, and both the AEC and the National Research Council (NRC) sent representatives to the ABCC site in Hiroshima in the months leading up to "the showdown in 1951." During this period, which overlapped with the negotiations for the peace treaty that would bring the occupation to a close in April 1952, Sams had become active in the Korean War and was spending more and more time in Korea; yet, as indicated by correspondence and interview notes, he met with representatives of the AEC and the NRC. After returning to Japan from Korea on 15 March 1951, Sams discussed the ABCC's "future scope of activities" with Dr. Ernest Goodpasture, Vice Chairman of the AEC Advisory Committee on Biology and Medicine, and later met with Dr. John C. Bugher, then Deputy Director of the AEC. Shields Warren to Crawford F. Sams, 22 March 1951, RG 331, Box 9350–56, NARA; Crawford F. Sams to Shields Warren, 31 March 1951, RG 331, Box 9350–56, NARA; Interview Notes, 5 October 1981. For an account of the reports by the NRC and AEC representatives and the debate over whether to continue funding the ABCC, see M. Susan Lindee, *Suffering Made Real*, 104–14.

11. In 1975, the ABCC became the Radiation Effects Research Foundation. For a summary of the organization and funding of this foundation, see M. Susan Lindee, *Suffering Made Real*, 250.

Chapter 17: Narcotics Control

1. Narcotics control was not one of the original organizational divisions of the PHW Section; however, SCAPIN 98, dated 6 October 1945, outlined the initial functions of narcotics control. General Headquarters, *Selected Data*, 192–94; Col. H.W. Allen, SCAPIN 98, 6 October 1945. See note 5 to chapter 1, above.

2. The spelling of Mr. Spears's name is uncertain. An alternative spelling appears on the back of a photograph taken by the U.S. Army Signal Corps. The photograph, dated 26 July 1949, shows five members of the Pharmaceutical Association Mission seated around

a table with five members of the PHW Section, including "W.L. Speer," chief of Narcotics Control. FEC-49-4736, CFS, Envelope F, HIA.

3. The eight regional offices of the Narcotics Section of the Ministry of Health and Welfare, which operated separately from the prefectural health offices, were located in the following cities: Sapporo; Sendai; Tokyo; Nagoya; Osaka; Hiroshima; Takamatsu; and Fukuoka. Public Health and Welfare Division, *Public Health and Welfare in Japan*, 3.

4. It is unclear (perhaps, intentionally) when this smuggling occurred or was discovered. Unclassified reports of narcotics control activities during the occupation do not mention involvement by communists. A report of the PHW Section, dated December 1949, states that "large amounts of narcotics . . . [were] intercepted either before reaching Japan or upon arrival from the Asiatic Continent" and that about 2000 people were arrested for narcotics violations in 1949, nearly one-fourth of whom were foreign nationals; but, it does not mention involvement by any political or ideological entity. Public Health and Welfare Section, *Mission and Accomplishments*, 33–34. Nor does a similar discussion in an article published in 1949 mention communist involvement. Crawford F. Sams, "Japan's New Public Health Program, Part Three," *Military Government Journal* 2 (Summer 1949): 12.

Chapter 18: Welfare

1. See the discussion of welfare activities and organizations in Public Health and Welfare Section, *Mission and Accomplishments*, 21–28.

2. Another advantage of the policy of dispersing refugees was to avert social unrest, which frequently accompanies retention in refugee camps. Public Health and Welfare Section, *Mission and Accomplishments*, 23.

3. Beginning in January 1946, SCAP directed the Japanese Government to restrict the movement of people from rural areas to cities of 100,000 or more population to alleviate health, economic, and welfare problems in the urban areas. SCAPIN 944 extended this order until 30 September 1946, because of the continuing shortage of housing and inadequate food distribution in the urban areas. Col. H.W. Allen, SCAPIN 563, "Control of Population Movements," 8 January 1946, RG 331, Box 9350–56, NARA; Brig. Gen. B.M. Fitch, SCAPIN 944, "Control of Population Movements," 11 May 1946, RG 331, Box 9350–56, NARA; Lt. Col. J.W. Mann, Memorandum on Information of General Application Pertaining to SCAPIN 944, 11 May 1946, RG 331, Box 9350–56, NARA.

4. SCAPIN 775 directed the Japanese Government to establish "a single National Governmental agency" to provide "through Prefectural and local governmental channels . . . adequate food, clothing, shelter, and medical care . . . to all indigent persons without discrimination or preferential treatment." SCAP placed "no limitation" on the amount of relief furnished, provided it was "within the amount necessary to prevent hardship." Brig. Gen. B.M. Fitch, SCAPIN 775, "Public Assistance," 27 February 1946, RG 331, Box 9350–56, NARA.

5. The Japanese interpretation of the concept of public assistance was one of "protection of the right to subsist" based upon Article 25 of the Constitution. Yoshitome Ushimaru, "Progress in Social Security," *Contemporary Japan* 23 (1955): 693–94. See the language of Article 25 in note 5 to chapter 6, above.

6. The criteria for the initial plans to distribute food and clothing were outlined in SCAPIN 352. Col. H.W. Allen, SCAPIN 352, "Reserve Supplies Held for Relief Distribution," 26 November 1945, RG 331, Box 9350–56, NARA.

7. See the discussion of the school lunch program in chapter 5.

Chapter 19: Social Security

1. For background on the various social insurance and health insurance laws and programs that constitute the social security system, see Public Health and Welfare Section, *Mission and Accomplishments*, 28–30, 39–40.

2. As Sams's noted in his opening comments in chapter 18, tuberculosis was a model for the integration of the four basic elements of a public health and welfare program. It presented challenges not only to the public health program but also to the welfare program. As treatment (and prevention) of tuberculosis improved and the tuberculosis death rate began to drop, the welfare program was challenged with meeting the medical costs of a chronic disease: Over half of the medical costs under the public assistance program were being spent for tuberculosis patients. By fiscal year 1953, the total annual medical payments under the public assistance program exceeded the total annual livelihood payments. Between fiscal year 1951 and 1954, the total annual livelihood payments had increased by over 25 percent, and the total annual medical payments had increased by nearly 125 percent. Yoshitome Ushimaru, "Progress in Social Security," 698–99.

Chapter 20: The Communist Activities

1. References to the events described in this chapter were not found in the unclassified reports of the PHW Section. The episodes Sams chose to include in this chapter strongly reflect the influence of selection factors in addition to the difficulties these episodes posed to the occupation.

2. From an analytical perspective based on Mary Douglas and Aaron Wildavsky's cultural theory of risk perception and their analysis of pollution, the Russian propaganda as well as Sams's comparisons of public health conditions in democratic and totalitarian societies exemplify how a normative sense of disease as "pollution"—not merely the physical risk of disease—is correlated with certain undesirable forms of political power or social control. Notice in this case that both sides used public health statistics either to blame or to absolve one side or the other, to uphold a social or political criticism of the other, and ultimately to justify their own "vision of the good society." Notice also that the "bungling" concerned tuberculosis, a disease that in every society has been profoundly related to social, political, and economic conditions. As Douglas and Wildavsky state, "Pollution ideas cluster thickest where cherished values conflict." Mary Douglas and Aaron Wildavsky, *Risk and Culture*. Berkeley: University of California Press, 1982, 6–7, 36–43. See also the discussions of Averting Catastrophe and Medical Intelligence in chapter 25. Note also the charges of "bacterial warfare" in the discussion of The Aftermath in chapter 30.

Following his return to the United States from his tour of duty in Japan and Korea, Sams continued to compare public health conditions in Japan with those in communist-held areas in Asia to illustrate the value of human life in a democracy:

> We've demonstrated that democracy holds human life as supremely valuable, and in the Far East this alone represents a real revolution.

Quoted in David Perlman, "Surgeon-Hero Gen. Sams, Ending Military Service, Tells of Disease-Ridden Red Armies," *San Francisco Chronicle*, 8 July 1951, 8.

3. See the discussion of Disaster Relief in chapter 18.
4. See the discussion of Food Relief and Propaganda in chapter 5.
5. See the discussion of Illicit Trade in chapter 17.

Chapter 21: The Big Question

1. Sams used variations on the term "democracy by demonstration" in numerous public statements, including a presentation at the annual meeting of the American Public Health Association in Boston in November 1948, to emphasize the unanticipated ways in which public health and welfare reforms were affecting the Japanese population. See Alta Mahoney, "Japan Health Plan Best in the World, U.S. Aide Says," *Boston Traveler*, 12 November 1948. See also Crawford F. Sams, "American Public Health Administration," 565.

From a comparative legal and cultural perspective, this term was also a rebuttal of the paradox of "democracy by fiat," which was a critical comment on the method of revising the Japanese Constitution, attributed to the legal scholar Minobe Tatsukichi. For a study of the ideas of Minobe Tatsukichi (1873–1948), who, during the occupation, was appointed to the Japanese privy council that was given the task of constitutional reform, and who, as an outspoken "conscience of democracy" in Japan, coined this paradox, see Frank O. Miller, *Minobe Tatsukichi: Interpreter of Constitutionalism in Japan*. Berkeley: University of California Press, 1965. *N.B.*, chapter VIII.

2. Infant mortality rates are another indicator of the health status of a population by which programs can be evaluated. From 1947 to 1950, infant mortality rates in Japan decreased from 76.7 deaths (per 1,000 live births) to 60.1, which was then the lowest rate reported in Japanese history. Ministry of Health and Welfare (*Kōseishō*), *Health and Welfare Services*, 72; Crawford F. Sams, "American Public Health Administration," 564.

3. Discussions of the population issue and the policy of the Far East Commission were not found in the unclassified reports of the PHW Section; however, Sams was quoted on the issue of population pressure and the policy of industrialization in David Perlman, 8 July 1951, 8.

4. For an account of the debate over birth control during the occupation by a participating proponent of Planned Parenthood, see Fumiko Y. Amano, "Family Planning Movement in Japan," *Contemporary Japan* 23 (1955): 752–65.

5. The marriage rate in Japan peaked in 1947 at 12.0 marriages per 1,000 population. Ministry of Health and Welfare (*Kōseishō*), *Health and Welfare Services*, 72.

6. Ministry of Health and Welfare (*Kōseishō*), *Health and Welfare Services*, 72.

Chapter 22: Summation of the Occupation

1. The intended sense of this statement is unclear without a specific reference, although Sams's allusion to "monuments . . . in the form of elaborate buildings" provides a clue. See Sams's criticism of attempts to improve health standards by financing, constructing, and equipping buildings in chapter 15 and his discussion of Doai Hospital in chapter 2. Note also the comments on "the largest part of the problem" of controlling disease being "advice, guidance and training" in Public Health and Welfare Section, *Mission and Accomplishments*, 35.

Chapter 23: Life in Japan

1. Having been a mounted officer in the army during the 1930s, Sams commented that, prior to World War II, horse mastership frequently distinguished the finest military commanders, as "the same principles used in training horses are the principles used in training men." The military pastime of polo then also required horse mastership, because the players had to train their own ponies. Crawford F. Sams, "Medic," 29–30, 41.

Chapter 24: 1945–1948

1. Compare this assignment with the scope of Sams's initial responsibility for educational reform in Japan, in addition to public health and welfare, and the proposal in November 1945 that he also serve as theater surgeon. See the discussions of the Public Health and Welfare Section and A Student of Organization in chapter 3.

2. Upon the establishment of the Republic of Korea in 1948, the military government's responsibility for civilian health and welfare formally ended. See Public Health and Welfare Division, *Public Health and Welfare in Japan*, 1–2.

3. Sams refers again to this epidemic in his discussions of cholera in chapters 8 and 25.

Chapter 25: 1950–1951

1. Public Health and Welfare Division, *Public Health and Welfare in Japan*, 2. See also note 1 to chapter 24, above.

2. Crawford F. Sams to Charles A. Willoughby, 9 December 1952, 2–3, CFS, Box 5, HIA.

3. See chapter 13 on the rehabilitation of the pharmaceutical and medical supply industry in Japan. See also note 2 to chapter 8, above.

4. Sams's explanation provides another example of how, in the context of the Korean War, the physical risks of disease among civilians and the efforts to control them acquired a value-laden meaning as a literal test of communism versus democracy. See note 2 to chapter 20, above.

Chapter 26: The Breakout

1. The Fourth Field Hospital had served in three of the same overseas combat areas with Sams. He first encountered it in the Middle East theater, where it was not only the first American hospital in that combat zone but also the first unit to take nurses into that combat zone. According to Sams, it was also the first "flying" hospital in U.S. military history. In 1943, it was moved by air from Tunisia to Malta; it was then flow into Sicily in the Mediterranean theater; from there it was flown to the European theater, where Sams encountered it in the winter of 1944–45. Following the Korean War, it was reactivated at Fort Devans, Massachusetts, where Sams revisited it in 1953. Crawford F. Sams, "Medic," 200–2, 238.

2. Crawford F. Sams to Charles A. Willoughby, 9 December 1952, 3.

3. These mobile army surgical hospitals later became known more popularly as M*A*S*H* units.

Chapter 27: North Korea

1. See Sams's brief account of civilian health and relief efforts during the occupation of North Korea from October to November 1950, in Crawford F. Sams to Charles A. Willoughby, 9 December 1952, 3–4.

Chapter 28: The New War

1. Samuel L.A. Marshall, *The River and the Gauntlet: Defeat of the Eighth Army by the Chinese Communist Forces, November 1950, in the Battle of the Chongchon River, Korea*. New York: William Morrow, 1953, 76.

2. Sams used various means and opportunities available to him to gather information about the events and circumstances surrounding the fate of Captain Struthers. See, for example, Crawford F. Sams to Thomas N. Page, 10 September 1953, CFS, Box 5, HIA.
3. For a similar account, see Crawford F. Sams to Charles A. Willoughby, 9 December 1952, 4.
4. Crawford F. Sams to Charles A. Willoughby, 9 December 1952, 4.

Chapter 29: A Complication

1. With regard to personnel, see Crawford F. Sams to Charles A. Willoughby, 9 December 1952, 3.

Chapter 30: A Korean Episode

1. Crawford F. Sams to Charles A. Willoughby, 9 December 1952, 5.
2. During Sams's mission in North Africa and the Middle East, one of his tasks was to ascertain the types of diseases that were present in those areas and their distribution, so troops that might be sent into combat there could be protected. In later writing about his reconnaissance of the countries, Sams notes that he first saw cases of bubonic plague in Haiffa and Jaffa, Palestine, in December 1941, where it was then endemic. Crawford F. Sams, "Medic," 175.
3. In the spring of 1941, Sams completed training as a paratrooper with the 501st Parachute Battalion, while serving as a medical instructor at the Infantry School at Fort Benning, Georgia. He was the first medical officer and one of the first line officers to qualify as a U.S. Army paratrooper. Concurrent with this training, Sams organized the medical service for injured or wounded paratroopers, tested the dropping of medical equipment as part of this program, developed screening tests for candidates for parachute training, developed empirical bases for reducing jump injuries, and evaluated policies for reducing time lost in training as a result of injuries. Crawford F. Sams, "Medic," 111–21.
4. An earlier account of this epidemiological intelligence mission in North Korea (which also includes discussions of the background and organization of the occupation of South Korea from 1945 to 1948; the situation in Korea following the communist invasion of the Republic of Korea in June 1950; the occupation of and withdrawal from North Korea in 1950–51; and the war involving Chinese Communists in North Korea in 1950–51) is contained in a letter to Maj. Gen. Charles A. Willoughby. Gen. Charles Andrew Willoughby (1892–1972) served as chief-of-staff of U.S. Army intelligence, Far East Command, from 1941 to 1951. In the fall of 1952, he had requested information from Sams for a book on the Pacific war, the occupation of Japan, and the Korean War. Except for Sams's official report on this mission, which was originally classified "secret," his letter to Willoughby of 9 December 1952 is believed to be the only other account of this mission written by Sams himself. This account adheres closely to the one in his letter. Crawford F. Sams to Charles A. Willoughby, 8 November 1952, CFS, Box 5, HIA; Crawford F. Sams to Charles A. Willoughby, 9 December 1952; Crawford F. Sams, Report on Special Operations in North Korea, 17 March 1951, CFS, Box 4, HIA.
5. The names of the participants in this classified mission appear as they were given in the original manuscript. They were not changed to correct the inconsistency in the manuscript, because that inconsistency, however unintentional, reflects the confusion that followed the media's exposure of this classified mission, which Sams discusses later in this chapter in The Aftermath.
Lt. Eugene F. Clark (USN) was the U.S. Navy lieutenant in this secret mission.

"Drake" was a fictitious name used in a radio script entitled, "Doctor Commando," written by Robert Anderson in 1952. Anderson's script was adapted from a popular article about Sams's mission, which was published in *Colliers* by Peter Kalisher in 1951. The radio script fictionally dramatized an epidemiological intelligence mission by an American military doctor in Korea during the war. Eugene F. Clark to Crawford F. Sams, 24 October 1951, CFS, Box 4, HIA; Robert Anderson, "Doctor Commando," 4 January 1952, CFS, Box 4, HIA.

6. "Commander E. Yun" was Commander Youn Joung. See Eugene F. Clark to Crawford F. Sams, 24 October 1951; Crawford F. Sams to Eugene F. Clark, 27 October 1951, CFS, Box 4, HIA.

7. Lieutenant Clark and Commander Youn, who were "forever and indelibly impressed" by Sams's determination, later dubbed this mission, "Operation SAMS." Eugene F. Clark to Crawford F. Sams, 24 October 1951.

8. Owing to the secrecy and sensitivity of this mission, the army intelligence report omitted the details of hand-to-hand combat "as a security measure," because it would disclose the presence of this covert group, whereas the enemy might otherwise attribute the results of the combat to enemy guerrillas. Eugene F. Clark to Crawford F. Sams, 24 October 1951. An undated statement attesting to the combat accompanied Clark's letter and was signed by Sams in order to properly credit Clark with combat service.

9. Sams later wrote that the communists themselves believed this disease was the plague. In the extreme situation, both the fear of disease and the lack of information contributed to the problem of calling different diseases by the same name, which Sams discussed in The Lessons of *Ikiri* in chapter 2.

10. Sams did not disclose how he determined this "clinical diagnosis." Based on his letter to Charles Willoughby, Sams apparently examined patients in Chilbo-ri:

> . . . we had to confine our activities to interrogation of the agents and first-hand information of what was happening in Chilbo-ri.

Crawford F. Sams to Charles A. Willoughby, 9 December 1952, 6.

11. In describing this "little episode" in his letter to Maj. Gen. Charles Willoughby, Sams commented on the article published by Peter Kalisher in 1951, as follows:

> So far as the episode in North Korea is concerned, the popularized version which you have read is more or less correct, with the exception that complete information was not released by G-2 to Kalisher as to the result of that episode.

Crawford F. Sams to Charles A. Willoughby, 9 December 1952, 5.

12. The term "bacterial warfare" reflects the escalation of the normative sense of disease as "pollution" in the highly charged lexicon of the cold war. See note 2 to chapter 20, above.

Chapter 31: The Relief of General MacArthur

1. See the enthusiastic comments—dateline Chicago, 19 May 1951—of Gen. James S. Simmons, then Dean of the Harvard School of Public Health, following his tour of Japan, Okinawa, and Korea, in "General Risked Life to Visit Red Hospital," *Boston Sunday Globe*, 20 May 1951.

2. A similar account of Sams's nomination as Surgeon General of the Army and his desire to retire upon his return to the United States is found in Sams's personal correspondence. Crawford F. Sams to Gus and Sally Ledfors, 7 January 1953, CFS, Box 5, HIA.

Chapter 32: The Twenty-second of April Offensive

1. See Sams's comment on the report on battle casualties in the discussion of Leaving Japan and his discussion of the Study of Korean War Casualties in the final chapter.
2. Sams applied for voluntary retirement from the army, after twenty-nine years of service, in the spring of 1951.
3. On 30 June 1951, the Public Health and Welfare Section of General Headquarters, SCAP, was disbanded; its functions were transferred to a newly designated Medical Section. The Public Health and Welfare Division of the Medical Section continued the public health and welfare activities with regard to the civilian population of Japan until the end of the occupation on 28 April 1952. See Public Health and Welfare Division, *Public Health and Welfare in Japan*, 1–2.

Chapter 33: Return to the United States

1. For Sams's letter of congratulations to the newly selected Surgeon General of the Army, see Crawford F. Sams to George E. Armstrong, 2 May 1951, CFS, Box 4, HIA. See also Sams's letter to the retiring Surgeon General of the Army. Crawford F. Sams to Raymond W. Bliss, 2 May, 1951, CFS, Box 4, HIA.
2. Note the reference to Sams's pending retirement in David Perlman, 8 July 1951, 8.
3. Sams was considered essential to the army but not as Surgeon General; his first request for retirement was denied. Some of Sams's personal correspondence dating from 1952 to 1953 indicates he felt disillusioned with the army and his current assignment. He wrote that he felt his "usefulness in the Army appeared to be ended" and that he wanted to "get out" of what had become "a corrupt organization." On 30 July 1952, he submitted his resignation from the army. By early December 1952, he was informed that his resignation would probably not be accepted under the current administration; hence, he wrote that he felt as if he were "a prisoner" in his own country. His resignation was turned down in January 1953. Crawford F. Sams to W.A. Beiderlinden, 27 February 1953, CFS, Box 5, HIA; Crawford F. Sams to Gus and Sally Ledfors, 7 January 1953; Crawford F. Sams to Charles A. Willoughby, 9 December 1952, 8; Crawford F. Sams to Marion E. Holstead, 7 January 1953, CFS, Box 5, HIA.
4. See note 5 to chapter 15, above.
5. Sams's reference to being "acutely aware" of the difficulties faced by young medics includes not only his direct observations in Korea, but also the loss of his son-in-law, Capt. Charles M. Struthers, in North Korea.
6. Sams's use of the term "our career" is assumed to be intentional and thus meant to include his wife. Elsewhere in the original manuscript, he referred to his wife as "the great soldier" and expressed his admiration for the "gallantry" of the wives of career officers in the military service. Crawford F. Sams, "Medic," 124.
7. See the discussion of Sams's last assignment in Korea in chapter 32.

Appendix I

1. James Atlas, "Choosing a Life," 22.
2. James Atlas, "Choosing a Life," 22, 23.
3. Crawford F. Sams, "Medic," 3.

Appendix I

Editorial Decisions

In abridging, annotating, and editing "Medic," the editor shares a sympathy with biographers. Biography, according to James Atlas, requires both "reticence" and "tenacity." "The biographer's job is to stay in the background, behind the scenes." Yet Atlas admits the biographer defies this undiscernible role:

> But of course the biographer is visible—in the selection of letters, documents and testimony from which he fashions his narrative; in his organization of this data; in the interpretation he puts on it; above all, in whom he chooses to write about.[1]

How does a biographer choose whom to write about? According to Atlas:

> Biographers themselves don't really know how they choose their subjects, any more than a poet knows how a particular image came into his head. . . . it all depends on finding the right subject, the one that induces biographical obsession.[2]

Unlike a biographer, an editor of autobiography chooses a manuscript and an author as well as a subject. These three elements constitute a framework for the editorial decisions.

On choosing "Medic," one discovers an autobiography of quest: a classical journey of adventure, transformation, danger, and service to society. The subject of this quest encounters the forces of history in bridging knowledge and cultures. He questions theories when experience cannot adequately be explained; he contributes to the solution of societal problems by his practical application of scientific methods; and he adapts his knowledge to the challenges of war and occupation. One also finds an author who, as a physician and a military officer, records his experiences with both factual honesty and guarded understatement; who, as a husband and a father, not only cherishes pleasant pastimes and experiences with his family but also preserves the privacy of his family life; and who, as a modern western hero, restates the classical theme that meaningful choices entail personal sacrifices:

> This drive to stand on my own feet and to be self-sufficient has been a major factor in my entire life. . . . It deprived me of many of the pleasures which I might have otherwise enjoyed, but it has also enabled me to accomplish things which others have said were impossible."[3]

Thus, in choosing "Medic," one of the more difficult decisions was how to abridge the manuscript for publication while preserving its core. The necessity of this decision arises owing to the manuscript's length. As discussed in the Introduction, this book includes parts IV and V of "Medic," which in length constitute over half of the manuscript and include what Sams considered his most significant work. This editor's attempts to fill gaps in the continuity, coherence, meaning, and context that arise from abridging the manuscript are found in the Introduction, in the Chronology, and in some of the notes.

The annotation is also intended to complement Sams's desire to provide a source for historical research and understanding and is based largely on archival sources and official documents. The emphasis of the notes varies according to the narrative content: The notes that accompany the chapters on Japan provide documentation and additional context for Sams's discussions of occupation policies and decisions; they also document rates of disease and other numerical information. In a few instances, the notes include analytical perspectives and cross-references to interpret nuances of Sams's statements and their context. The notes that accompany the chapters on Korea serve to corroborate, amplify, or add to the plausibility of his discussion.

Because editing requires a degree of consistency and adherence to form as well as reticence, certain editorial changes were made in the organization of parts IV and V of "Medic," as they appear in this book. The changes are considered minor in that they are not believed to have altered the context or the meaning of Sams's narrative in a substantive way, or in a direction other than which Sams intended; however, readers who are concerned with the authenticity of the text may wish to note the editor's decisions and make an independent judgment. These editorial changes are described below. The first four changes pertain only to the chapters on Japan; the last two pertain throughout this book.

1. The order of certain chapters was changed for purposes of coherence. The order in which a number of the chapters on Japan appear in the original manuscript generally follows the order in which they are discussed in the official reports of the PHW Section. Their order is also similar to the organizational structure of the PHW Section of SCAP, with a chapter devoted to each division.

In the manuscript, the chapters on The Reorganization of Health and Welfare and on Statistics follow the discussion of the preventive medicine program. Here, these two chapters (6 and 7) precede the chapters on the preventive medicine program. Sams's references to the health centers in his discussion of the preventive medicine program indicated the need for this change. In addition, his discussion of the use of statistical information by the district health officer in chapter 7 on Statistics relates to the discussion of the health center system in chapter 6 on The Reorganization of Health and Welfare; so these two chapters were retained in the original sequence but their order in relation to the preventive medicine chapters was reversed.

2. Two of the longer chapters in the manuscript were subdivided into shorter chapters in this book. Chapters 8, 9, and 10 on the preventive medicine program in Japan constitute a single chapter in the manuscript. Owing to its length, this chapter was subdivided and the material was regrouped according to the subject matter: namely, the nature of the diseases, their causes, and the methods of their control and treatment. This reorganization resulted in three shorter chapters of approximately equal length. The sequence in which the diseases are discussed differs slightly from the order in which they are presented in the manuscript.

The two chapters on Medicine and Dentistry (chapter 12) and on Hospitals (chapter 15) constitute a single chapter, entitled "Medical Care," in the manuscript. Owing to its length as well as the number of topics it covered, this single chapter was subdivided into two chapters and retitled.

3. In two instances, the content was reorganized between chapters for purposes of clarity and coherence. First, Sams's discussion of the reorganization of the Japanese Government under the Constitution of 1947 appears in the manuscript in the chapter on The Decision: SCAP. In this book, it appears in chapter 6 on The Reorganization of Health and Welfare to clarify the context of that discussion. Second, Sams's discussion of the separation of the professions of medicine, dentistry, and pharmacy appears in the manuscript in the chapter on Medical Care. In this book, it appears in chapter 13 on Pharmacy and Pharmaceutical Affairs, because the effects of SCAP's decision to separate the professions are more fully explained in the discussion of the pharmacy profession.

4. Deletions were made primarily to eliminate certain types of redundancies. For example, a discussion of the estimated number of domestic animals that could be raised in Japan was deleted in chapter 5 on Food Relief and Nutrition but retained in chapter 11 on The Veterinarians. Other redundancies that suggest the strength of Sams's attitudes and opinions by means of their repetition have been retained throughout this book.

5. All subheadings within chapters of this book were added and a few of the chapters on Japan were retitled. No subheadings appear in the manuscript regardless of the length of a chapter.

6. The spelling of a person's name was changed only when it could be confirmed. It was not possible to confirm the names of all individuals mentioned in the text. Also, the order of Japanese and Korean names in the text and in captions to the photographs follows oriental conventions: The family name is followed by the given name. An exception is made in the notes with bibliographical references: In these notes, the names follow conventions for bibliographical entries regardless of the origin of the name.

—ZZ

Appendix II

Photographs

Photographs have many uses. They can invite interest and curiosity. They can serve as a memorial of events and people. They can, with careful documentation, even serve as a source of validation for elements of an historical record.

The photographs in this book have been added as visual references to portray in a somewhat representative way some of the people and activities that Sams wrote about in "Medic" as well as to depict aspects of the setting that might now be difficult to imagine. All of the photographs have been selected from the Crawford F. Sams Collection at the Hoover Institution Archives and are published with permission of Stanford University. This discussion of the photographs is intended to invite awareness of the selection processes that resulted in their inclusion in this book.

The selection of photographs occurred in three stages, two of which preceded the determination of which photographs to include in this book. The first stage involved all of the highly complex choices and constraints that a given photographer negotiates in taking a particular photograph. The second stage involved all of the factors in Sams's personal decisions to save certain photographs along with his papers and later to include them in a collection at the Hoover Archives. The third stage involved procedures to screen and to select photographs from the Crawford F. Sams Collection to accompany his narrative.

The Crawford F. Sams Collection at the Hoover Archives includes over nine hundred photographs of which more than six hundred depict people and scenes from the occupation of Japan. The procedure to screen photographs for possible inclusion in this book began with two criteria for acceptability: First, the photograph had to be in a reproducible condition. Second, there had to be some form of documentation of or means of identifying the pictorial contents of the photograph. None of the photographs in Sams's collection that include documentation depict aspects of the occupation of Korea or the Korean War; others could not be identified as such with certainty. Consequently, all of the photographs in this book portray people, scenes, and activities from the occupation of Japan.

The acceptable photographs were then screened according to a third criterion: The photograph had to depict some aspect of health and welfare activities during the occupation of Japan that Sams discussed in "Medic." This process narrowed the selection to forty-two photographs, each of which depicted one or more such aspects. These photographs were then sorted into eleven categories based upon their depiction of people, activities, events, scenes, or organizations mentioned in the manuscript. Some photographs could be classified in more than one category.

These photographs were then reviewed within each category and between each category to select a total of twenty-two photographs that were optimally representative of the people and activities and the setting. At this stage, certain additional factors were considered desirable in selecting the set of photographs: the depiction of activities at the national and local levels; the depiction of the interaction of Americans and Japanese; the depiction of Sams's range of activities; and the inclusion of photographs by various photographers, not only whether professional or amateur, named or anonymous, but also within the U.S. Army Signal Corps. The final selection of photographs included at least one photograph from each of the eleven categories.

The photographs attributed to the U.S. Army Signal Corps have two apparent advantages: They usually carry documentation about the date, place, and people depicted in the photograph. They may also include permission to reproduce and use the photograph. Certain journalistic tendencies of the Signal Corps photographers are also discernible from Sams's collection of photographs from the occupation of Japan: The Signal Corps photographers covered occupation activities for official purposes of SCAP and the Far East Commission. They documented events or activities that were then believed to be politically, if not historically, important, such as the promulgation of the Japanese Constitution in 1947. Their photographs are likely to represent the positive side of the occupation from the perspective of the occupation forces. Their work is also more likely to have been released to the press and to have been previously published. These tendencies can be advantages or disadvantages depending on the use of a given photograph.

I would like to acknowledge the permission of the Hoover Archives to publish the photographs in this book as well as the permission of the Radiation Effects Research Foundation to publish Figure 19. Remy Squires was particularly helpful in accommodating my requests for the reproduction of photographs.

I also wish to acknowledge the courtesies of the following people and organizations who helped to confirm the identification of individuals and events depicted in the photographs: Yvonne Johns, Patricia Dwyers, Jim Zoble, Amy Evans, Virginia M. Ohlson, Dorothy Toom Pollock, Hashimoto Michio, Hashimoto Masami, M. Susan Lindee, Margaret Irwin, James V. Neel, William J. Schull, Louise P. Cavagnaro, Carl F. Tessmer, Herman Wigodsky, and Iwamura Tatsuro and the *Asahi Shimbun*. Their contributions added valuable documentation to the photographs.

—ZZ

Index

A

Acupuncture, 130–31
Adler, Elmer, 9
Ainu, 50–51, 196–97
Allied Council, 178
Almond, Edward M. (Ned), 38, 209, 223, 229, 240
Alt, Grace, 140
  photo, 142
Alvery, Sir, 198
American Medical Association, 123, 129, 171, 255
Antibiotics.
  penicillin, 103, 107, 136
  streptomycin, 113, 136–37, 232
Aoki, Hideo.
  photo, 162
Armstrong, George, 258, 262
Armstrong, Harry, 255
Assay of biological products.
  for animals, 115–16
  for people, 76, 102, 137
Atomic Bomb Casualty Commission, 150–52, 284n.1, 284n.3
  photo, 151
  See also Radiation Effects Research Foundation

B

Bacillus Calmette-Guerin vaccine. See BCG
Band, Doctor, 138
Bantu Hotel, 225–26
Barrows, David Prescott, xiii
BCG, 110–12, 178, 179–80
Beechwood, Doctor, 115
Bethea, James, 195
Biederlinden, Bill, 209
"Big question," 183
Biological warfare, 254, 293n.12
Birth rates (in Japan), 187
  in demographic trends, 184
  reduction of, 185, 186
Black death. See Plague
Bliss, Raymond, 39, 255
  photo, ii
Bliss report, 39–41
Bradley, Sladen, 239, 259
Brugger, Florence.
  photo, 162
Burroughs, General, 263

C

CARE, 164
Catholic Church, 185–86
Chamberlain, Steve, 37, 38
Champaney, Colonel, 232
Censorship.
  military, 264n.4
  of classified information, 293n.8, 293n.11
Cheslak, Walter.
  photo, 151
Chichibu, Prince, 197
Chichibu, Princess, 197
Cholera, 21–22

Cholera *(continued)*
  in Japan, 89–91
  in Korea, 91, 207, 217–18
  See also Ikiri
Chosen Hotel, 225–26, 237
Chosen Reservoir, 238, 241, 246
Chou, Minister, 214, 226, 229, 230
Civil Information and Education Section (of SCAP), 34, 63, 124
Clark, Eugene F., 248, 250, 252, 253, 292–93n.5
Clay, General, 33
Cold War, xi, xii, 10, 43, 67, 241, 267n.4, 291n.4
Collins, Selwyn T., 79
Communist activities (in Japan).
  methods of operation, 155–56, 176, 181
  narcotics smuggling, 155–56
  propaganda, 60, 62, 174, 179–81
  and tuberculosis rates, 178–79, 289n.2
  sabotage of BCG program, 179–80
  sources of, 174–76
Connor, Pete, 194
Constitution.
  of Japan, 68–70, 163, 271n.1, 272n.2–4, 272n.7
  Article 25, x, 69, 272n.5, 288n.5
  promulgation of (photos), 69, 70
  of Republic of Korea, 234–35
Cooperative Agencies for Remittances to Europe, Inc., *See* CARE
Coulter, John B., 223
Council on Medical Education (of Japan), 124
Cox, Herald R., 85
Currency (of Japan).
  foreign exchange of, 65, 139, 215
  inflation, 94, 169–71
    and employment, 170
    and public assistance, 159
  stabilization of, 94, 169
Crist, William, 11, 24

D

Dai Ichi building, 25, 30
Davall, Colonel, 213, 228
DDT.
  in Japan, 14, 84–85, 87, 94, 138, 215, 277n.9
  in Korea, 215, 218, 234
Dean, Bill, 211, 229–30, 231
Death rates (in Japan).
  crude, 102, 183
Denit, Guy, 39, 138
Dentistry (in Japan).
  economic incentives, 132–33
  reform of, 131, 133–34
Democracy by demonstration, 183, 290n.1
Diphtheria.
  in Japan, 102–3, 279n.3, 280n.4
  in Korea, 207, 213, 217, 228, 234, 241
Disaster relief (in Japan), 29, 165–66, 180
Dixon, Oness, 115
Dodge, Joseph, 94, 169
Dogs, 118–19
  Akita, 191
Drake, Lieutenant. *See* Clark, Eugene F.
Draper, Doctor, 139
Drugs.
  hexylresorcinol, 136
    demonstration of efficacy, 135–36
  paraminosalicylic acid, 136–37
  sulfanilamide, 94, 103
  See also Antibiotics
Dryvenko, General, 174, 178–79, 181
Dulles, John Foster, 260
Dwyer, Dale, 220
Dwyer, Patricia (Patsy), xvi, 190–91, 220, 264
Dykes, Ken, 34
Dysenteries (in Japan), 31, 92, 94, 95, 278n.1, 278–79n.8, 279n.9

E

Economic Cooperation Administration, 209, 213, 225

Economics and Scientific Section (of SCAP), 34, 60, 63, 135, 138, 159, 167, 170
  Labor Division of, 171, 175, 177
Education, Ministry of (of Japan), 23, 33, 63, 76, 124, 141
Eichelberger, General, 5
Eighth Army, 5, 11, 19, 25, 37–38, 213, 219, 227, 231, 232, 235, 238, 241, 242, 249, 258, 259
Eisenhower, Dwight D., 33
Environmental factors and disease, 88, 92, 96–98, 100–1, 114, 218
Evans, Milton J., 285n.4–5
  photo, 198

F

Family system (of Japan), 48, 77, 79, 158
  devotion to children, 65
  self-sufficiency of, 170–71
Far East Command, ix, 33, 39, 141, 204, 211
Far East Commission, 32, 183–84, 185
Farrell, Thomas F., 19–20
First Army, 5, 263
Flanagan, Father, 161
Food deficit (in Japan), 46–47, 54–55, 270n.1
  supplies for SCAP, 46–47, 117
  See also Nutrition
Foreign nationals (in Japan).
  health and welfare of, 18
  hospitals for, 18–19, 29, 269n.1
Forestry and Agriculture, Ministry of (of Japan), 65, 115
Fourth field hospital, 224, 291n.1
Fox, Alonzo P. (Pat), 38, 209
Friendship.
  as a theme of "Medic", xi, xv
  between nations, 23, 43, 67, 139, 188, 210, 256, 257, 259
  between persons, 3, 21, 76, 96, 193, 194, 198, 204, 211, 224, 227, 230, 239, 255, 259, 262, 264

Friendship *(continued)*
  within the military services, 14, 41, 221, 225, 228, 248, 252, 263
Fukuzumi, Doctor.
  photo, 86

G

GARIOA, 60, 64, 86, 117
Gascoigne, Lady, 198
Gay, Hobart R. (Hap), 224
General Sams Cup, 193
Geneva Conventions, 15, 19, 28, 130–31, 244, 268n.2
Germany.
  Japanese views of, 42
  occupation of, 32–33, 58, 174, 185, 204
Gorby, Vi, 227, 241
Gordon, Colonel, 105
Government and Relief in Occupied Areas. *See* GARIOA
Government Section (of SCAP), 34, 145

H

Hammond, William, 97
Hara, Taiichi.
  photo, 162
Harada, Colonel, 21–24, 28
Harrison, Colonel R.
  photo, 61
Hashimoto, Masami, 273n.10
  photo, 74
Hashimoto, Michio, x
Hays, Silas, 264
Health and Welfare Laws. *See* Laws
Health and Welfare, Ministry of.
  of Japan, 23, 31, 33, 42, 63, 65, 70–71, 76, 78, 79, 115, 124, 136, 137, 145, 151, 154, 161, 177, 260
  of Republic of Korea, 208
Health centers (in Japan), 60, 71–73, 79, 94, 115, 131
  model, 72–73, 74, 112, 141, 146, 273n.10
  photos, 61, 74, 112
  prewar, 71, 78
Health insurance (in Japan), 167–69

Health insurance *(continued)*
  financial stability of, 169
  issue of compulsion, 168, 171
  principles of, 168–69, 172
Henderson, Elmer, 255
Herring, Bud, 228
Hickey, Doyle O. (Tom), 38, 253
Hirohito, Emperor, 197
  photo, 70
  respect for, 23, 197
Hiroshima.
  bombing of, ix, 9
  studies of effects of, 20, 150
  See also Atomic Bomb Casualty Commission
  See also International Red Cross Committee
Hiyashi, Doctor, 111
Hodges, Courtney, 5
Hodges, John, 204, 205, 230
Honseki, 77
Hoover, Herbert, 57, 63
Hoover Institution Archives, x
Hospitals.
  in Japan, 12, 15, 17, 23, 28–29, 122, 140, 144–45
  demilitarization of, 145–46
  destruction of, 28, 144
  communicable disease, 23, 50, 82–83, 110, 146, 183
  foreign national, 18–19, 29, 269n.1
  model hospitals, 29, 141, 146
  modern standards of administration, 143, 146, 148
  photo, 99
  school of hospital administration, 29, 146, 284n.4
  in Korea, 206, 208, 215, 224, 227–28, 231–32, 233, 248, 252, 255
  equipment and supplies for, 206, 213, 215, 227–28, 232, 241–42
  military hospitals, 224, 227–28, 241
  See also MASH
  See also Missionaries
Hume, Edgar Erskine, 219, 255, 258, 262
  photo, ii

I

Ikiri, 21–23
Imaoka, Keniichiro.
  photo, 162
Imperial Hotel, 25, 27, 54, 189, 192, 255, 261
Inchon, 216, 219, 223, 224, 227, 229
Industrialization.
  policies on, 184, 185
  effect on population stabilization, 186
  social hazards of, 167
Infant mortality (in Japan), 183, 290n.2
Institute of Infectious Diseases, 76
  photos, ii, 86
Institute of Public Health (of Japan), 75, 115, 129, 131, 141, 186, 272–73n.8, 274n.13–16, 278n.4
Instructions, Supreme Commander for the Allied Powers. See SCAPIN
International Red Cross Committee, 19–20, 165, 244
Ito, Canada.
  photo, 74
Iwashita–san, 192

J

Jackson, Doctor, 136
Japan Antituberculosis Association, 197
Japan Dental Association, 131
Japan Medical Association, 128–29, 136, 261
Japan Pharmaceutical Association, 132, 261
Japanese B encephalitis, 96–99
  photo, 99
  in relation to poliomyelitis, 99–100
Johns, Yvonne, xvi, 190, 195, 199, 220, 237, 238, 249, 262, 264
Johnson, Harry, 125
Juno, Doctor, 19–20

K

Katayama, Tsuneo.
  photo, 74
Kaufman, Warren, 75

INDEX   305

Keeney, Paul, 205
Kelser, Ray, 96
Keller, Helen, 160
Kelly, Harry.
   photo, 151
Kido, Colonel, 192–93
Kitasato, Doctor.
   photo, ii
Kittredge, Tracy B.
   photo, 61
Koenig, Nathan.
   photo, 61
Korea, 203
   Allied occupation of, 204–8, 209
      organization of health and welfare, 205, 206–8
   Japanese occupation of, 203, 205, 206–7
   North
      hydroelectric power system, 207, 236–37
      military build up of, 209–10
      oil refineries, 207, 232, 233
      U.N. occupation of, 234–35, 236
   Republic of, 205, 208
      invasion of, 209, 212, 214
      organization of civilian relief, 211–13, 215–17, 226–29, 231–32
      rice harvest, 216, 229
   See also Thirty-eighth parallel
Korean War, 198, 209, 211, 218–19, 221, 223–30, 231, 234–35, 258–59
   Chinese military involvement, 236–39
   enemy infiltration, 214, 218–19, 221–22
   medical intelligence, 217–18, 241, 246–47
   reasons for controlling disease, 217
   U.S. military casualties, 221, 240, 241, 258, 262, 263
   hazards of being road bound, 221
   soldiers missing-in-action, 239–40, 258
   U.S. troop strength, 211
      shortage of U.S. medical personnel, 213, 219–20
   withdrawal of U.N. forces, 240–42
   See also Hospitals
   See also Korea

Kōseishō. *See* Health and Welfare, Ministry of (of Japan)
Koseki, 77
Koya, Yoshio, 75
Kramer, Colonel, 34
Kramer, Dutch, 239
Krueger, Walter, 5
Kusama, Yoshio, 124

L

LARA, 64, 163–64
Laws, health and welfare (of Japan), 42
   Article 25 of the Constitution, x, 69, 272n.5, 288n.5
   Child Welfare Law, 79, 161
   Daily Life Security Law, 64, 79, 159, 161, 168
   Dental Practitioners Law, 133
   Health Center Law, 72, 273n.9
   Medical Service Law, 146–47
   Medical Practitioners Law, 124–25, 133
   on medical examiner system, 126
   on narcotics control, 154
   on nursing education and licensure, 142
   Pharmaceutical Affairs Law, 132–34, 137, 282n.1
   Preventive Vaccination Law, 103, 279n.10
   Venereal Disease Prevention Law, 107
League of Red Cross Societies, 244
Lee, Doctor Y.S., 208
Licensed Agencies for Relief in Asia. *See* LARA
Life expectancy (in Japan), 183
Lowe, Frank E., 225–26
Luykx, Henrik.
   photo, 151

M

MacArthur, Douglas, 5, 17, 225
   as U.N. Commander, 211, 216, 231, 234, 235, 244–45, 253, 254
   as U.S. Far East Commander, ix, 33, 204, 209, 211

MacArthur, Douglas *(continued)*
  as SCAP, 32, 40–41, 42, 58, 59, 85, 107, 145, 158, 171, 177–78, 185, 190
  dealings with the Japanese, 24
  dealings with the Russians, 174
  relief of, 255–57, 258, 261
McCoy, Frank, 32, 185
McCoy, Oliver R., 75
MacDonald, Doctor, 205
Mallahan, Colonel, 223
Manabe, Mitsuta, 28, 44–46, 50, 51
Manufacture of drugs and medical supplies (in Japan).
  DDT, 85, 138
  hexylresorcinol, 136
  penicillin, 136
  paraminosalicylic acid, 137
  streptomycin, 136–37
  vaccines
    BCG, 111–12
    diphtheria toxoid, 102
    smallpox, 81–83
    typhoid and paratyphoid, 95
    typhus, 86–87
  for use in Korea, 85, 138, 215
  wartime production, 134–35
  X-ray film, 138
Marquat, Bill, 34, 138, 177
Martin, Joe, 138, 195, 262
MASH, xi, 227, 259
Maxwell, Russell, ix
"Medic," x-xi, xii
Medical care (in Japan).
  fees and economic incentives, 122–23, 132–34
  organization of, 122
  prewar medical education, 120–21
  reform of medical care and education, 123–31
    Council on Medical Education, 124
    internships, 125–26, 281*n*.5
    licensure, 124–25
    medical examiner system, 126
    publications, 129, 282*n*.8

Medical care (in Japan) *(continued)*
  separation of medicine, dentistry, and pharmacy, 132–34
  specialties, 127–28
  teaching missions, 126–27
  See also Japan Medical Association
Medical and Pharmaceutical Deliberation Council (of Japan), 133
Medical Field Service Schools.
  at Carlisle Barracks, xi
  at Fort Sam Houston, 252
Milburn, Frank W. (Shrimp), 223, 259
Miller, Lieutenant (USN), 249
Miller, Paul, 38
Missionaries.
  in Japan, 28, 140
  in Korea, 208, 227, 231, 233–34
Missouri, U.S.S., 7
Mobile Army Surgical Hospitals. *See* MASH
Morgenthau Doctrine, 185
Morgenthau, Henry, 185
Moolten, Sylvan E. 125
Mount Fuji, 6
Moxacautery, 130
Muccio, Ambassador, 212

N

Nagako, Empress, 197
  photos, 70, 198
Nagasaki.
  bombing of, ix, 9
  studies of effects of, 150
Narcotics.
  addiction to, 153–55
  control of, 153–54, 156
  medical uses of, 153
  smuggling of, 155–56, 288*n*.4
    financing of Communist party, 155–56, 181
National Hygienic Laboratory (of Japan), 137
National Institute of Health (of Japan), 75–76, 137, 151
Natural Resources Section (of SCAP), 34, 60, 65, 98

Neff, Nelson, 166
Newsweek, 253
Nippon Times, 24, 279n.3
North Korea. *See* Korea
Notestein, Frank W., 184
Noyes, Ed, 262
Nugent, Don, 34
Nursing (in Japan).
  hospital patient care, 140, 143, 148
  midwifery, 141–42
  photos, 142, 198
  public health nursing, 141–43
  reform of nursing care and education, 140–43, 165
    licensure and registration, 142
    model nursing schools, 140–41
    Nursing Education Council, 140
    texts and journals, 141
Nutrition (in Japan).
  education, 59–60
  patterns of, 54–56, 62
    role of animal husbandry in, 65–66, 117–18
  photo, 61
  qualitative versus quantitative needs, 47, 57, 59, 60
  ration system, 18, 30, 58
  role in medical care, 145
  role in tuberculosis, 54, 58, 109
  seasonal food shortages, 47, 56–57, 59, 270–71n.2
  survey of nutritional status, 14, 47, 55–56, 58, 59, 62
  See also School lunch program

O

O'Donnell, Agnes.
  photo, 61
Officer Personnel Act of 1947, 41
Ohata, Tane.
  photo, 162
Ohlson, Virginia M., 283n.4, 285n.4
  photo, 198
Okada, Doctor, 111

Operation SAMS, 248–51, 251–52, 292n.4, 293n.7

P

Paratyphoid fever.
  in Japan, 92, 94–95, 278n.1
  in Korea, 216
Parran, Thomas (Tom), 89
Pate, Maurice, 57, 63
Paul, John R., 97, 99–100
Pets, 118–19
  Taisa, 191
Pharmacy (in Japan), 132–34
  See also Medical care
Phelps, Leonard, 77, 80, 275n.1
Plague, 247–48, 252, 253
  in the Middle East, 247, 292n.2
Planned Parenthood, 185
Pneumonia, 103, 280n.5
Policies (of SCAP).
  abrogating licensed prostitution, 107
  against preferential treatment of Japanese veterans, 145, 283–84n.3
  on American families in occupied Japan, 189–90, 199
  on distribution of international relief supplies, 164
  on economic stabilization, 169–70
  on exchanging gifts, 53
  on food sources for occupation personnel, 46–47, 117, 281n.4
  on imports of supplies, 81, 85–87, 135, 138, 139, 276n.2
  on industrialization of Japan, 184, 185
  on instituting democracy in Japan, 183–84
  on labor and management relations, 177–78
  on methods of implementing reforms, 133
  on population movement, 158
  on purge of military personnel, 145–46
  on treatment of foreign nationals, 18
  on zaibatsu, 192
  See also Far East Commission

308 INDEX

Policies *(continued)*
  See also State, War, and Navy
    Coordinating Committee
Poliomyelitis, 92, 99–101, 279*n*.13
  moral dilemmas of, 100–1
Population growth (in Japan).
  the "big question," 183
  stabilization of, 55, 185–86
  See also Birth rates
Population movement.
  in Japan, 30, 45, 157
    control of, 158
  in Korea, 206, 207, 211, 224, 233, 241, 242
  role in spreading disease, 81, 85, 87, 89, 207, 213
Potsdam Declaration, xiv, 24
Press, 9, 24, 171, 186, 187, 244, 253–54, 256, 290*n*.3, 293*n*.1
  role in health promotion, 60, 87
  See also Newsweek
  See also Nippon Times
Propaganda, 60, 62, 174, 178–82, 183
  charges of biological warfare, 254, 293*n*.12
  disease control as counterpropaganda, 217
Prostitution.
  in Japan, 17, 105–7
  in Korea, 105–6
  in the Middle East, 105
  U.S. military policies on, 103–4, 106
  See also Venereal diseases
Public Health and Welfare Section (of SCAP), x, xiv, 25, 33–36, 37, 163, 260, 269*n*.1, 294*n*.2
  Dental Division, 44, 131
  Medical Affairs Division, 125
  Narcotics Control Division, 153, 287*n*.1
  Nursing Affairs Division, 140
  Statistical Division, 77
  Supply (Pharmaceutical) Division, 138
  Veterinary Division, 115
  weekly bulletin of, 37–38
Public health train, 273–74*n*.11

Purge of military personnel. *See* Hospitals, demilitarization of
  See also Disaster relief
  See also Red Cross, of Japan, reorganization of

Q

Quarantine services, 89–91, 277*n*.11–12

R

Rabies, 118–19
Radiation Effects Research Foundation, iv, 287*n*.11
Randol, Marshall, xiii
Red Cross.
  of Japan, 140, 165, 197, 208
    hospitals, 140, 176
    photo, 198
    reorganization of, 165
  of Republic of Korea, 208
    hospital, 208, 227
  role in Korean War, 243–45
  See also International Red Cross Committee
Republic of Korea. *See* Korea
Rhee, Syngman, 205, 210–11, 212, 234, 245
Ridgely, Dale, 44, 45, 50, 51, 131
Ridgeway, Matthew, 242, 254, 258, 260
Riordan, Bernard, 138
Riordan, Ralph, 166
Rispler, Doctor, xiii
Rockefeller Foundation, 75, 85, 129, 148, 274*n*.14, 274*n*.16
Rockefeller, John D., Jr., 260
Rosenthal, Saul, 110

S

Sachs, Ernest, xiii
Sams, Crawford F.
  as advisor for health and welfare, South Korea, 205–6
  as chief of health, education, and welfare, USAFP, 10, 33

Sams, Crawford F. *(continued)*
  as chief of health and welfare, U.N. Command, 212, 213, 244–45, 253
  as chief of public health and welfare, SCAP, 34, 212, 260
  as honorary "Admiral of the Navy," 249
  career decisions, xii-xiv, 33, 39–41, 190, 264
  concept of responsibilities, 44
  nomination as Surgeon General of the Army, 255
  photos, ii, 26, 40, 46, 47, 61, 74, 99, 142, 151, 198
  shortcomings as a bureaucrat, 39
  views and opinions
    on abortion, 186–87
    on codes of conduct, 16–17, 41
    on communism, 179, 180, 181
    on demonstration of ideas, 64, 135–36, 183, 262, 284n.5
    on effects of disease on military operations, 217, 254
    on extension of social security benefits, 172–73
    on factors in underdevelopment, 67, 188
    on horses, 2, 79, 115, 116, 130, 192–93, 290n.1
    on integration of health and welfare programs, 157, 172
    on Japanese norms and customs, 45–46, 50–53, 79, 195
    on language barriers and culture, 21–22
    on lessons in conduct, 24, 28, 51
    on maintaining face or prestige, 23–24, 25, 95, 253
    on medical specialists, 127–28
    on organization, 33, 39–40
    on overall mission, 147–49, 188, 208, 260, 264
    on pleasures of a Japanese garden, 191–92
    on prevention versus treatment, 113, 147–48
    on private welfare organizations, 163
    on psychology of respect for strength, 43, 210, 214–15, 226, 256

Sams, Crawford F. *(continued)*
    on recreation and travel in Japan, 192–97
    on religious beliefs and health, 48–49, 63
    on research, xiii, xiv
    on role of veterinarians in human health, 114, 280–81n.1
    on scientific progress and nationalism, 96, 136
    on socialized state medicine, 168–69
    on standards of medical care, 122–21
    on termination of the Korean War, 257
    on U.S. military support of free nations, 210
    on weapons of destruction, 9–10
    on worth of the individual, xv, 182, 183, 188, 241
Sams, Elva Viola Allen, 190–92, 194–96, 199, 220, 238, 249, 261, 262, 264, 294n.6
Sanitary engineers, 75, 93, 278n.4
Sanitary standards.
  for milk supplies, 62
  in Japan, 92, 115–17
    era of new sanitation, 116
    seafood inspection, 116–17
  in Korea, 213, 218
Sanitary teams.
  in Japan, 93–95
  in the Middle East, 93
  in Panama, 93
SCAP, General Headquarters, 25
  formation of, 33, 34–35
  method of operation, 35–38
  See also Civil Information and Education Section
  See also Economics and Scientific Section
  See also Government Section
  See also MacArthur, Douglas
  See also Natural Resources Section
  See also Policies
  See also Public Health and Welfare Section
  See also SCAPIN

310 INDEX

SCAPIN, 20–21, 36
  SCAPIN 48, "Public Health Measures," 268–69n.5, 270n.3, 275n.3, 281n.2, 282–83n.3, 283n.1
  SCAPIN 93, "Removal of Restrictions on Political, Civil and Religious Liberties," 270n.2, 278n.3
  SCAPIN 97, "Release of Surplus Japanese Army and Navy Medical Supplies for Civilian Use" 282–83n.3
  SCAPIN 98, "Information on Japanese Public Health," 268–69n.5, 275n.3, 287n.1
  SCAPIN 106, "Manufacture of DDT in Japan," 277n.9
  SCAPIN 214, "Information on Japanese Animal Disease Control" 280–81n.1
  SCAPIN 273, "Relief Board for Veterans," 283–84n.3
  SCAPIN 304, "Imperial Japanese Army and Navy Hospitals," 283–84n.3
  SCAPIN 331, "Prevention and Control of Typhus Fever in Japan," 276–77n.5
  SCAPIN 352, "Reserve Supplies Held for Relief Distribution," 288n.6
  SCAPIN 368, "Prevention and Control of Typhus Fever in Japan," 276–77n.5
  SCAPIN 561, "Inequitable Distribution of Supplies to Reception Centers," 277n.12
  SCAPIN 563, "Control of Population Movements," 288n.3
  SCAPIN 731, "Deficiencies Noted at Reception Centers in Japan," 277n.12
  SCAPIN 775, "Public Assistance," 288n.4
  SCAPIN 781, "Unsatisfactory Conditions Aboard Repatriation Vessels," 277n.12
  SCAPIN 791, "Medical Supplies for Repatriation Program," 277n.10
  SCAPIN 920, "Appointment of Insect and Rodent Control Officers," 278n.5

SCAPIN *(continued)*
  SCAPIN 921, "Vaccination Against Smallpox," 276n.3
  SCAPIN 922, "Manufacture of DDT in Japan," 277n.9, 278n.5
  SCAPIN 944, "Control of Population Movements," 288n.3
  SCAPIN 945, "Reorganization of Governmental Public Health and Welfare Activities," 273n.9
Scawthorne, Colonel, 115
Schenk, Hubert (Hugh) G., 34
School lunch program, 62–64, 65, 117
Schwictenberg, Al, 255
Scobey, J.W.
  photo, 61
Shepard, Whitfield, 38
Shiga, Kiyoshi.
  photo, ii
Shimadzu, Prince, 176, 197
Simmons, James Stevens, 96, 255, 265n.2, 293n.1
  as mentor, x, xiii, 3
  photos, ii, 74
Sixth Army, 5, 37, 227
Smallpox.
  in American soldiers, 83–84
  in Japan, 30, 31, 81–84
  in Korea, 83–84, 206, 207, 213, 216, 228, 234, 241, 246, 247, 248, 250, 252
  hemorrhagic, 252
  in the Middle East, 83
Smith, Kingsbury, 243
Social security (in Japan).
  effects of anti-inflationary measures on, 170
  financial stability of, 168, 169
  study of, 171
  origin of modern concept of, 167
  principles of, 157, 167, 169, 172
Social work (in Japan), 161–62
  photos, 112, 162
  See also Welfare
South Korea. *See* Korea

INDEX 311

Spears, W.L., 153, 287–88n.2
Standlee, Earl, 264
State, War, and Navy Coordinating Committee. *See* SWNCC
Statistics.
 health, 77–78
 vital, 77, 79
 welfare, 79
Stillwell, General, 5
Strahler, Marguerita, 19, 165
Struthers, Charles M., 1, 199, 220–21, 237–39
Struthers, Yvonne. *See* Johns, Yvonne
Sturgeon. *See* Sturgis, U.S.S. *General S.D.*
Sturgis, U.S.S. *General S.D.*, 5–7, 9, 10, 19, 267–68n.1
Suginami Health Center.
 photo, 112
Supreme Commander for the Allied Powers. *See* SCAP
 See also MacArthur, Douglas
Sutherland, General, 38
Swing, Joe, 180
SWNCC, 18, 32, 183

T

Takamatsu, Nobuhito, 141, 197
 photo, 198
Takamatsu, Princess, 141, 197
Taylor, Grant, 150
Taylor, Tommy, 194
Tenrikyo ("Teaching of the Heavenly Truth"), 48, 50
Tenth Army, 5, 203
Tessmer, Carl F., 150,
 photo, 151
Thirty-eighth parallel, 203, 204, 205, 206, 207, 209, 236, 244, 256, 257, 258
 See also Korea
Thompson, Warren S., 184
Tokugawa clan, 41
Tokugawa shrine, 44, 47
Tokyo Health Department, 176–77
Toyonaka Health Center.
 photo, 74

Truman, Harry, 175, 225, 255
Tsukahara, Kunio.
 photo, 112
Tuberculosis (in Japan), 109–13, 280n.8, 280n.10
 and integration of health and welfare programs, 112, 157
 photo, 112
 postwar mortality, 110
Tuck, W. Hallam.
 photo, 61
Turner, Thomas B. (Tommy), 107, 108
Typhoid fever, 22, 62
 in Japan, 30, 31, 92, 94–95, 278n.1, 279n.11
 in Korea, 207, 213, 216, 228, 234, 241, 246, 248, 252
Typhus, 22
 in Japan, 30–31, 84–88, 277n.8
 research, 87–88
 photos, 86, 87
 in Korea, 206, 207, 213, 216, 228, 234, 241, 246, 247, 248, 250, 252
 in the Middle East, 22, 85, 88

U

UNICEF, 64, 164–65
Unitarian Service Committee. *See* Medical care, teaching missions
United Nations, 211, 234–35, 243–45
 Civil Assistance Command, 232, 243
 objective to reunite Korea, 234, 243, 256
United Nations International Children's Emergency Fund. *See* UNICEF
United Nations Security Council, 211
U.S. Food Mission.
 photo, 61
U.S. Public Health Service, 79, 89, 277n.12
U.S. Typhus Commission, 85, 277n.4, 277n.7
Utsunomiya, 45
Uyeno station, 30, 44–45, 54

V

Van Fleet, General, 258–59
Venereal diseases.
  in Japan, 105–8
    reporting of, 107, 275n.5
  in Korea, 105, 108
  in the Middle East, 105, 280n.6
  in U.S. military forces, 103–5, 109
  moral issues in controlling, 103, 107, 109
Veterinarians, 114–18, 280–81n.1
Volk, Herbert.
  photo, 86
Voorhies, Tracy, 57

W

Waksman, Doctor, 137
Walker, Walton, 213, 219, 224, 237, 238, 242
War crimes. *See* Geneva Conventions
Warren, Shields, 150
Warren, Stafford, 150
Water supply systems.
  in Japan, 27, 92, 278n.2
  in Korea, 225, 228, 231
Welfare.
  in Japan
    administrative units, 162
    child welfare, 160–61
    concept of public assistance, 159, 288n.5

Welfare *(continued)*
    international relief agencies, 163–65
    photo, 198
    policies, 158, 159–60, 164
    private welfare organizations, 62–63, 163
    rehabilitation programs, 160
    scope of relief, 30–31, 157
    social work, 161–62
  in Korea
    child welfare, 208
    organization of relief, 211, 212–13
    personnel, 212
Wheeler, Speck, 85, 98
Whelpton, Doctor, 184
Whitman, Ross H.
  photo, 61
Whitney, Courtney, 34, 145, 177, 256
Willoughby, Charles A., 253, 256, 292n.4
World Health Organization, 190
Wright, Frank Lloyd, 27
Wright, Pinky, 209

Y

Yasuda, Kazuo.
  photo, 74
Yoshida, Shigeru, 66, 261, 271n.5
Youn, Joung, 249, 250, 252, 253, 293n.6
Yun, Commander E. *See* Youn, Joung

Z

Zaibatsu, 169, 192

About the Editor

Zabelle Zakarian is an M.P.H. graduate of the University of Illinois. She attended the Paul H. Nitze School of Advanced International Studies at The Johns Hopkins University and holds an Sc.D. from The Johns Hopkins School of Public Health. She lives in Washington, D.C.